# Handbook *of* Pharmaceutical Technology

# Handbook *of* Pharmaceutical Technology

**Poonam Kushwaha**
M Pharm, PhD (Pharmaceutics)
Assistant Professor
Faculty of Pharmacy, Integral University
Lucknow, Uttar Pradesh, India

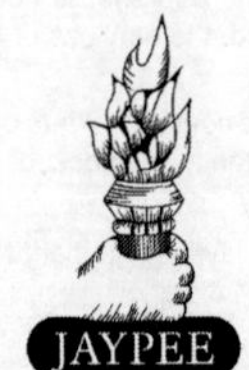


**JAYPEE BROTHERS MEDICAL PUBLISHERS**
*The Health Sciences Publisher*
New Delhi | London

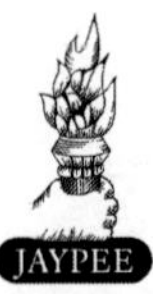

**Jaypee Brothers Medical Publishers (P) Ltd**

**Headquarters**
EMCA House
23/23-B, Ansari Road, Daryaganj
New Delhi - 110 002, India
Landline: +91-11-23272143, +91-11-23272703
+91-11-23282021, +91-11-23245672
E-mail: jaypee@jaypeebrothers.com

**Corporate Office**
4838/24, Ansari Road, Daryaganj
New Delhi - 110 002, India
Phone: +91-11-43574357
Fax: +91-11-43574314
E-mail: jaypee@jaypeebrothers.com

**Overseas Office**
J.P. Medical Ltd
83 Victoria Street, London
SW1H 0HW (UK)
Phone: +44 20 3170 8910
E-mail: info@jpmedpub.com

**EU GPSR** Authorised Representative
Logos Europe, 9 rue Nicolas Poussin
17000, La Rochelle, France
Phone: +33 (0) 6 67 93 73 78
E-mail: contact@logoseurope.eu

Website: www.jaypeebrothers.com
Website: www.jaypeedigital.com



**Inquiries for bulk sales may be solicited at:** jaypee@jaypeebrothers.com

***Handbook of Pharmaceutical Technology***

*First Edition*: 2015
*Reprint*: **2026**
ISBN 978-93-5152-774-9

*Printed at: Samrat Offset Pvt. Ltd.*

# Preface

Pharmaceutical technology involves the rational design and manufacture of dosage forms to ensure that the required biological and physical performances of the therapeutic agent are attained. The formulation scientist is, therefore, expected to have knowledge of several scientific disciplines, including physical pharmaceutics, pharmaceutical chemistry, and biopharmaceutics. Pharmaceutical technology may, therefore, be correctly viewed as an essential and unique component of the pharmaceutical sciences and, accordingly, the pharmacy undergraduate degree. Due to the interdisciplinary nature, pharmaceutical technology is often considered difficult and challenging to most of the students. This textbook aims to ease the perceived difficulties of this subject and shall illustrate the significance of pharmaceutical formulations.

The content of this text aims to deliver the essential information concerning the formulation of the dosage forms in a format that will surely aid the understanding and, hence, remove the complexities of the various topics which students normally face. The reader will observe that, in addition to the required theoretical aspects, each chapter contains information regarding the various types of excipients that are used commonly in the formulation of dosage forms. It is the author's opinion that this information is essential to ensure that the reader is able to bridge the information gap between the theory and practice of dosage form design. In understanding the physicochemical properties of excipients (and indeed therapeutic agents), the student will be able to optimize the prepared dosage form and, in addition, will be able to answer examination questions with the appropriate depth which is essential for attaining a good percentile.

This book consists of 7 chapters; the chapters describe the various categories of dosage form. Chapters 1 and 2 describe the formulation of solid-dosage forms (tablets and capsules) with particular emphasis on the excipients and methods used to prepare them. Chapter 3 describes pharmaceutical importance and techniques of microencapsulation. Chapter 4 describes parenteral formulations and, in particular, illustrates strategies for the successful formulation of parenteral products. Chapter 5 concisely describes the theoretical aspects, carrier(s) and approaches used for designing novel drug delivery systems. Chapter 6 describes the function, purpose and control of pharmaceutical packaging materials. Finally, Chapter 7 describes the types of surgical materials and their manufacture. The major objective of writing this book is to present the information in a lucid, condensed and cohesive form, to cater specifically the needs of undergraduate and graduate students of pharmacy.

I am thankful to my family for their sincere support, patience and sparing me of responsibilities. I thankfully acknowledge various sources for basic ideas, landmark contribution, and contents. I welcome suggestions from students and teachers which will help improving the volume in future.

**Poonam Kushwaha**

# Contents

# Chapter 1

# Tablets

## INTRODUCTION

Tablets are solid unit dosage form in which one usual dose of drug has been accurately placed. They are solid; round, oblong or unique in shape; thick or thin; large or small in diameter; flat or convex, engraved or imprinted with an identifying symbol; coated or uncoated; colored or uncolored; one, two or three layered. They are the most widely used solid dosage form of medicament. There are several types of tablet solid dosage forms that are designed to optimize the absorption rate of the drug, increase the ease of administration by the patient, control the rate and site of drug absorption and mask the taste of a therapeutic agent. Because of their advantages, their popularity is increasing continuously day-by-day.

### Advantages

1. Tablets are unit dosage forms that provide an accurate, stable dose with greatest precision and least content variability.
2. Tablets are easy to use, handle and carry by the patient.
3. Tablets are attractive and elegant in appearance.
4. Tablets are the most stable dosage form with respect to their physical, chemical and microbiological attributes.
5. The manufacturing cost of tablets is low as compared to other dosage forms and their manufacturing speed is also quite high.
6. The packaging and shipping of tablets is comparatively easy and cheap.
7. The unpleasant taste and odor of medicament(s) can be easily masked by sugar coating.

8. The incompatibilities of medicament(s) and their deterioration due to environmental factors are less in case of tablet.
9. Whenever a fractional dose is required, tablets are divided into halves and quarters by drawing lines during manufacturing to facilitate breakage.
10. They are more suitable for large scale production than other oral dosage forms.
11. Tablets provide administration of even minute dose of drug in an accurate amount.
12. Their identification is probably the easiest because of variety of shapes and colors.
13. Tablets are formulated with certain special release profile products such as enteric or delayed release products.
14. They are economical as their cost is lowest as compared to other oral dosage forms.

## Disadvantages

1. Drugs that are amorphous in nature or have low density character are difficult to compress into tablet.
2. Hygroscopic drugs are not suitable candidates for compressed tablets.
3. Drugs having poor wetting properties, slow dissolution profile and high optimal gastrointestinal absorption are difficult or impossible to formulate as a tablet.
4. Drugs having bitter taste and objectionable odor requires special treatment like coating or encapsulation which may increase their production cost.
5. Drugs that are sensitive to oxygen or may also require certain treatment like special coating as well as packaging which may increase the overall manufacturing cost.
6. High dose drugs are difficult to formulate as tablet dosage form.
7. Some drugs which preferably get absorbed from the upper part of GIT may cause bioavailability problem in tablet dosage form.
8. Drugs that are liquid in nature are difficult to formulate as a tablet.
9. Swallowing of tablets specially by children and critically ill-patients is very difficult.

### Desired characteristics of tablet

1. The objective of formulation and fabrication of tablet is to deliver the correct amount of drug in proper form at or over proper time.
2. Tablet should be elegant having its own identity and free from defects such as cracks, chips, contamination, discoloration, etc.
3. It should have chemical and physical stability to maintain its physical integrity over time.
4. It should be capable to prevent any alteration in the chemical and physical properties of medicinal agent(s).
5. It should be capable of withstanding the rigors of mechanical shocks encountered in its production, packaging, shipping and dispensing.
6. An ideal tablet should be able to release the medicament(s) in body in predictable and reproducible manner.

## TYPES AND CLASSES OF TABLETS

### I. Oral tablet for ingestion

*A. Compressed tablets (Fig. 1.1)*

These are uncoated tablets made by compression of one or more active ingredients with or without excipients by employing any of three basic methods of tablet manufacturing. Tablets in this category, are usually intended to provide rapid disintegration and drug release. These drugs are typically water-insoluble and include therapeutic categories such as adsorbents and antacids. These tablets also contain diluents, binders, disintegrants, glidants and organoleptic agents. The compressed tablets are usually prepared on large scale production methods whereas the molded tablets are prepared extemporaneously on a small scale.

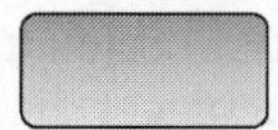

FIGURE1.1: Compressed tablet

*B. Multiple compressed tablets*

Multiple compressed tablets are prepared by compressing the fill material more than once. They are also known as multiple layered tablets or a tablet within the tablet. Layered tablets are prepared by the initial compaction of a portion of fill material in a die followed by additional fill material and compression to form two or more layered tablets depending upon number of separate fills. Each layer contains different medicinal agent(s) separated from another to minimize physical and chemical incompatibilities.

The tablets in this category are prepared for two reasons: 1. To separate physically or chemically incompatible ingredients, 2. To produce repeat action/prolonged action tablet.

The tablet manufacturing machine is generally operated at relatively lower speed than for standard compression tablet. There are three categories under this class:

### I. Multilayered tablets (Fig. 1.2)

When two or more active pharmaceutical ingredients are needed to be administered simultaneously and they are incompatible, the best option for the formulation pharmacist would be to formulate multilayered tablet. It consists of several different granulations that are compressed to form a single tablet composed of two or more layers and usually each layer is of different color to produce a distinctive looking tablet. Each layer is fed from separate feed frame with individual weight control. Dust extraction is essential during compression to avoid contamination. Therefore, each layer undergoes light compression as each component is laid down. This avoids granules intermixing if the machine vibrates.

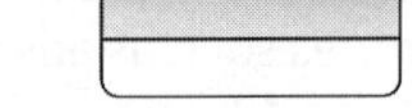

FIGURE 1.2: Multilayered tablet

### II. Compression coated tablets (Fig. 1.3)

This type of tablet has two parts—Internal core and surrounding coat. The core is small porous tablet and prepared on one turret. For preparing final tablet, a bigger die cavity in another turret is used in which first the coat material is filled to half and then core tablet is mechanically transferred, again the remaining space is filled with coat material and finally compression force is applied. This tablet readily lend itself into a repeat action tablet as the outer layer provides the initial dose while the inner core release the drug later on. But, when the core quickly releases the drug, entirely different blood level is achieved with the risk of over dose toxicity. To avoid immediate release of both the layers, the core tablet is coated with enteric polymer so that it will not release the drug in stomach while the first dose is added in outer sugar coating.

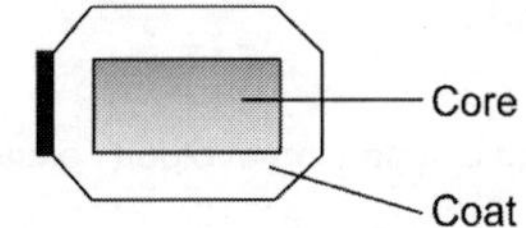


FIGURE 1.3: Compression coated tablet

III. Inlay tablets (Fig. 1.4)

In case of layered tablet instead of core tablet being completely surrounded by coating, top surface is completely exposed. During preparation, only the bottom of the die cavity is filled with coating material and core is placed upon it. When compression force is applied, some coating material is displaced to form the sides and compress the whole tablet. It has some advantages over compression coated tablets:

i. Less coating material is required
ii. Core is visible, so coreless tablets can be easily detected
iii. Reduction in coating forms a thinner tablet and thus freedom from capping of top coating.

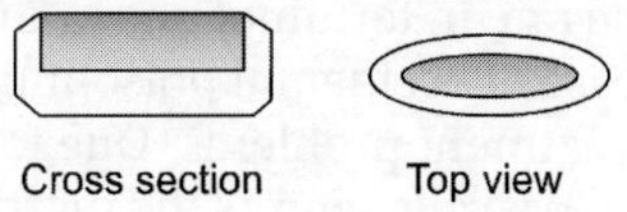


FIGURE 1.4: Inlay tablets

### *C. Modified release tablets (Fig. 1.5)*

The main aim behind formulation of this dosage form is to release the medicament slowly for long time duration after administration of a single tablet. Moreover, these types of formulations are generally used to target the site specific releases.

A widespread use of this type of tablet is seen in present scenario, as well as many researchers have concentrated their attention in this direction. This is mainly because of improvement in patient's compliance as the dosage frequency is reduced, patient can take

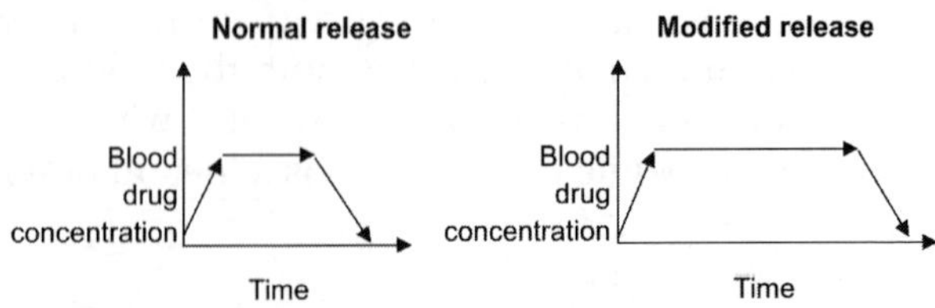


FIGURE 1.5: Graphical comparison of blood concentration versus time

an undisturbed sleep at night, it's also beneficial for psychiatric patients who forget to take their tablets regularly and the dose-related side effects and toxicities are reduced. Any adjuvant that can alter water uptake rate, swelling and gelling characteristics of matrixing agents can alter the release rate of API, e.g. electrolytes in HPMC matrix tablet. It's also possible to achieve pulsed drug release. Weakly-basic drugs exhibit good solubility at low pH while less soluble at high pH conditions, which can result in incomplete drug release for sustained release formulations. The drug release can be modified by providing suitable microenvironmental pH in the tablet, e.g. acidic polymer, succinic acid, etc. Similarly, inclusion of alkaline polymers results in desirable drug release of acidic drugs. On the other hand, formulation of this type of dosage form presents challenge for the formulator—Increases the cost of manufacturing, chances of burst drug release and drop in drug release rate in terminal phase and thus incomplete release on API. In case of accidental poisoning, the doctor has to deal with special treatment problems. Due to large size, patient may feel difficulties in swallowing as the matrixing agent to drug ratio is high. Classic approaches are usually based on adaptation of either film coated or multiparticulate technologies or those involving slow release matrices.

### *D. Delayed action and enteric coated tablets*

They are tablets with a coating that resist dissolution or disruption in the gastric fluid (stomach) but readily disintegrate in the intestinal fluid to release the drug, thus rendering them delayed release features. Enteric coating is generally employed when the drug substance is unstable in gastric fluid and may get destroyed or where it may cause irritation to the gastric mucosa or in cases where the bypassing the stomach would result in the enhancement of drug absorption from the intestine to a significant extent. The coating materials are primarily mixed with acid functionality and acid ester functionally synthetic or modified natural polymers. Cellulose acetate phthalate (CAP) is the most commonly used enteric coating polymer. Other materials are polyvinyl acetate phthalate (PVAP) and hydroxypropyl methylcellulose phthalate (HPMCP).

### *E. Film coated tablets*

Film coated tablets are the compressed tablets coated with a thin layer of suitable polymer capable of forming a skin like film over the tablet. The polymeric substances most commonly used are hydroxypropyl cellulose, hydroxypropyl methylcellulose and ethylcellulose. The film is usually colored and has the advantage over sugar coating in that it is more durable, less bulky and less time consuming to apply. The film coating protects the medicament from atmospheric effects. By its composition the coating is designed to rupture and expose the core tablet at the desired location within the GIT.

### *F. Chewable tablets*

Chewable tablets are the tablets which are required to be broken and chewed in between the teeth before ingestion. These tablets are given to the children who have difficulty in swallowing and to the adults who dislike swallowing. A number of antacid tablets and multivitamin tablets are prepared as chewable tablets. Chewable tablets are to be chewed in the mouth and broken into smaller pieces prior to swallowing and are not intended to be swallowed intact. In this way, the time required for disintegration is reduced and the rate of absorption of the medicament may increase. For the preparation of chewable tablets, mannitol is used as a base. These tablets should have very acceptable taste and flavor. They should disintegrate in a short time and produce cool sweet taste. Chewable tablets can be taken at any place even if water is not available.

Important considerations in the formulation of these types of tablets are the incorporation of the pleasant diluents such as mannitol, sorbitol and sucrose, etc. for the taste and the mouth feel. Disintegrants are usually not required for these tablets. Such types of tablets are commonly employed in the preparation of multivitamins, antacids and antibiotics, specially for children and elderly patients. The most common chewable tablets in the market are chewable aspirin tablets for children.

## II. Tablet used in oral cavity

### *A. Buccal and sublingual tablets*

These tablets are required to be placed below the tongue (sublingual) or in the side of the cheek (buccal) where they release their medicament for absorption directly through the oral mucosa into the systemic circulation bypassing the GIT and liver. Nitroglycerin and mannitol hexanitrate buccal tablets dissolve in 1–2 minutes to produce immediate effect. Drugs administered by this route are intended to produce systemic drug effect and consequently they must have good absorption properties through the oral mucosa. Generally, these types of tablets contain those drugs which are destroyed, inactivated or not absorbed in the GIT but are directly absorbed through the mucosal tissues of the oral cavities. These tablets contain large proportions of sweetening agents like mannitol, sorbitol, xylitol to impart sweetness. One unique effect of using mannitol is that it has a negative heat of solubility that feels like a cooling sensation as the tablet dissolves. These tablets should be formulated with bland excipients which do not stimulate salivation.

### *B. Troches and lozenges (Figs 1.6A and B)*

These are uncoated tablets containing medicaments in a sweetened and flavored base intended to dissolve slowly in the mouth. They are used in oral cavities where they are required to exert a local effect in the mouth or throat. Such tablets are

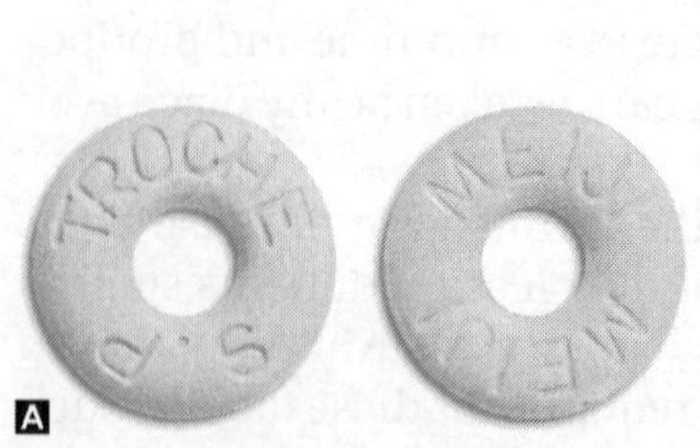


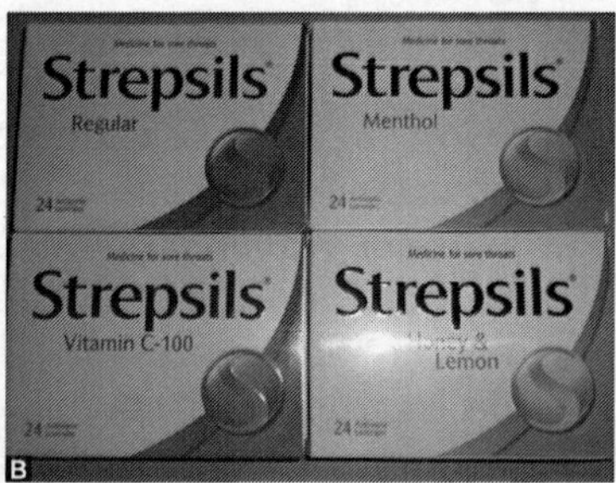


FIGURES 1.6A and B: A: Troches and B: Lozenges

commonly used to treat sore throat or to control coughing in common cold. They generally contain anesthetics, various antiseptics, antibacterial agents, demulcents, astringents and antitussives agents. The choice of diluents is very important and the chosen material should produce a smooth texture and pleasant taste in the mouth.

*C. Dental cones (Fig. 1.7)*

Dental cones are relatively minor tablet that are designed to be placed in the empty socket remaining after tooth extraction. These tablets slowly release antibacterial compounds to prevent the growth of the bacteria in the empty socket following tooth extraction. They may also be used to reduce the bleeding by containing an astringent or coagulant. The vehicles commonly used are sodium bicarbonate, sodium chloride or an amino acid.

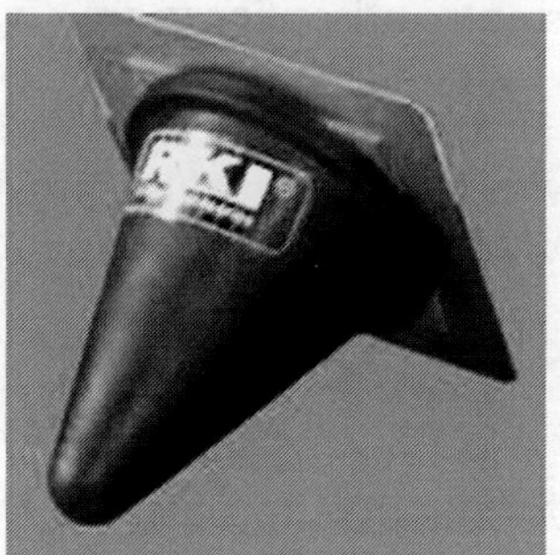

FIGURE 1.7: Dental cones

## III. Tablet administered by other routes

*A. Implantation tablets*

Implantation or depot tablets are small tablet meant for insertion under the skin by giving a small surgical cut into the skin which is stitched after insertion of the tablet. A special injector utilizing a hollow needle and plunger may be used to administer rod-shaped tablet. These are designed for subcutaneous implantation in animal or man. Their purpose is to provide prolonged drug effect ranging from month to year. Since, these tablets are implanted intramuscularly or subcutaneous, therefore, they must be sterile. They must be prepared under aseptic conditions and packed in unit dose sterile container. These tablets are more commonly used in veterinary than human medicine. They can also be used for birth control in human beings. Generally steroidal hormone like testosterone, stilbestrol, etc. are formulated as implants. These tablets have been largely replaced by other dosage forms such as diffusion controlled silicone tubes filled with drug or biodegradable polymers that contain entrapped drug in variety of forms.

*B. Vaginal tablets*

Vaginal tablets are compressed tablets meant for insertion into vaginal cavity and designed to undergo slow dissolution and drug release in the cavity. Sometimes, vaginal suppositories or pessaries are prepared by compression which is known as vaginal tablets. These are usually ovoid or almond in shape to facilitate the retention in vagina. It is used to release antibacterial agents, astringents and antiseptics to treat vaginal infection or possibly to release steroids for systemic absorption. Soluble additives are used for the preparation of these tablets. These are often formulated with buffering agent to provide favorable pH to stimulate the action of the given medicament(s).

## IV. Tablets used to prepare solution

*A. Effervescent tablets*

The oral dosage forms are the most popular way of taking medication despite having some disadvantages like slow absorption and thus onset of action is prolong. This can be overcome by administering the drug in liquid form but, many APIs have limited level of stability in liquid form. So, effervescent tablets acts as an alternative dosage form. The tablet is added into a glass of water just before administration and the drug solution or dispersion is to be drunk immediately. The tablet is quickly broken apart by internal liberation of $CO_2$ in water due to interaction between tartaric acid and citric acid with alkali metal carbonates or bicarbonates in presence of water.

Due to liberation of $CO_2$ gas, the dissolution of API in water as well as taste masking effect is enhanced. To manufacture these tablets, either wet fusion or heat fusion is adopted. The tablets are compressed soft enough to produce an effervescent reaction that is adequately rapid. Water soluble lubricants are used to prevent an insoluble scum formation on water surface. To add sweetness to the formulation, saccharin is added since sucrose is hygroscopic and add too much of bulk to the tablet. The manufacturing shall be done under controlled climatic condition to avoid effervescent reaction. Today, the most commonly used effervescent tablet is aspirin tablet.

### *B. Soluble tablets*

Water soluble tablets are intended for application after dissolution in water and contain an active ingredient which should be totally soluble in water at used concentrations. All the excipients used to formulate these tablets are required to be completely soluble in water including the glidants, binders, etc. So, manufacturing of this kind of tablets are challenge for the formulator.

### *C. Dispensing tablets*

Dispensing tablets are molded tablets containing a small dose of a potent medicament along with soluble excipients. These are intended to be added to a given volume of water by the pharmacist or the consumer to produce a solution of a given drug concentration. Materials that are commonly used are mild silver proteinate, dichloride of mercury and quaternary ammonium compound. These tablets are less commonly used. Another difficulty is that some of the components previously used in this dosage form are highly toxic and extremely hazardous and even lethal.

### *D. Hypodermic tablets*

Hypodermic tablets are soft molded tablets containing soluble ingredients and were originally used for extemporaneous preparation of solution for injection in sterile water or water for injection. A major limitation of these tablets was an attainment of sterility required for injection preparation. These tablets are not of much used in the modern day practice because of availability of stable liquid injections and powder for injection.

### *E. Tablet triturates*

These are small, cylindrical, molded or compressed tablets. They provide an extemporaneous method of preparation by the pharmacist. They are rarely used nowadays that is why they are obsolete today. The employed drugs in such types of products are quite potent and are mixed with lactose and possibly a binder such as powdered acacia.

## FORMULATION OF TABLETS

I. Active pharmaceutical ingredients (API)
II. Excipients.

### I. Active pharmaceutical ingredients (API)

*Ideal properties of API for formulating tablets*

1. High purity

API has to be in pure form otherwise impurities can catalyze series of chemical reactions, e.g. in case of hydrocortisone impurity of cupric ion causes oxidation of ketone functional group. API should meet specifications given in the respective pharmacopoeia.

2. High stability

The API should be stable against photolysis, oxidation, hydrolysis, etc. to keep the formulation a simple one. Sensitive particles require careful handling during manufacturing.

3. Good compatibility with excipients

In order to formulate a tablet one need to add excipient along with API. There should not be any kind of interaction between excipient and API. Excipients have to be inert in nature. However, there are some reported examples of API-excipient interactions like lisinopril reacts with lactose and undergoes browning reaction leading to darkening on storage. So, avoid the use of lactose and use other fillers for API containing primary amine. To ascertain drug and excipient interaction, 1:1 mixture is prepared and stored under accelerated/ICH conditions. The amount of drug degraded shall be determined to select the most suitable excipient.

4. Optimum bulk powder properties

Bulk powder properties have to be optimum to:

i. Prevents segregation.
ii. Have optimum size tablet particularly for low potency-low density API.
iii. Have good flow.

*5. Optimum and uniform particle size distribution*

API should have uniform particle size and close particle size distribution because it has pronounced effect on uniformity of content, uniformity of weight, disintegration time, granule friability, drying rate kinetics of wet granulation, flowability, compressibility, stability, dissolution, bioavailability, etc. The flow and compression characteristics are important from the viewpoint of industrial pharmacist. Strong tablets are obtained if fine particles are used due to increase in surface area and surface energy.

*6. Spherical shape*

The shape of particles decides flowability. Spherical-shaped particles exhibit good flow as compared to needle-shaped particles. Particles with irregular shape may exhibit hindered-flow due to interlocking between particles. This point is very important since it is directly related with weight of tablet and uniformity.

*7. Good flowability*

Flow is important for having uniformity of weight and uniformity of drug content. It can be measured using angle of repose, Carr's index and Hausner's ratio.

The methods used to improve flow are summarized below:

i. Addition of glidants.
ii. Addition of fines—Addition of fines upto certain extent improves flow. This is because of filling of void space and decrease in surface roughness.
iii. By wet granulation—Wet granulation gives regular sphere-shaped granules and removes static charge if present on particle surface. Thus, flow property improved.
iv. By densification with help of slugging.

*8. Optimum moisture content*

Moisture content has to be optimum because of the following reasons:

i. Total lack of moisture results into brittle tablet.
ii. Moisture affects flow, which in turn affects uniformity of content.

iii. High amount of moisture gives stickiness, which will affect compaction.
iv. Picking/sticking may be observed.

Moisture content can be controlled by:

i. Use of anhydrous salts.
ii. Use of nonaqueous solvent.
iii. Optimum drying time.
iv. Addition of finely powdered adsorbent like magnesium oxide.

*9. Good compressibility*

API should exhibit good compressibility. However, this depends upon its intrinsic nature like:

A. Elasticity

The particles deform under the effect of pressure in a die but they revert back to original state on removal of applied pressure, i.e. on ejection. Such tablets may exhibit capping and/or lamination. The intrinsic nature of particle can be changed by:

i. Wet massing.
ii. Precompression.
iii. Plastic tabulating matrix (micro, crystalline cellulose) elastic material is less suitable for direct compression.

B. Plasticity

Plastic material gets bonded after viscoelastic deformation. Viscoelastic deformation is time dependent. Hence, the crushing strength is dependent on the time that tablet spends in a die. Changing the turret speed can change dwell time. Plastic materials may exhibit viscoelastic deformation.

C. Brittle fracture

A particle fractures into small particles on application of pressure in a die. Brittle fracture also promotes tableting. Brittle materials are less lubricant sensitive as compared to plastic materials. A blend of lactose and MCC is widely used in industry to get advantages of brittle materials and plastic materials.

*10. Absence of static charge on surface*

It is important because of the following reasons:

i. It affects uniformity of dose and weight variation (flow worsen if attractive forces generated).

ii. During mixing, it may cause segregation and lead to non-uniformity of content if API and excipients are charged.
iii. Charged API may adhere to feed frame and result into serious damage to tablet equipment.

In order to remove charge certain treatments can be given like granulation, addition of diluents or lubricant, surface coating with help of colloidal silica, etc.

*11. Good organoleptic properties*

Many API are unpalatable and unattractive in their natural form. In such cases, tablet formulations require certain care. API has to be checked for color and taste.

A. Color

Ideally API should be colorless. For colored API, the following steps shall be considered:

i. Select appropriate excipient to avoid mottling.
ii. Incorporate API in smallest particle size.
iii. Incorporate color in dry form along with binder and activate mixture by addition of water or other activator.
iv. Coating can be applied to conceal nonuniform color (sugar coated multivitamin tablet).

B. Taste

It is very important for tablets because they come in contact with taste buds. Ideally API should have no taste. But sometimes it might have unpleasant taste like bitter, e.g. Chloramphenicol, Clindamycin, etc. The following taste masking options can be tried:

i. Use of prodrug to decrease API solubility in saliva or to reduce affinity for taste receptor, e.g. Chloramphenicol palmitate.
ii. Sugar coating or film coating.
iii. Addition of sweeteners like mannitol in cause of fast dissolving tablet or chewable tablet.
iv. Use of drug-ion exchange adsorbent in formulation.
v. Drug β-cyclodextrin complex may exhibit good taste profile and good compressibility as well.

Miscellaneous points

i. API should not exhibit sublime characteristics.

ii. Liquid APIs are less suitable for tablet formulation. One of the options is conversion of liquid in pseudosolid (mix liquid API with adsorbents). A combination of valproic acid and sodium valproate is a typical example of converting a liquid into pseudosolid.
iii. BCS class IV drugs are difficult to formulate if dissolution and bioavailability requirements are to meet as per regulatory agencies.

## II. Excipients

Excipient means any component other than the active pharmaceutical ingredient(s) intentionally added to the formulation of a dosage form. Many guidelines exist to aid in selection of nontoxic excipients such as IIG (Inactive Ingredient Guide), GRAS (Generally Regarded as Safe), Handbook of Pharmaceutical Excipients and others.

While selecting excipients for any formulation following things should be considered wherever possible—keep the excipients to a minimum in number to minimize the quantity of each excipients and multifunctional excipients may be given preference over unifunctional excipients.

Excipients play a crucial role in designing the delivery system, determining its quality and performance. Excipients though usually regarded as nontoxic. There are examples of known excipient induced toxicities which include renal failure and death from diethylene glycol, osmotic diarrhea caused by ingested mannitol, hypersensitivity reactions from lanolin and cardiotoxicity induced by propylene glycol.

Excipients are chosen in tablet formulation to perform a variety of functions like:

i. For providing essential manufacturing technology functions (binders, glidants, lubricants may be added).
ii. For enhancing patient acceptance (flavors, colorants may be added).
iii. For providing aid in product identification (colorants may be added).
iv. For optimizing or modifying drug release (disintegrants, hydrophilic polymers, wetting agents, biodegradable polymers may be added).
v. For enhancing stability (antioxidant, UV absorbers may be added).

Substances other than active ingredients are commonly referred as excipients. The commonly used excipients are diluents, binders and adhesives, disintegrants, lubricants, anti-adherents, glidants, fillers, colors and sweeteners, etc. Tablet excipients must meet certain criteria in the formulation such as:

i. They must be nontoxic and acceptable to the regulatory agencies in all countries where the product is to be marketed.
ii. They must be commercially available in an acceptable grade in all countries where the product is to be manufactured.
iii. Their cost must be acceptably low.
iv. They must be physiologically inert.
v. They must be physically and chemically stable by themselves and in combination with the drug(s) and other tablet components.
vi. They must be free of any unacceptable microbiologic load.
vii. They must be color compatible (not producing any off-color appearance).
viii. If the drug product is also classified as a food (e.g. certain vitamins products), the diluents and other excipient must be approved direct to food additives.
ix. They must have no deleterious effect on the bioavailability of the drug(s) in the product.

*Various excipients used in tablet formulation and their functionalities:*

1. Diluents

These are the inert substances which are added to increase the bulk to make the tablet of a practical size for compression. Diluents like mannitol, lactose, sorbitol, sucrose and inositol when present in sufficient quantity can impart properties to some compressed tablets that permit disintegration in the mouth by chewing (chewable tablet). In the formulation, the incompatibility of diluents must be considered (calcium salts used as diluents for the broad spectrum antibiotics like Tetracycline have been shown to interfere with the drug absorption from GIT. Microcrystalline cellulose (Avicel® usually is used as an excipient in direct compression formula. Hydroxypropyl methylcellulose (HPMC or Pharmacoat®) is used to prolong the release of active ingredient from tablet and also as a film former in tablet coating.

In order to facilitate tablet handling during manufacture and to achieve targeted content uniformity, the tablet size should be kept above 2–3 mm and weight of tablet above 50 mg. Many potent drugs have low dose (e.g. diazepam and clonidine hydrochloride) in such cases diluents provide the required bulk of the tablet when the drug dosage itself is inadequate to produce tablets of adequate weight and size. Usually, the range of diluent may vary from 5%–80%. Diluents are also synonymously known as fillers. Diluents are often added to tablet formulations for secondary reasons like to provide better tablet properties such as:

i. To provide improved cohesion
ii. To allow direct compression manufacturing
iii. To enhance flow
iv. To adjust weight of tablet as per die capacity.

No matter for what purpose they (diluents) are added, they must meet certain basic criteria for satisfactory performance in tablet dosage form. They are as follows:

i. Diluents should not react with the drug substance and moreover it should not have any effect on the functions of other excipients.
ii. It should not have any physiological or pharmacological activity of its own.
iii. It should have consistent physical and chemical characteristics.
iv. It should neither promote nor contribute to segregation of the granulation or powder blend to which they are added.
v. It should be able to be milled (size reduced) if necessary in order to match the particle size distribution of the active pharmaceutical ingredient.
vi. It should neither support microbiological growth in the dosage form nor contribute to any microbiological load.
vii. It should neither adversely affect the dissolution of the product nor interfere with the bioavailability of active pharmaceutical ingredient.
viii. It should preferably be colorless or nearly so.

*Classification of diluents (Table 1.1)*

Tablet diluents or fillers can be divided into following categories:

i. Organic materials—Carbohydrate and modified carbohydrates.

ii. Inorganic materials—Calcium phosphates and others.
iii. Co-processed diluents.

Carbohydrate substances such as sugars, starches and celluloses may also function as binders during wet granulation process, whereas when used in direct compression system they serve as the diluent. The inorganic diluents, do not exhibit binding properties when used in wet granulation and direct compression.

Tablet diluent or filler may also be classified on the basis of their solubility in water as soluble and insoluble.

**Table 1.1**: Classification of diluents on the basis of their solubility

| *Insoluble tablet fillers or diluents* | *Soluble tablet fillers or diluents* |
|---|---|
| Starch | Lactose |
| Powdered cellulose | Sucrose |
| Microcrystalline cellulose | Mannitol |
| Calcium phosphates | Sorbitol |

Selection of diluent should be done after considering properties of diluent such as: compactibility, flowability, solubility, disintegration qualities, hygroscopicity, lubricity and stability.

I. Organic diluents

A. Sugar and sugar alcohols

Lactose: α-lactose monohydrate, spray dried lactose and anhydrous lactose are widely used as diluent.

**α-lactose monohydrate (hydrous)**:

- Lactose monohydrate is not directly compressible and therefore it is suitable for use in wet granulation.
- It has poor flow properties
- α-lactose monohydrate is water soluble
- It produces a hard tablet and the tablet hardness increases on storage.
- Disintegrant is usually needed in lactose containing tablets.
- Drug release rate is usually not affected.
- It is usually unreactive, except for discoloration when formulated with amines and alkaline materials (i.e. browning or maillard reaction).

- It contains approximately 5% moisture and hence is a potential source of instability specially with moisture sensitive drugs.
- It is inexpensive.
- It is commercially available under the trade name of Pharmatose® and Respitose® manufactured by DMV International.

**Lactose spray dried**

- It is directly compressible diluent.
- It exhibits free flowing characteristics.
- It needs high compression pressure in order to produce hard tablets.
- Its compressibility is adversely affected if dried below 3% moisture.
- It has high dilution potential.
- It is more prone to darkening in the presence of excess moisture, amines and other compounds due to the presence of a furaldehyde.
- Usually, neutral or acid lubricant should be used when spray dried lactose is employed.
- Expensive compared to anhydrous and hydrous lactose.
- It is commercially available as spray process 315® manufactured by Foremost Farms USA.

**Lactose anhydrous**

- Lactose anhydrous is a directly compressible diluent.
- It does not exhibit free flowing property.
- It can pick up moisture at elevated humidity as a result of which changes in tablet dimensions may occur.
- It does not undergo a maillard reaction to the extent shown by spray dried lactose, although this may occur in some cases to a slight degree.
- It is inexpensive.
- It is commercially available as Pharmatose® DCL 21 manufactured by DMV Pharma.

**Sucrose**

- It requires high machine pressures, specially in cases with over wetted granulations.

- It is water-soluble.
- It possesses good binding properties.
- It is slightly hygroscopic.
- It is inexpensive.
- It produces gritty mouth feel (i.e. it is not free from grittiness).

**Mannitol**

- Mannitol a sugar alcohol is an optical isomer of sorbitol.
- It exhibits poor flow properties.
- It requires high lubricant content.
- It is probably the most expensive sugar used as a tablet diluent and is water-soluble.
- It is widely used in chewable tablets because of its negative heat of solution, its slow solubility and its mild cooling sensation in mouth.
- It can be used in vitamin formulation, where moisture sensitivity may create a problem.
- It is comparatively nonhygroscopic.
- It is free from grittiness.
- It possesses low caloric value and is noncariogenic.
- It is commercially available under the brand names Pearlitol® and Mannogem®.

**Sorbitol**

- Sorbitol is often combined with mannitol formulations in order to reduce diluent cost.
- It is highly compressible diluent and is water soluble.
- It is hygroscopic in nature.
- It has good mouth feel and sweet cooling taste.
- It is free from grittiness.
- It possesses low caloric value and is noncariogenic.
- It is commercially available as Sorbifin® and Neosorb®.

Poorly absorbed sugar alcohols such as sorbitol and mannitol can decrease small intestinal transit time. Therefore, absorption may be altered for the drugs that are preferentially absorbed from this region.

B. Celluloses

**Powdered cellulose**

- Powdered cellulose products consist of finely divided amorphous and crystalline α-cellulose particles.
- Powdered cellulose may be used alone or together with other fillers such as lactose, calcium phosphates, dextrans and others.
- It possesses poor compressibility and exhibits poor flow properties.
- It has poor binding properties and low dilution potential.
- It is water-insoluble.
- It possesses some degree of inherent lubricity.
- It is inexpensive.
- It is commercially available under the trade name of Elcema®G-250 manufactured by Degussa Corporation.

**Microcrystalline cellulose**

- Microcrystalline cellulose (MCC) is highly compressible and is perhaps the most widely used direct-compression tablet diluent.
- Hard tablets at low compression pressures are usually obtained when MCC is used as tablet diluent.
- It undergoes plastic deformation on compression and hence it is more sensitive to lubricants.
- It exhibits fair flowability.
- It exhibits binding properties.
- It also possesses disintegrant activity and thus promotes fast tablet disintegration.
- It is water-insoluble.
- It is commercially available under the trade name of Emcocel® manufactured by Penwest Pharmaceutical Co.

II. Inorganic diluents

**Calcium phosphates**

- They are granular-insoluble materials.
- They are widely used both as wet granulation and direct compression diluents in tablet formulation.
- Bulk density of calcium phosphates is higher than that of organic fillers.

- They are used extensively in vitamin and mineral preparations.
- They are directly compressible and are characterized by brittle fracture on compression during tableting process.
- Hard tablets are produced when calcium phosphates are used as diluents. They exhibit good flow properties.
- They are nonhygroscopic.
- They are inexpensive.
- They are abrasive in nature and hence can cause wear of tablet tooling. Sometimes, their alkalinity is a major source of drug instability.

Calcium phosphates includes here—The dihydrate and anhydrous form of dibasic calcium phosphate and tribasic calcium phosphate.

A. Dibasic calcium phosphates
  - Dibasic calcium phosphate dihydrate is also known as dicalcium phosphate, calcium hydrogen phosphate dihydrate and secondary calcium phosphate dihydrate.
  - Dibasic calcium phosphate is available commercially under the trade name Di-Tab® (manufactured by Rhone-Poulenc).

B. Tribasic calcium phosphates
  - Tribasic calcium phosphate is also commonly referred as tricalcium phosphate, tricalcium orthophosphate and hydroxyapatite.
  - Tribasic calcium phosphate is available under the trade name Tri-Tab®.

III. Co-processed diluents (Table 1.2)

- Co-processing involves combining two or more materials by an appropriate process.
- The products so formed are physically modified in such a special way that they do not lose their chemical structure and stability. Nowadays direct compression technique has been one of the well-accepted methods of tablet manufacture.
- An extensive range of materials from various sources have been developed and marketed as directly compressible diluents such as lactose, starch, cellulose derivatives,

inorganic substance, polyalcohols, and sugar-based materials.

- In addition to the development of directly compressible excipients by modifying just a single substance, co-processing of two or more components has been applied to produce composite particles or co-processed excipients.
- The composite particles or co-processed excipients are introduced in order to provide better tableting properties than a single substance or the physical mixture.

**Table 1.2:** List of co-processed excipients used to achieve better tableting properties

| *Trade name* | *Description* |
|---|---|
| Fast flo lactose® | It is spray processed lactose which is a mixture of crystalline α-lactose monohydrate and amorphous lactose |
| Microcellac® | 75% lactose and 25% MCC (microcrystalline cellulose) |
| Ludipress® | 93% α-lactose monohydrate, 3.5% polyvinylpyrrolidone, and 3.5% Crospovidone |
| Nu-Tab® | Sucrose 95%–97%, invert sugar 3%–4% and magnesium stearate 0.5% |
| Di-Pac® | Sucrose 97% and modified dextrins 3% |
| Sugartab® | Sucrose 90%–93% and invert sugar 7%–10% |
| Emdex® | Dextrose 93%–99% and maltose 1%–7% |
| Cal-Tab® | Calcium sulfate 93% and vegetable gum 7% |
| Cal-Carb® | Calcium carbonate 95% and maltodextrins 5% |
| Calcium 90® | Calcium carbonate (minimum) 90% and starch, NF (maximum) 9% |

2. Binders

Binder is one of an important excipient to be added in tablet formulation. In simpler words, binders or adhesives are the substances that promote cohesiveness. It is utilized for converting powder into granules through a process known as granulation.

Types of binders (Tables 1.3–1.5)

Direct compression (DC) binders (Table 1.6)

Due to ease of manufacture, product stability and high efficiency, the use of direct compression for tableting has increased. For direct compression, directly compressible binders are required which should exhibit adequate powder compressibility and flowability. Direct compression binders should be selected on the basis of compression behavior, volume reduction under applied pressure and flow behavior in order to have optimum binding performance. The choice and selection of binders is extremely critical for direct compression tablets.

**Table 1.3**: Classification of binders

| *Sugars* | *Natural binders* | *Synthetic/semisynthetic polymers* |
|---|---|---|
| Sucrose | Acacia | Methylcellulose |
| Liquid glucose | Tragacanth | Ethylcellulose |
| | Gelatin | Hydroxy propyl methylcellulose (HPMC) |
| | Starch paste | Hydroxypropylcellulose |
| | Pregelatinized starch | Sodium carboxymethyl cellulose |
| | Alginic acid | Polyvinylpyrrolidone (PVP) |
| | Cellulose | Polyethylene glycol (PEG)<br>Polyvinyl alcohols<br>Polymethacrylates |

**Table 1.4**: Commonly used binders

| *Binders* | *Category* |
|---|---|
| Starch 1500 | Partially pregelatinized maize starch |
| Methocel | Hydroxypropyl methylcellulose |
| Walocel | Hydroxypropyl methylcellulose |
| Luvitec | Polyvinylpyrrolidone |
| Luvicross | Polyvinylpyrrolidone |
| Luvicaprolactam | Polyvinylcaprolactam |

**Table 1.5**: Characteristics of commonly used binder

| *Binders* | *Specified concentration* | *Comments* |
|---|---|---|
| Starch paste | 5%–25% w/w | – Freshly prepared starch paste is used as a binder<br>– Its method of preparation is very crucial |

*Contd...*

*Contd...*

| *Binders* | *Specified concentration* | *Comments* |
|---|---|---|
| Pregelatinized starch (PGS) | 5%–10% w/w (direct compression) | It is starch that have been processed chemically and/or mechanically to rupture all or part of the granules in the presence of water and subsequently dried |
| [Partially and fully PGS] | 5%–75% w/w (wet granulation) | – It contains 5% free amylose, 15% free amylopectin and 80% unmodified starch<br>– It is obtained from maize, potato or rice starch<br>– It is multifunctional excipient used as a tablet binder, diluent, disintegrant and flow aid<br>– They enhance both flow and compressibility and can be used as binders in direct compression as well as wet granulation<br>– High purity PGS allow simplified processing as they swell in cold water and therefore reduce time/costs compared with traditional starch paste preparation |
| Hydroxypropyl methyl cellulose (HPMC) | 2%–5% w/w | – It is comparable to methylcellulose<br>– It is used as a binder in either wet or dry granulation processes |
| Polyvinyl pyrrolidone (PVP) | 0.5%–5% w/w | – It is soluble in both water and alcohol<br>– It is used in wet granulation process<br>– It is also added to powder blends in the dry form and granulated in situ by the addition of water, alcohol or hydroalcoholic solution<br>– Valuable binder for chewable tablets<br>– The drug release is not altered on storage |
| Polyethylene glycol (PEG) 6000 | 10%–15% w/w | – It is used as a meltable binder<br>– Anhydrous granulating agent where water or alcohol cannot be used<br>– It may prolong disintegration time when concentration is 5% or higher<br>– It improves the plasticity of other binders |

3. Lubricants

Lubricants are the substances which prevents adhesion of the tablet material to the surface of the dies and punches, reduce interparticle friction, facilitate an easy ejection of tablets from the die cavity and improves rate of flow of tablet granulation. Commonly used lubricants are talc, magnesium stearate, calcium stearate, stearic acid, hydrogenated vegetable oil and PEG. The method of adding lubricant is an important factor for satisfactory results. The quantity of lubricant significantly varies from 0.1%–5%. The additions of lubricant to granules in the form of emulsion or suspension are used to reduce the processing time. The primary problem in the preparation of water soluble tablet is the selection of satisfactory lubricant. Soluble lubricants include sodium benzoate, sodium acetate, sodium chloride and Carbowax 4000.

**Table 1.6:** Commonly used DC binders

| *DC binders* | *Class* |
|---|---|
| Avicel (PH 101) | MCC[a] |
| SMCC (50) | SMCC[b] |
| Uni-pure (DW) | Partially PGS[c] |
| Uni-pure (LD) | Low density starch |
| DC lactose | DC lactose anhydrous |
| DI tab | DC-DCPD[d] |

a—Microcrystalline cellulose, b—Silicified microcrystalline cellulose, c—Pregelatinized starch, d—Dibasic calcium phosphate dihydrate

4. Glidants

A glidant is a substance that improves the flow characteristics of a powder mixture. These materials are always added in the dry state just prior to compression. The most commonly used glidants are colloidal silicon dioxide (Cabosil® and Cabot®) and asbestos free talc. They are used in concentration less than 1%. Talc is also used and may serve the dual purpose of lubricant/glidant.

### 5. Disintegrants

Disintegrants are the substance or a mixture of substances added to a tablet to facilitate its break up or disintegration after administration. Starches, clays, cellulose and cross-linked polymers are most commonly used disintegrants. The oldest and still the most popular disintegrants are corn and potato starch. Other ingredients like veegum, methylcellulose, agar, bentonite, cellulose, citrus pulp and CMC are also used. They are mostly added into two portions, one part is added prior to granulation and the remainder is mixed with the lubricant and finally both are mixed just before the compression.

Bioavailability of a drug depends in absorption of the drug, which is affected by solubility of the drug in gastrointestinal fluid and permeability of the drug across gastrointestinal membrane. The drugs solubility mainly depends on physical-chemical characteristics of the drug. However, the rate of drug dissolution is greatly influenced by disintegration of the tablet.

The drug will dissolve at a slower rate from a nondisintegrating tablet due to exposure of limited surface area to the fluid. The disintegration test is an official test and hence a batch of tablet must meet the stated requirements of disintegration.

Disintegrants, an important excipient of the tablet formulation, are always added to tablet to induce breakup of tablet when it comes in contact with aqueous fluid and this process of desegregation of constituent particles before the drug dissolution occurs, is known as disintegration process and excipients which induce this process are known as disintegrants.

The objectives behind addition of disintegrants are to increase surface area of the tablet fragments and to overcome cohesive forces that keep particles together in a tablet.

#### Methods of addition of disintegrants

The method of addition of disintegrants is also a crucial part. Disintegrating agent can be added either prior to granulation (intragranular) or prior to compression (after granulation, i.e. extragranular) or at the both processing steps. Extragranular fraction of disintegrant (usually, 50% of total disintegrant requires) facilitates breakup of tablets to granules and the intragranular addition of disintegrants produces further erosion of the granules to fine particles.

*Types of disintegrants (Table 1.7)*

i. Starch

Starch was the first disintegrating agent widely used in tablet manufacturing. Before 1906 potato starch and corn starch were used as disintegrants in tablet formulation. However, native starches have certain limitations and have been replaced by certain modified starches with specialized characteristics.

The mechanism of action of starch is wicking and restoration of deformed starch particles on contact with aqueous fluid releases certain amount of stress which is responsible for disruption of hydrogen bonding formed during compression.

The concentration of starch used is also very crucial part. If it is below the optimum concentration then there are insufficient channels for capillary action and if it is above optimum concentration then it will be difficult to compress the tablet.

ii. Pregelatinized starch

Pregelatinized starch is produced by the hydrolyzing and rupturing of the starch grain. It is a directly compressible disintegrants and its optimum concentration is 5%–10%. The

**Table 1.7:** List of disintegrants

| *Disintegrants* | *Concentration in granules (% w/w)* | *Special comments* |
|---|---|---|
| Starch | 5–20 | Higher amount is required, poorly compressible |
| Starch 1500 | 5–15 | - |
| Avicel® (PH 101, PH 102) | 10–20 | Lubricant properties and directly compressible |
| Solka-Floc® | 5–15 | Purified wood cellulose |
| Alginic acid | 1–5 | Acts by swelling |
| Na alginate | 2.5–10 | Acts by swelling |
| Explotab® | 2–8 | Sodium starch glycolate, superdisintegrant |
| Polyplasdone®(XL) | 0.5–5 | Cross-linked PVP |
| Amberlite® (IPR 88) | 0.5–5 | Ion exchange resin |
| Methylcellulose, Na CMC, HPMC | 5–10 | - |
| AC-DI-Sol® | 1–3 | Direct compression |

main mechanism of action of pregelatinized starch is through swelling.

iii. Modified starch

To have a high swelling properties and faster disintegration, starch is modified by carboxy methylation followed by cross-linking, which is available in market as cross-linked starch. Sodium starch glycolate and low substituted carboxymethyl starches (marketed under the trade name of Promogel and Explotab) are used as modified starches.

Mechanism of action of this modified starches are rapid and extensive swelling with minimum gelling. And its optimum concentration is 4%–6%. If it goes beyond its limit, then it produces viscous and gelatinous mass which increases the disintegration time by resisting the breakup of tablet. They are highly efficient at low concentration because of their greater swelling capacity.

iv. Cellulose and its derivatives

Sodium carboxy methylcellulose (NaCMC and Carmellose sodium) has highly hydrophilic structure and is soluble in water. But when it is modified by internally cross-linking, we get modified cross-linked cellulose, i.e. Cross Carmellose sodium which is nearly water insoluble due to cross-linking. It rapidly swells to 4–8 times its original volume when it comes in contact with water.

v. Microcrystalline cellulose (MCC)

MCC exhibits very good disintegrating properties because MCC is insoluble and act by wicking action. The moisture breaks the hydrogen bonding between adjacent bundles of MCC. It also serves as an excellent binder and has a tendency to develop static charges in the presence of excessive moisture content. Therefore, sometimes it causes separation in granulation. This can be partially overcome by drying the cellulose to remove the moisture.

vi. Alginates

Alginates are hydrophilic colloidal substances which has high sorption capacity. Chemically, they are alginic acid and salts of alginic acid. Alginic acid is insoluble in water, slightly acidic in reaction. Hence, it should be used in only acidic or neutral granulation. Unlike starch and MCC, alginates do not retard flow and can be successfully used with ascorbic acid, multivitamin formulations and acid salts of organic bases.

vii. Ion-exchange resin

Ion-exchange resin (Amberlite®IPR-88) has higher water uptake capacity than other disintegrating agents like starch and sodium CMC. It has tendency to adsorb certain drugs.

viii. Miscellaneous

This miscellaneous category includes disintegrants like surfactants, gas producing disintegrants and hydrous aluminium silicate. Gas producing disintegrating agents is used in soluble tablet, dispersible tablet and effervescent tablet.

Polyplasdone®XL and Polyplasdone®XLIO act by wicking, swelling and possibly some deformation recovery. Polyplasdone®XL does not reduce tablet hardness, provide rapid disintegration and improved dissolution. Polyplasdone® as disintegrating agent has small particle size distribution that imparts a smooth mouth feel to dissolve quickly. Chewable tablet does not require addition of disintegrant.

Superdisintegrants (Table 1.8)

As day passes, demand for faster disintegrating formulation is increasing. So, pharmacist needs to formulate disintegrants i.e. superdisintegrants which are effective at low concentration and have greater disintegrating efficiency and they are more effective intragranularly. But, they have one drawback, i.e. hygroscopic therefore, are not used with moisture sensitive drugs.

And this superdisintegrants act by swelling and due to swelling pressure exerted in the outer direction or radial direction, it causes tablet to burst or the accelerated absorption of water leading to an enormous increase in the volume of granules to promote disintegration.

### *Factors affecting disintegration*

A. Effect of fillers

The solubility and compression characteristics of fillers affect both rate and mechanism of disintegration of tablet. If soluble fillers are used then it may cause increase in viscosity of the penetrating fluid which tends to reduce effectiveness of strongly swelling disintegrating agents and as they are water-soluble, they are likely to dissolve rather than disintegrate. Insoluble diluents produce rapid disintegration with adequate amount of disintegrants.

**Table 1.8:** List of superdisintegrants

| *Superdisintegrants* | *Example* | *Mechanism of action* | *Special comment* |
|---|---|---|---|
| Cross carmellose®<br>Ac-Di-Sol®<br>Nymce ZSX®<br>Primellose®<br>Solutab®<br>Vivasol® | Cross-linked cellulose | Swells 4–8 folds in < 10 seconds<br>Swelling and wicking both | Swells in two dimensions.<br>Direct compression or granulation |
| Crospovidone<br>Crospovidone M®<br>Kollidon®<br>Polyplasdone® | Cross-linked PVP | Swells very little and returns to original size after compression but act by capillary action | Water insoluble and spongy in nature so get porous tablet |
| Sodium starch glycolate<br>Explotab®<br>Primogel® | Cross-linked starch | Swells 7–12 folds in < 30 seconds | Swells in three dimensions and high level serve as sustain release matrix |
| Alginic acid NF<br>Satialgine® | Cross-linked alginic acid | Rapid swelling in aqueous medium or wicking action | Promote disintegration in both dry or wet granulation |
| Soy polysaccharides<br>Emcosoy® | Natural super disintegrant | | Does not contain any starch or sugar. It is Used in nutritional products. |
| Calcium silicate | | Wicking action | Highly porous,<br>Light weight<br>Optimum concentration is between 20%–40% |

B. Effect of binder

As binding capacity of the binder increases, disintegrating time of tablet increases and this counteract the rapid disintegration. Even the concentration of the binder can also affect the disintegration time of tablet.

C. Effect of lubricants

Mostly, lubricants are hydrophobic and they are usually used in smaller size than any other ingredient in the tablet formulation. When the mixture is mixed, lubricant particles may adhere to the surface of the other particles. This hydrophobic coating inhibits the wetting and consequently tablet disintegration.

Lubricant has a strong negative effect on the water uptake if tablet contains no disintegrants or even high concentration of slightly swelling disintegrants. On the contrary, the disintegration time is hardly affected if there is some strongly swelling disintegrants are present in the tablet. But there is one exception like sodium starch glycolate whose effect remains unaffected in the presence of hydrophobic lubricant unlike other disintegrants.

D. Effect of surfactants

Sodium lauryl sulfate increased absorption of water by starch or had a variable effect on water penetration in tablets. Surfactants are only effective within certain concentration ranges. Surfactants are recommended to decrease the hydrophobicity of the drugs because the more hydrophobic the tablet the greater the disintegration time. It is claimed that disintegration time of granules of water-soluble drugs does not seem to be greatly improved by the addition of nonionic surfactant during granulation, but the desired effect of a surfactant appears when granules are made of slightly soluble drugs. The speed of water penetration is increased by the addition of a surfactant.

6. Coloring agents

Colors in compressed tablet are used to impart aesthetic appearance to the dosage form. Color helps the manufacturer to control the product during its preparation as well as serves as a means of identification to the user. One of the basic requirements concerning the use of colorant in pharmaceuticals is that it must be approved and certified by the FDA. Colorants can be used in solution form or in suspension form. Proper distribution of suspended colorants in the coating solution requires the use of the powdered colorants (<10 microns).

Most commonly used colorants in use are certified FD & C or D & C colorants. These are synthetic dyes or lakes. Lakes are choice for sugar or film coating as they give reproducible results. Concentration of colorants in the coating solutions depends on the color shade desired, the type of dye, and the concentration of opaquant-extenders. If very light shade is desired, concentration of less than 0.01% may be adequate on the other hand, if a dark color is desired a concentration of more than 2.0% may be required. The inorganic materials (e.g. iron oxide) and the natural coloring materials (e.g. anthocyanins, carotenoids, etc.) are also used to prepare coating solution. Anthocyanin magenta red dye is nonabsorbable in biologic system and resistant to degradation in the gastrointestinal tract.

7. Flavoring agents

Flavors are usually limited to chewable tablets or other tablets intended to dissolve in the mouth. In general flavors that are water soluble have been found little acceptance in manufacturing of tablets because of their poor stability. Flavoring agents do not affect any physical characteristics of the tablet granulation. Flavors are incorporated either as solids (spray dried flavors) or oils or aqueous flavors. Solids that are dry flavors, are easier to handle and generally more stable than oils.

8. Sweetening agents

Sweeteners are added to tablet formulation to improve the taste of chewable tablets. One has to be careful in deciding the nature and concentration of the sweeteners as most of them may produce undesirable taste and some may be carcinogenic.

*Some commonly used sweeteners in tablet formulations are:*

**Natural sweeteners**: Mannitol, lactose, sucrose and dextrose
**Artificial sweeteners**: Saccharine, cyclamate and aspartame

Saccharine is 500 times sweeter than sucrose. Its major disadvantages are, that it has a bitter after taste and is carcinogenic. Even cyclamate is carcinogenic. Aspartame is about 180 times sweeter than sucrose. The primary disadvantage of aspartame is its lack of stability in the presence of moisture. List of Excipient with their functions given in Table 1.9:

**Table 1.9:** Excipient with their functions in tablet formulation

| *Excipients* | *Functions* |
|---|---|
| Diluents or fillers | Diluents make the required bulk of the tablet when the drug dosage itself is inadequate to produce tablets of adequate weight and size |

*Contd...*

*Contd...*

| *Excipients* | *Functions* |
|---|---|
| Binders or granulating agents or adhesives | Binders are added to tablet formulations to add cohesiveness to powders, thus providing the necessary bonding to form granules, which under compaction form a cohesive mass or a compact which is referred to as a tablet |
| Disintegrants | A disintegrant is added to most tablet formulations to facilitate a breakup or disintegration of the tablet when placed in an aqueous environment |
| *Antifrictional agents*: | |
| Lubricants | Lubricants are intended to reduce the friction during tablet formation in a die and also during ejection from die cavity |
| Antiadherents | Antiadherents are added to reduce sticking or adhesion of any of the tablet granulation or powder to the faces of the punches or to the die wall |
| Glidants | Glidants are intended to promote the flow of tablet granulation or powder mixture from hopper to the die cavity by reducing friction between the particles |
| Miscellaneous Wetting agents | Wetting agents are added to tablet formulation to aid Water uptake during disintegration and assist drug dissolution |
| Dissolution retardants | Dissolution retardants as the name suggest, retards the dissolution of active pharmaceutical ingredient(s) |
| Dissolution enhancers | Dissolution enhancers as the name suggest, enhance the dissolution rate of active pharmaceutical ingredient(s) |
| Adsorbents | Adsorbents are capable of retaining large quantities of liquids without becoming wet; this property of absorbent allows many oils, fluid extracts and eutectic melts to be incorporated into tablets |
| Buffers | Buffers are added to provide suitable microenvironmental pH to get improved stability and/or bioavailability |
| Antioxidants | Antioxidants are added to maintain product stability, they act by being preferentially oxidized and gradually consumed over shelf life of the product |
| Chelating agents | Chelating agents are added to protect against autoxidation; they act by forming complexes with the heavy metal ions which are often required to initiate oxidative reactions |
| Preservatives | Preservatives are added to tablet formulation in order to prevent the growth of micro-organisms |
| Colors | Colors are added to tablet formulation for following purposes: to disguise off color drugs, product identification and for production of more elegant product |

*Contd...*

*Contd...*

| *Excipients* | *Functions* |
|---|---|
| Flavors | Flavors are added to tablet formulation in order to make them palatable enough in case of chewable tablet by improving the taste |
| Sweeteners | Sweeteners are added to tablet formulation to improve the taste of chewable tablets |

## GRANULATION

Granulation may be defined as a size enlargement process which converts small particles into physically stronger and larger agglomerates.

Powders/granules intended for compression into tablets must possess two essential properties—flow property and compressibility. Flow property/fluidity is required to produce tablets of a consistent weight and uniform strength. Compressibility is required to form a stable, intact compact mass when pressure is applied. These two objectives are obtained by adding binder to tablet formulation and then proceeding for granulation process. Granules so formed should possess acceptable flow property and compressibility. Some drugs exhibit poor fluidity and compressibility. In such cases, binders have to be added for improving flow property and compressibility. Other reasons for granulation process are to improve appearance, mixing properties, to avoid dustiness, to densify material, to reduce segregation, in general either to eliminate undesirable properties or to improve the physical and chemical properties of fine powders.

### Granulation processes

The standard methods frequently used today in tablet manufacturing are granulation and direct compression. Granulation technique includes wet granulation and dry granulation/slugging methods wherein binders are added in solution/suspension form and in dry form respectively. In direct compression, binders possessing direct compressibility characteristics are used. Binder when used in liquid form gives better binding action as compared to when used in dry form.

## Mechanism of granule formation (Fig. 1.8)

*Granules are formed in three stages:*

i. **Nucleation**: Here, the particles adhere due to liquid bridges which are the initiation step of granulation. These adhered particles play a role of nucleus for further enlargement of granules.
ii. **Transition**: Enlargement of nucleus takes place by two possible mechanisms. Individual particle adhere to the nucleus or two or more nuclei combine among themselves.
iii. **Ball growth or enlargement of the granule**: Ball growth occurs either by coalescence or breakage or abrasion transfer or layering. In coalescence, a larger granule is formed when two or more granules are united. In breakage, granules break and the fragments of granule adhere to other granules. This forms a layer of material over intact granules. In abrasion transfer, granule materials are abraded through attrition by the agitation of granule bed and abraded material adheres to other granules resulting into enlarged granules. In layering, particles adhere to the already formed granules and increasing their size.

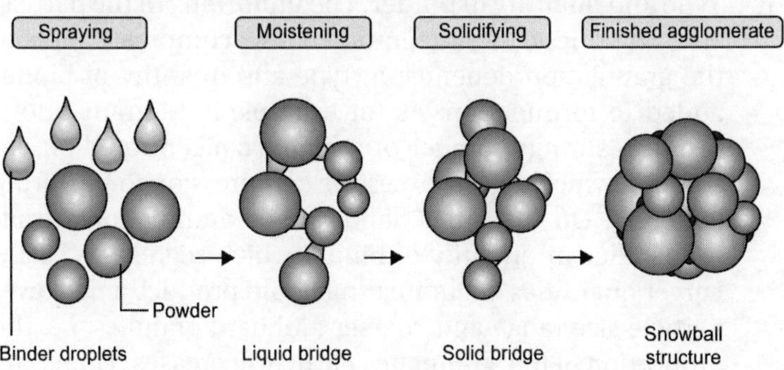


FIGURE 1.8: Stages of granule formation

## Factors to be considered in granulation

i. **Compatibility**: The primary criteria are the compatibility of binder with the API and other tablet components. This is traditionally found by choosing appropriate stability study design. Currently, differential scanning calorimetry (DSC) is used to ascertain compatibility.

ii. **Characteristics of drugs and other excipients**: The drugs characteristics like its compressibility, particle size, surface area, porosity, hydrophobicity, solubility in binder are important while fixing a granulation process. The drug that exhibits poor compressibility requires the use of a strong binder (liquid glucose, sucrose, etc.) while the drugs that exhibit good compressibility can be successfully handled using a weak binder ( starch paste, etc.). Fine and porous particles require higher amount of liquid binder as compared to coarse particles. Hydrophilic drug/excipients exhibiting absorption characteristics require higher volume of binder as compared to hydrophobic drug/ excipients. The granule quality (size, friability) is governed by the solubility of the drug in the granulation solution.

iii. **Spreading of binder**: Spreading of binder/granulation solution on the powder blend is of paramount importance in successful granulation. A binder that spreads easily on particles, is superior as compared to that which shows poor wetting quality. HPMC is a superior binder for paracetamol as compared to PVP.

iv. **Type and quantity of binder**: The uniformity of the particle size, hardness, disintegration and compressibility of the granulation depends on type and quantity of binder added to formulation. As for example hard granulations result to stronger binder or a highly concentrated binder solution which require excessive compression force during tableting. On the other hand, fragile granulations result to insufficient quantity of binder which segregates easily. Larger quantities of granulating liquid produce a narrower particle size range and coarser and hard granules, i.e. the proportion of fine granulates particle decreases. Therefore, the optimum quantity of liquid needed to get a given particle size should be known in order to keep a batch to batch variations to a minimum.

v. **Temperature and viscosity**: The temperature and viscosity of binder are also important. Fluid (less viscous) binders exhibit good spreading behavior.

vi. **Method of addition of binder**: The method of addition of binder is also important. PVP can be used as solution as a binder or it may be dry blended with powders and later activated by adding water. Distribution of binder is favored if it is dispersed instead of pouring it.

vii. **Mixing time**: The mixing time also determines quality of granules. If the wet massing time is higher (resulting into hard granules), the tablets may fail the dissolution test in certain cases since drug release from hard granules is altered.

viii. **Material of construction of granulator**: The material of construction of granulator determines the volume of binder required as well as granule size distribution. Any vessel walls which are wetted easily by binder demand the need of higher volume of binder. As for example, vessel wall made up of stainless steel requires higher volume of binder as compared to vessel made up of plastics (PMMA–polymethylmethacrylate and PTFE–polytetrafluoroethylene, i.e. Teflon). In case of PMMA and PTFE due to high contact angle, all granulating liquid is forced immediately into the powder bed and gives narrow particle size distribution.

ix. **Type of granulator**: Fluidized bed granulator produces porous granules as compared to high shear granulators.

x. Process variables: Higher degree of densification of the granules results to higher impeller speed as well as longer wet massing time. And also there is tendency of agglomeration since liquid saturation increases. Consequently, impeller speed and wet massing time affect the granule size.

xi. **Apparatus variables**: The apparatus variables in high shear mixer have a larger effect on granule growth than in fluidized bed granulators because the shear forces are dependent on the mixer construction. The size and shape of the mixing chamber, impeller and chopper vary in different high shear mixers.

xii. **Impeller movement**: Adhesion of wetted mass to the vessel is less if impeller movement is helical. This gives a narrower granule size and few lumps. In case of high shear mixers, adhesion of wetted mass to the vessel is a problem which can be reduced by proper construction of the impeller or by coating the vessel with polytetrafluoroethylene, i.e. Teflon.

## Ideal characteristics of granules

The ideal characteristics of granules include uniformity, good flow, and compactibility. These are usually accomplished through creation of increased density, spherical shape, narrow particle size distribution with sufficient fines to fill void spaces between granules, adequate moisture (between 1%–2%), and incorporation of binder, if necessary.

The effectiveness of granulation depends on the following properties:

i. Particle size of the drug and excipients.
ii. Type of binder (strong or weak).
iii. Volume of binder (less or more).
iv. Wet massing time (less or more).
v. Amount of shear applied to distribute drug, binder and moisture.
vi. Drying rate (hydrate formation and polymorphism).

## Evaluation tests for binders/granules

Compactness, physical and chemical stability, rapid production capability, efficacy are some of the characteristics that make tablet a ruling dosage form. These characteristics depend on the quality of granules from which it is made. The characteristics of granules produced are affected by formulation and process variables. So, it becomes essential to evaluate the granule characteristics to monitor its suitability for tableting.

A. **Particle size and particle size distribution**: The particle size of granules affect the average tablet weight, tablet weight variation, disintegration time, granule friability, granulation flowability and the drying rate kinetics of wet granulations. Therefore, the effects of granule size and size distribution on the quality of tablet should be determined by formulator. The methods usually adopted for measurement of particle size and particle size distribution includes microscopy, sieving, sedimentation and conductivity test.
B. **Surface area**: Surface area of the drug effects upon dissolution rate specially in cases where drug have limited water solubility. The two most common methods for surface area determination are gas adsorption and air permeability.
C. **Density**: Granule density, true density, bulk density may influence compressibility, tablet porosity, flow property, dissolution and other properties. Higher compression load is required in case of dense and hard granules which in turn

increases the tablet disintegration and drug dissolution times. Density is usually determined by pycnometer.

D. **Percentage compressibility**: Compressibility is the ability of powder to decrease in volume under pressure. Compressibility is a measure that is obtained from density determinations.

Percentage compressibility = (tapped density – bulk density/tapped density) × 100

Compressibility measures gives idea about flow property of the granules as per Carr's Index Relationship between Carr's index and flow property is shown in Table 1.10.

**Table 1.10**: Relationship between Carr's index and flow property

| *% compressibility* | *Flow description* |
|---|---|
| 5–15 | Excellent |
| 12–16 | Good |
| 18–21 | Fair |
| 23–28 | Poor |
| 28–35 | Poor |
| 35–38 | Very poor |
| > 40 | Extremely poor |

E. **Flow properties**: It is very important parameter to be measured since it affects the mass of uniformity of the dose. It is usually predicted from Hausner's ratio and angle of repose measurement. Relationship between Hausner's ratio and flow property is shown in Table 1.11.

Hausner's ratio

Hausner's ratio = tapped density/bulk density.

**Table 1.11**: Relationship between Hausner's ratio and flow property

| *Hausner's ratio* | *Type of flow* |
|---|---|
| Less than 1.25 | Good flow |
| 1.25–1.5 | Moderate |
| More than 1.5 | Poor flow |

Angle of repose (Φ)

Angle of repose (Φ) is the maximum angle between the surface of a pile of powder and horizontal plane. It is usually determined by fixed funnel method and is the measure of the flowability of powder/granules. Relationship between angle of repose and flow property is shown in Table 1.12:

$$\Phi = \tan^{-1} (h/r)$$

Where, h = height of heap of pile
r = radius of base of pile

**Table 1.12**: Relationship between angle of repose and flow property

| *Angle of repose (Φ)* | *Type of flow* |
|---|---|
| < 25 | Excellent |
| 25 – 30 | Good |
| 30 – 40 | Passable |
| > 40 | Very poor |

F. **Friability**: Friability is important since it affects in particle size distribution of granules affecting compressibility into tablet, tablet weight variation, granule flowability. Friability is determined carrying out tumbler test or using friability tester (Roche Friabilator) and % loss is determined.

G. **Moisture content**: It affects the granule flowability, compressibility as well as the stability of moisture sensitive drug and therefore, should be determined to evaluate the quality of granule.

## METHOD OF TABLET PREPARATION

There are three general methods of tablet preparation—

### 1. Direct compression method

The method consists of compressing tablets directly from powdered material without modifying the physical nature of the materials itself. This method of tablet making is of special interest for small group of crystalline chemicals having the entire physical characteristic necessary for the formulation of a good tablet. Substances like chlorides, chlorates, bromides, iodides, nitrates and permanganates, salts of potassium, ammonium chloride and methanamine, etc. are manufactured by direct compression as they have cohesive properties. Advantages of this method are simplicity of process, absence of granulating steps, avoidance of moisture and drying step, minimum material handling and rapidity of the total process. The limitations of this method are that only a few crystalline drugs can be directly compressed. Otherwise this process has no other major limitation.

In early days, most of the tablets require granulation of the powdered active pharmaceutical ingredient (API) and excipients. The availability of new excipients or modified form of old excipients and the invention of new tablet machinery or modification of old tablet machinery provides an ease in manufacturing of tablets by simple procedure of direct compression.

Amongst the techniques used to prepare tablets, direct compression is the most advanced technology. It involves only blending and compression, thus offering advantage particularly in terms of speedy production. Because it requires fewer unit operations, less machinery, reduced number of personnel and considerably less processing time along with increased product stability.

The term "direct compression" is defined as the process by which tablets are compressed directly from powder mixture of API and suitable excipients. No pretreatment of the powder blend by wet or dry granulation procedure is required.

### Merits

- Direct compression is more efficient and economical process as compared to other processes, because it involves only dry blending and compaction of API and necessary excipients.
- The most important advantage of direct compression is economical process. Reduced processing time; reduced labor costs, fewer manufacturing steps, and less number of equipments is required, less process validation, reduced consumption of power.
- Elimination of heat and moisture, thus increasing not only the stability but also the suitability of the process for thermolabile and moisture sensitive API's.
- Particle size uniformity.
- Prime particle dissolution. In case of directly compressed tablets after disintegration, each primary drug particle is liberated. While in the case of tablets prepared by compression of granules, small drug particles with a larger surface area adhere together into larger agglomerates; thus decreasing the surface area available for dissolution.

- The chances of batch-to-batch variation are negligible, because the unit operations required for manufacturing processes is fewer. Chemical stability problems for API and excipient would be avoided.
- It provides stability against the effect of aging which affects the dissolution rates.

*Merits over wet granulation process*

The variables faced in the processing of the granules can lead to significant tableting problems. Properties of granules formed can be affected by viscosity of granulating solution, the rate of addition of granulating solution, type of mixer used and duration of mixing, method and rate of dry and wet blending. The above variables can change the density and the particle size of the resulting granules and may have a major influence on fill weight and compaction qualities. Drying can lead to unblending as soluble API migrates to the surface of the drying granules.

### Demerits

a. Excipient related
   i. Problems in the uniform distribution of low dose drugs.
   ii. High dose drugs having high bulk volume, poor compressibility and poor flowability are not suitable for direct compression. For example, aluminium hydroxide, magnesium hydroxide.
   iii. The choice of excipients for direct compression is extremely critical. Direct compression diluents and binders must possess both good compressibility and good flowability.
   iv. Many active ingredients are not compressible either in crystalline or amorphous forms.
   v. Direct compression blends may lead to unblending because of difference in particle size or density of drug and excipients. Similarly the lack of moisture may give rise to static charges, which may lead to unblending.
   vi. Nonuniform distribution of color, specially in tablets of deep colors.
b. Process related
   i. Capping, lamination, splitting, or layering of tablets are sometimes related to air entrapment during direct

compression. When air is trapped, the resulting tablets expand. When the pressure of tablet is released, and resulting in splits or layers in the tablet.

ii. In some cases require greater sophistication in blending and compression equipments.
iii. Direct compression equipments are expensive.

*Steps involved in direct compression*

i. Milling of drug and excipients
ii. Mixing of drug and excipients
iii. Tablet compression.

*Direct compression excipients*

Direct compression excipients mainly include diluents, binders and disintegrants. Generally, these are common materials that have been modified during the chemical manufacturing process, in such a way that it improves compressibility and flowability of the material. The physicochemical properties of the ingredients such as particle size, flowability and moisture are critical in direct compression tableting. The success of direct compression formulation is highly dependent on functional behavior of excipients.

**An ideal direct compression excipient should possess the following attributes:**

i. It should have good compressibility.
ii. It should possess good hardness after compression, that is material should not possess any deformational properties; otherwise this may lead to capping and lamination of tablets.
iii. It should have good flowability.
iv. It should be physiologically inert.
v. It should be compatible with wide range of API.
vi. It should be stable to various environmental conditions (air, moisture, heat, etc.).
vii. It should not show any physical or chemical change in its properties on aging.
viii. It should have high dilution potential, i.e. able to incorporate high amount of API.
ix. It should be colorless, odorless and tasteless.
x. It should accept colorants uniformity.
xi. It should possess suitable organoleptic properties according to formulation type, i.e. in case of chewable

tablet diluent should have suitable taste and flavor. For example, mannitol produces cooling sensation in mouth and also sweet taste.

xii. It should not interfere with bioavailability and biological activity of active ingredients.

xiii. It should be easily available and economical in cost.

## 2. Dry granulation method

This process of granulation is also known as slugging, double compression or recompression method. This process of tablet preparation is commonly used when the tablet ingredients are sensitive to moisture or are unable to withstand elevated temperature during drying. Under such conditions, dry granulation is the method of choice provided the tablet ingredients have sufficient inherent binding or cohesive properties. The essential steps are weighing, mixing, slugging, dry screening, lubrication and compression. For the formation of a cohesive slug, spray dried or powdered binders such as acacia or microcrystalline cellulose may be added to the dry powder. Lubricants are added to reduce powder adhesion to the punches and to facilitate ejection of intact slugs from the dies. Initially, large slugs are obtained by compressing powdered material containing excipients. The slugs are then forced through mesh screen breaking them into granules. The remaining lubricant is added to the granulation with gentle blending and the resulting material is compressed into tablet.

### Advantages

The main advantages of dry granulation or slugging are that it uses less equipments and space. It eliminates the need for binder solution, heavy mixing equipment and the cost and time consuming drying step required for wet granulation. Slugging can be used for advantages in the following situations:

i. For moisture sensitive material
ii. For heat sensitive material
iii. For improved disintegration since powder particles are not bonded together by a binder.

### Disadvantages

i. It requires a specialized heavy duty tablet press to form slug.

ii. It does not permit uniform color distribution as can be achieved with wet granulation where the dye can be incorporated into binder liquid.
iii. The process tends to create more dust than wet granulation, increasing the potential contamination.

*Steps in dry granulation*

i. Milling of drugs and excipients
ii. Mixing of milled powders
iii. Compression into large, hard tablets to make slug
iv. Screening of slugs
v. Mixing with lubricant and disintegrating agent
vi. Tablet compression.

*Dry granulation process*

In dry granulation process the powder mixture is compressed without the use of heat and solvent. It is the least desirable of all methods of granulation. The two basic procedures are to form a compact of material by compression and then to mill the compact to obtain a granules. Two methods are used for dry granulation. The more widely used method is slugging, where the powder is precompressed and the resulting tablet or slug are milled to yield the granules. The other method is to precompress the powder with pressure rolls using a machine such as chilosonator.

A. Slugging process

Granulation by slugging is the process of compressing dry powder of tablet formulation with tablet press having die cavity large enough in diameter to fill quickly. The accuracy or condition of slug is not too important. Only sufficient pressure to compact the powder into uniform slugs should be used. Once slugs are produced they are reduced to appropriate granule size for final compression by screening and milling.

Factors which determine how well a material may slug are:

i. Compressibility or cohesiveness of the matter
ii. Compression ratio of powder
iii. Density of the powder
iv. Machine type
v. Punch and die size
vi. Slug thickness
vii. Speed of compression
viii. Pressure used to produce slug

B. Roller compaction (Fig. 1.9)

The compaction of powder by means of pressure roll can also be accomplished by a machine called chilsonator. Unlike tablet machine, the chilsonator turns out a compacted mass in a steady continuous flow. The powder is fed down between the rollers from the hopper which contains a spiral auger to feed the powder into the compaction zone. Like slugs, the aggregates are screened or milled for production into granules.

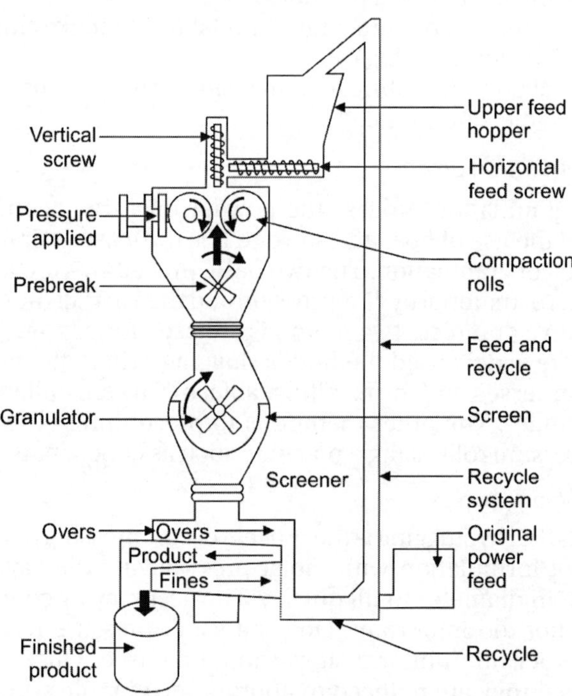


FIGURE 1.9: Chilsonator roller compactor

Excipients required for dry granulation

The excipients used for dry granulation are basically same as that of wet granulation or that of direct compression. With dry granulation, it is often possible to compact the active ingredient with a minor addition of lubricant and disintegrating agent. Fillers that are used in dry granulation include the following examples: Lactose, dextrose, sucrose, MCC, calcium sulfate, Sta-Rx®, etc.

### 3. Wet granulation method

This is the oldest and the most widely used method of tablet preparation. The powdered and mixed tablet ingredients are converted into a moist coherent mass and then into granules before compression into tablets. The essential steps that are involved during the preparation of tablet are weighing, mixing, granulation, screening the dump mass, drying, dry screening, lubrication and finally compression. This method is time consuming. The process involves the blending and mixing of active ingredients, diluents and disintegrant. The mixed material is then sifted through a screen of suitable mesh to remove or break the lumps. The sifted material is converted into a damp mass by adding and mixing with the binder solution. The damp mass is forced through 6–8 mesh screens for granulation. The wet granules are dried in an oven; particles may agglomerate and forms lumps and therefore dry screening operation is often required after drying. To the dried granules is then added the remaining quantity of disintegrant and lubricant. Finally, the granules are compressed into tablets.

*Steps involved in the wet granulation*

i. Mixing of the drug(s) and excipients.
ii. Preparation of binder solution.
iii. Mixing of binder solution with powder mixture to form wet mass.
iv. Coarse screening of wet mass using a suitable sieve (6–12 no. sieve).
v. Drying of moist granules.
vi. Screening of dry granules through a suitable sieve (14–20 no. sieve).
vii. Mixing of screened granules with disintegrant, glidant, and lubricant.

*Limitation of wet granulation*

i. The greatest disadvantage of wet granulation is its cost. It is an expensive process because of labor, time, equipment, energy and space requirements.
ii. Loss of material during various stages of processing.
iii. Stability may be major concern for moisture sensitive or thermolabile drugs.

iv. Multiple processing steps add complexity and make validation and control difficult.
v. An inherent limitation of wet granulation is that any incompatibility between formulation components is aggravated.

*Special wet granulation techniques*

i. High shear mixture granulation
ii. Fluid bed granulation
iii. Extrusion-spheronization
iv. Spray drying.

## i. High shear mixture granulation

High shear mixture has been widely used in pharmaceutical industries for blending and granulation. Blending and wet massing is accompanied by high mechanical agitation by an impeller and a chopper. Mixing, densification and agglomeration are achieved through shear and compaction force exerted by the impeller.

*Advantages*

A. Short processing time.
B. Less amount of liquid binders required compared with fluid bed.
C. Highly cohesive material can be granulated.

## ii. Fluid bed granulation

Fluidization is the operation by which fine solids are transformed into a fluid like state through contact with a gas. At certain gas velocity the fluid will support the particles giving them free mobility without entrapment.

Fluid bed granulation is a process by which granules are produced in single equipment by spraying a binder solution onto a fluidized powder bed. The material processed by fluid bed granulation are finer, free flowing and homogeneous.

## iii. Extrusion and spheronization

It is a multiple step process capable of making uniform sized spherical particles. It is primarily used as a method to produce multi-particulates for controlled release application.

*Advantages*

A. Ability to incorporate higher levels of active components without producing excessively larger particles.
B. Applicable to both immediate and controlled release dosage form.

### iv. Spray drying granulation

It is a unique granulation technique that directly converts liquids into dry powder in a single step. This method removes moisture instantly and converts pumpable liquids into a dry powder.

*Advantages*

A. Rapid process
B. Ability to be operated continuously
C. Suitable for heat sensitive product.

Lists of equipments for wet granulation

A. High shear granulation:
   i. Little ford lodgie granulator
   ii. Little ford MGT granulator
   iii. Diosna granulator
   iv. Gral mixer.
B. Granulator with drying facility:
   i. Fluidized bed granulator
   ii. Day nauta mixer processor

**Table 1.13**: Typical unit operation involved in wet granulation, dry granulation and direct compression

| *Wet granulation* | *Dry granulation* | *Direct compression* |
|---|---|---|
| Milling/screening | Milling/screening | Milling/screening |
| Preblending | Preblending | Blending |
| Addition of binder | Slugging/roller compaction | Compression |
| Screening of wet mass | Dry screening | |
| Drying of the wet granules | Blending of lubricant | |
| Screening of dry granules | Compression | |
| Blending of lubricant (and disintegrant) | | |
| Compression | | |

iii. Double cone or twin shell processor
iv. Topo granulator.

C. Special granulator:
i. Roto granulator
ii. Marumerizer.

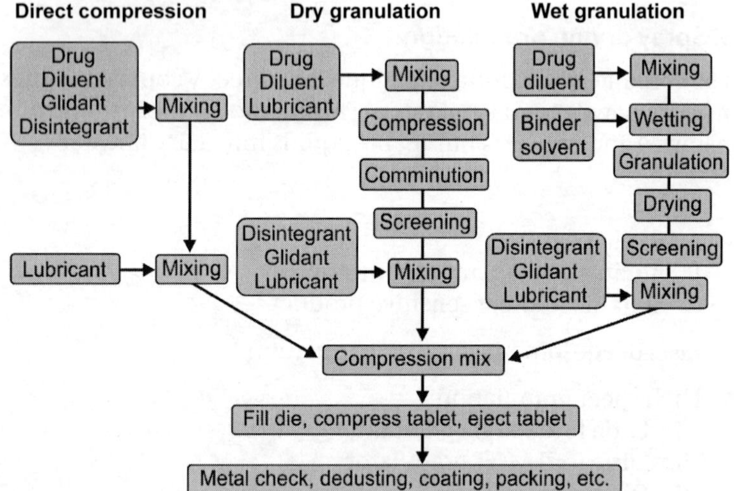


FIGURE 1.10: Typical unit operation involved in wet granulation, dry granulation and direct compression

**Table 1.14**: Comparative features of wet granulation, dry granulation and direct compression

| *Wet granulation* | *Dry granulation* | *Direct compression* |
|---|---|---|
| • Improved flow by increasing particle size and sphericity | • Improved flow by increasing particle size | • Fewer processing steps – blending and compression. hence, reduced processing time |
| • Uniform distribution of API, color, etc.– improved content uniformity | • Improved uniformity of powder density | • Processing without moisture and heat – fewer stability problems |
| • Good for bulky powders, less dust and environmental contamination | • Improved cohesion during compression | • Rapid and most direct method of tablet compression |
| • Lower compression pressure, less wear and tear on tooling | • Granulation without addition of liquid | • Changes in dissolution less likely on ageing since there are less formulation variables |

## ADVANCEMENT IN GRANULATIONS

### A. Steam granulation

It is modification of wet granulation. Here steam is used as a binder instead of water. Its several benefits includes higher distribution uniformity, higher diffusion rate into powders, more favorable thermal balance during drying step, steam granules are more spherical, have large surface area hence increased dissolution rate of the drug from granules, processing time is shorter, therefore, more number of tablets are produced per batch, compared to the use of organic solvent water vapor is environmentally friendly, no health hazards to operators, no restriction by ICH on traces left in the granules, freshly distilled steam is sterile and therefore the total count can be kept under control, lowers dissolution rate so can be used for preparation of taste masked granules without modifying availability of the drug. But the limitation is that it is unsuitable for thermolabile drugs. Moreover, special equipments are required and are unsuitable for binders that cannot be later activated by contact with water vapor.

### B. Melt granulation/thermoplastic granulation

Here granulation is achieved by the addition of meltable binder. That is binder is in solid state at room temperature but melts in the temperature range of 50°–80°C. Melted binder then acts like a binding liquid. There is no need of drying phase since dried granules are obtained by cooling it to room temperature. Moreover, amount of liquid binder can be controlled precisely and the production and equipment costs are reduced. It is useful for granulating water sensitive material and producing sustained release granulation or solid dispersion. But this method, is not suitable for thermolabile substances. When water soluble binders are needed, polyethylene glycol (PEG) is used as melting binders. When water insoluble binders are needed, stearic acid, cetyl or stearyl alcohol, various waxes and mono-, di- and triglycerides are used as melting binders.

### C. Moisture activated dry granulation (MADG)

It involves minimal moisture addition, distribution and agglomeration. No drying step is required. Water distribution is via high-shear mixer, or low-shear mixer with highly atomized water spray. Tablets prepared using MADG method has better content uniformity than direct compression. This method utilizes very little granulating fluid and requires no drying, since any excess moisture is absorbed by hydrophilic polymers such as cellulose or silica added to the moist preblend. It produces granules with excellent flowability and uniformity, and is applicable to controlled release.

### D. Moist granulation technique (MGT)

It involves addition of small amount of granulating fluid to activate dry binder and to facilitate agglomeration. Then a moisture absorbing material like microcrystalline cellulose (MCC) is added to absorb any excess moisture. By adding MCC in this way, drying step is not necessary. It is applicable for developing a controlled release formulation.

### E. Thermal adhesion granulation process (TAGP)

It is applicable for preparing direct tableting formulations. TAGP is performed under low moisture content or low content of pharmaceutically acceptable solvent by subjecting a mixture containing excipients to heating at a temperature in the range from about 30°C to about 130°C in a closed system under mixing by tumble rotation until the formation of granules. This method utilizes less water or solvent than traditional wet granulation method. It provides granules with good flow properties and binding capacity to form tablets of low friability, adequate hardness and have a high uptake capacity for active substances whose tableting is poor.

### F. Foam granulation

Here liquid binders are added as aqueous foam. It has several benefits over spray (wet) granulation such as it requires less binder than spray granulation, requires less water to wet granulate, rate of addition of foam is greater than rate of addition of sprayed liquids, no detrimental effects on granulate, tablet, or in-vitro drug dissolution properties, no plugging problems since use of spray nozzles is eliminated, no overwetting, useful for granulating water sensitive formulations, reduces drying time, uniform distribution of binder throughout the powder bed, reduce manufacturing time, less binder required for immediate release (IR) and controlled release (CR) formulations.

## OPERATIONS INVOLVED IN TABLET MANUFACTURING

The manufacture of oral solid dosage forms such as tablets is a complex multistage process under which the starting materials change their physical characteristics a number of times before the final dosage form is produced. Traditionally, tablets have been made by granulation, a process that imparts two primary requisites to formulate: compatibility and fluidity. Both wet granulation and dry granulation (slugging and roll compaction) are used. Regardless of whether tablets are made by direct compression or granulation, the first step, milling and mixing, is the same; subsequent steps differ. Numerous unit processes are involved in making tablets, including particle size reduction and sizing, blending, granulation, drying, compaction, and (frequently) coating. Various factors associated with these processes can seriously affect content uniformity, bioavailability, or stability.

### i. Dispensing

Dispensing is the first step in any pharmaceutical manufacturing process. Dispensing is one of the most critical steps in pharmaceutical manufacturing; as during this step, the weight of each ingredient in the mixture is determined according to dose.

Dispensing may be done by purely manual by hand scooping from primary containers and weighing each ingredient by hand on a weigh scale, manual weighing with material lifting assistance like vacuum transfer and bag lifters, manual or assisted transfer with automated weighing on weigh table, manual or assisted filling of loss-in weight dispensing system, automated dispensaries with mechanical devices such as vacuum loading system and screw feed system.

Issues like weighing accuracy, dust control (laminar air flow booths, glove boxes), during manual handling, lot control of each ingredient, material movement into and out of dispensary should be considered during dispensing.

### ii. Sizing

The sizing (size reduction, milling, crushing, grinding, pulverization) is an important step (unit operation) involved in the tablet manufacturing.

In manufacturing of compressed tablet, the mixing or blending of several solid ingredients of pharmaceuticals is easier and more uniform if the ingredients are approximately of same size. This provides a greater uniformity of dose. A fine particle size is essential in case of lubricant mixing with granules for its proper function.

Advantages associated with size reduction in tablet manufacture are as follows:

i. It increases surface area, which may enhance an active dissolution rate and hence bioavailability.
ii. Improved the tablet-to-tablet content uniformity by virtue of the increased number of particles per unit weight.
iii. Controlled particle size distribution of dry granulation or mix to promote better flow of mixture in tablet machine.
iv. Improved flow properties of raw materials
v. Improved color and/or active ingredient dispersion in tablet excipients.
vi. Uniformly sized wet granulation to promote uniform drying. There are also certain disadvantages associated with this unit operation if not controlled properly. They are as follows:
vii. A possible change in polymorphic form of the active ingredient, rendering it less or totally inactive, or unstable.
viii. A decrease in bulk density of active compound and/or excipients, which may cause flow problem and segregation in the mix.
ix. An increase in surface area from size reduction may promote the adsorption of air, which may inhibit wettability of the drug to the extent that it becomes the limiting factor in dissolution rate.

A number of different types of machine may be used for the dry sizing or milling process depending on whether gentle screening or particle milling is needed. The ranges of equipment employed for this process includes fluid energy mill, colloidal mill, ball mill, hammer mill, cutting mill, roller mill, conical mill, etc.

### iii. Powder blending

The successful mixing of powder is acknowledged to be more difficult unit operation because, unlike the situation with liquid, perfect homogeneity is practically unattainable.

In practice, problems also arise because of the inherent cohesiveness and resistance to movement between the individual particles. The process is further complicated in many system, by the presence of substantial segregation influencing the powder mix. They arise because of difference in size, shape, and density of the component particles.

The powder/granules blending are involved at stage of pregranulation and/or postgranulation stage of tablet manufacturing. Each process of mixing has optimum mixing time and so prolonged mixing may result in an undesired product. So, the optimum mixing time and mixing speed are to be evaluated. Blending step prior to compression is normally achieved in a simple tumble blender. The blender may be a fixed blender into which the powders are charged, blended and discharged. It is now common to use a bin blender which blends.

In special cases of mixing a lubricant, over mixing should be particularly monitored.

The various blenders used include blender, oblicone blender, container blender, tumbling blender, agitated powder blender, etc. commonly used blenders are shown in Figure. 1.11.

But nowadays to optimize the manufacturing process, particularly in wet granulation the various improved equipments which combine several processing steps (mixing, granulation and/or drying) are used. They are high-shear mixing equipments.

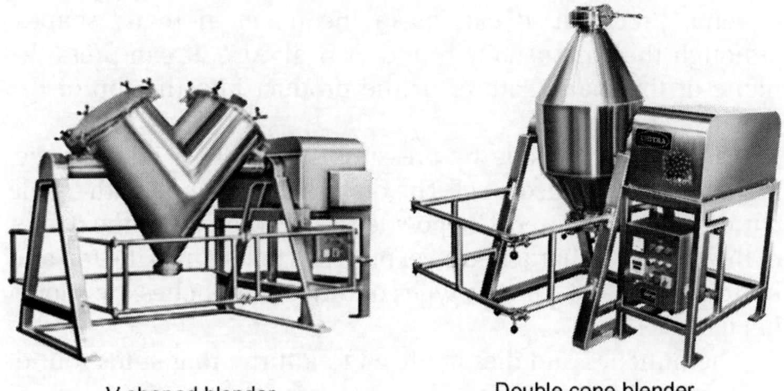

V-shaped blender　　Double cone blender

FIGURE 1.11: Commonly used blenders

### iv. Granulation

Following particle size reduction and blending, the formulation may be granulated, which provides homogeneity of drug distribution in blend.

### v. Drying

Drying is a most important step in the formulation and development of pharmaceutical product. It is important to keep the residual moisture low enough to prevent product deterioration and ensure free flowing properties. The commonly used dryer includes fluidized bed dryer, vacuum tray dryer, microwave dryer, spray dryer, freeze dryer, turbo - tray dryer, pan dryer, etc.

## TABLET COMPRESSION

After the preparation of granules (in case of wet granulation) or sized slugs (in case of dry granulation) or mixing of ingredients (in case of direct compression), they are compressed to get final product. The compression is done either by single punch machine (stamping press) or by multistation machine (rotary press).

The tablet press is a high-speed mechanical device. It 'squeezes' the ingredients into the required tablet shape with extreme precision. It can make the tablet in many shapes, although they are usually round or oval. Also, it can press the name of the manufacturer or the product into the top of the tablet.

Each tablet is made by pressing the granules inside a die, made up of hardened steel. The die is a disk shaped with a hole cut through its center. The powder is compressed in the center of the die by two hardened steel punches that fit into the top and bottom of the die. Various types of dies and punches are shown in Figure 1.12.

The punches and dies are fixed to a turret that spins round. As it spins, the punches are driven together by two fixed cams—an upper cam and lower cam. The top of the upper punch (the punch head) sits on the upper cam edge. The bottom of the lower punch sits on the lower cam edge.

The shapes of the two cams determine the sequence of movements of the two punches. This sequence is repeated over and over because the turret is spinning round.

The force exerted on the ingredients in the dies is very carefully controlled. This ensures that each tablet is perfectly formed. Because of the high speeds, they need very sophisticated lubrication systems. The lubricating oil is recycled and filtered to ensure a continuous supply.

## Parts of tablet compression machines

- Hopper for holding and feeding granulation to be compressed
- Dies that define the size and shape of the tablet
- Punches for compressing the granulation within the dies
- Cam tracks for guiding the movement of the punches
- Feeding mechanisms for moving granulation from the hopper into the dies.

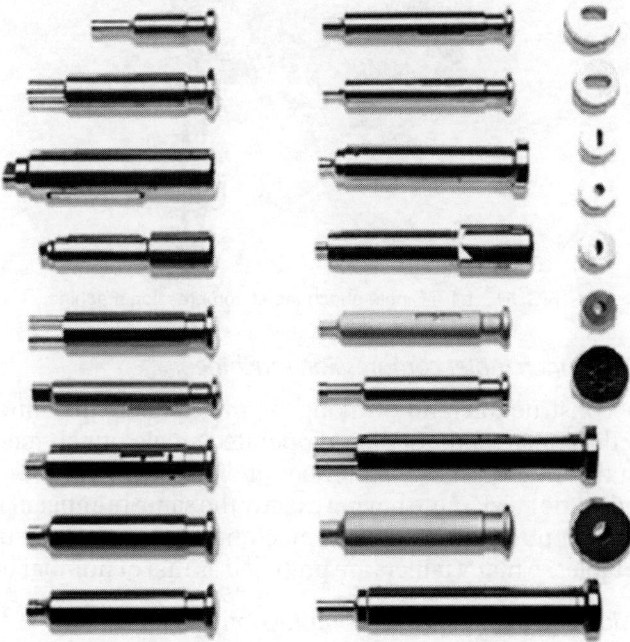

FIGURE 1.12: Types of punches and dies

## Types of tablet compression machines

i. Single punch tablet compression machine
ii. Multiple punch tablet compression machine
iii. Rotary tablet compression machine
iv. Multilayered rotary tablet compression machine.

### *i. Single punch tablet compression machine (Fig. 1.13)*

In these types of machines, one set of die and punch is fitted and only one tablet can be compressed at one time. They are used when small quantity of tablets is to be prepared. They are hand operated or power operated and with these machines 60–90 tablets/min can be prepared.

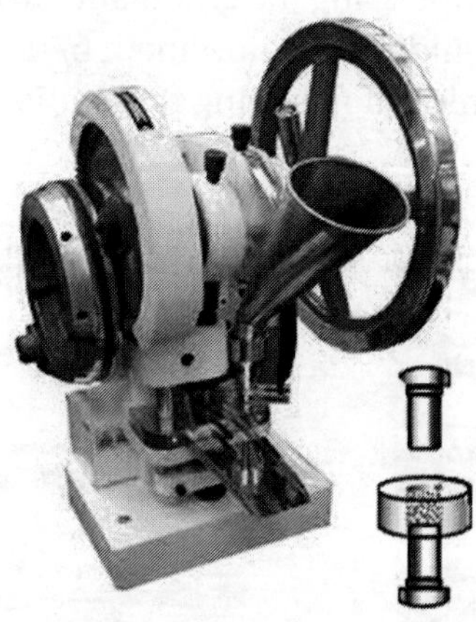

FIGURE 1.13: Single punch tablet compression machine

### *ii. Multipunch tablet compression machine*

The construction and working of multipunch machines are exactly similar as that of hand operated single punch machine, with the difference that a number of dies varying from 2–12 are fitted in the steel frame having exactly the same number of upper and lower punches. With these machines, in one cycle instead of one tablet so many tablets are prepared as that of number of dies.

### *iii. Multilayed rotary tablet compression machine*

With this machine tablets having one, two or three layers can be produced. They have the advantage that in compatible drugs can be compressed in different layers and separating these layers with an inert material.

*iv. Rotary tablet compression machine (Fig. 1.14)*

For large scale production, rotary tablet compression machines are used. The high speed rotary machine is fitted with as many as 70 sets of dies and punches and can produce upto 10,000 tablets/min. In a rotary machine, the head of the tablet machine that holds the upper punches, dies and lower punches in place rotates. As the head rotates, the punches are guided up and down by fixed cam tracks, which control the sequence of filling, compression and ejection. The portions of the head that hold the upper and lower punches are called the upper and lower turrets respectively. The portion holding the dies is called the die table.

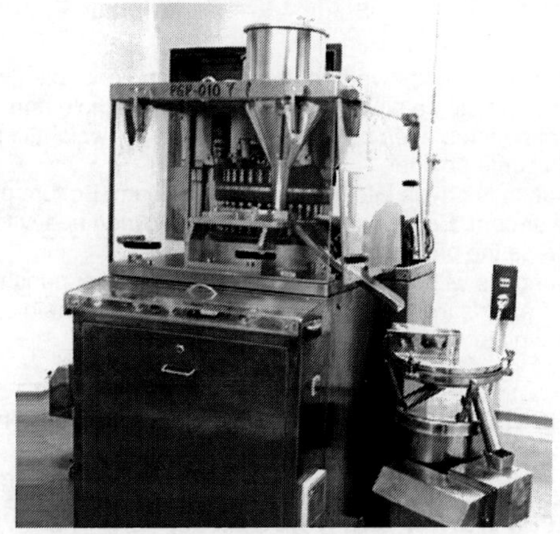

FIGURE 1.14: Rotary tablet compression machine

## Compression cycle

Stages occurring during compression are shown in Figure 1.15. At the start of the compression cycle, granulation stored in a hopper, empties into the feed frame which has several interconnected compartments. These compartments spread the granulation over a wide area to provide time for the dies to fill. The pull down cam guides the lower punches to the bottom, allowing the dies to overfill. Punches then pass over a weight-control cam, which reduces the fill in the dies to the desired amount. A swipe off blade at the end of the feed frame removes the excess

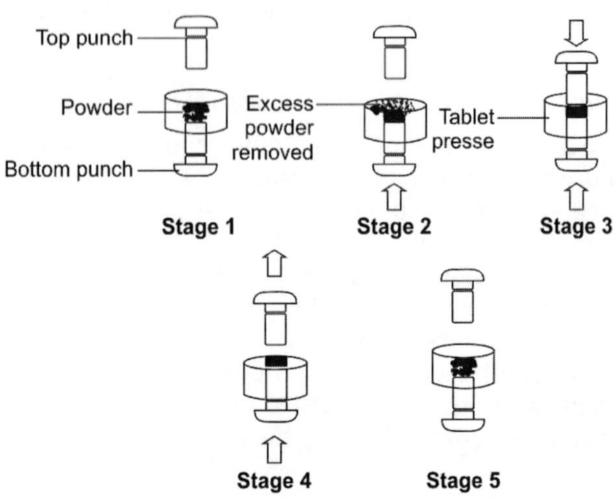


Stage 1: Top punch is withdrawn from the die by the upper cam. Bottom punch is low in the die so powder falls in through the hole and fills the die.
Stage 2: Bottom punch moves up to adjust the powder weight, it raises and expels some powder.
Stage 3: Top punch is driven into the die by upper cam. Bottom punch is raised by lower cam. Both punch heads pass between heavy rollers to compress the powder.
Stage 4: Top punch is withdrawn by the upper cam. Lower punch is pushed up and expels the tablet. Tablet is removed from the die surface by surface plate.
Stage 5: Return.

FIGURE 1.15: Stages occurring during compression

granulation and directs it around the turret and back into the front of the feed frame. The lower punches travel over the lower compression roll while simultaneously the upper punches ride beneath the upper compression roll. The upper punches enter a fixed distance into the dies, while the lower punches are raised to squeeze and compact the granulation within the dies. After the moment of compression, the upper punches are withdrawn as they follow the upper punch raising cam. The lower punches ride up the cam which brings the tablets slightly above the surface of the dies. The tablets strike a sweep off blade affixed to the front of the feed frame and slide down a chute into a receptacle. At the same time, the lower punches re-enter the pull down cam and the cycle is repeated. Tablet compression cycle is shown in Figure 1.16.

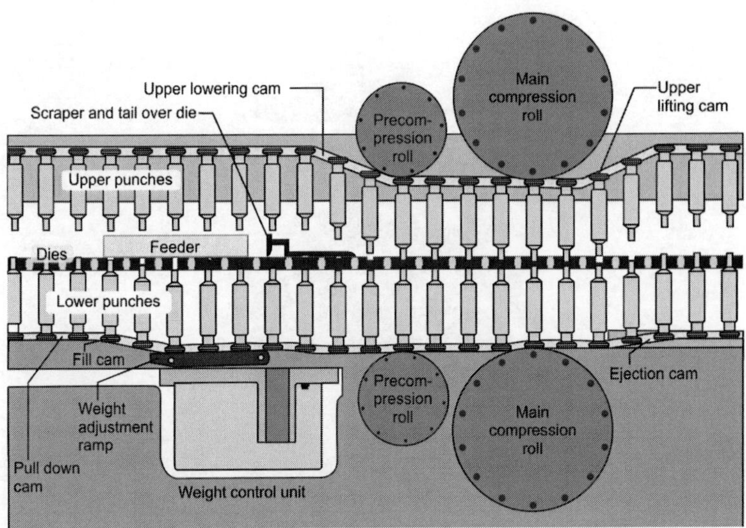


FIGURE 1.16: Tablet compression cycle

## AUXILIARY EQUIPMENTS

### i. Feeding device

In many cases, speed of die table is such that the time of die under feed frame is too short to allow adequate or consistent gravity filling of die with granules, resulting in weight variation and content uniformity. To avoid these problems, mechanized feeder can employ to force granules into die cavity.

### ii. Tablet weight monitoring devices

High rate of tablet output with modern press requires continuous tablet weight monitoring with electronic monitoring devices like Thomas Tablet Sentinel, Pharmakontroll and Killan control system-MC. They monitor force at each compression station by strain gauge technology which is then correlated with tablet weight.

### iii. Tablet deduster (Fig. 1.17)

In almost all cases, tablets coming out of a tablet machine bear excess powder on its surface and are run through the tablet deduster to remove that excess powder.

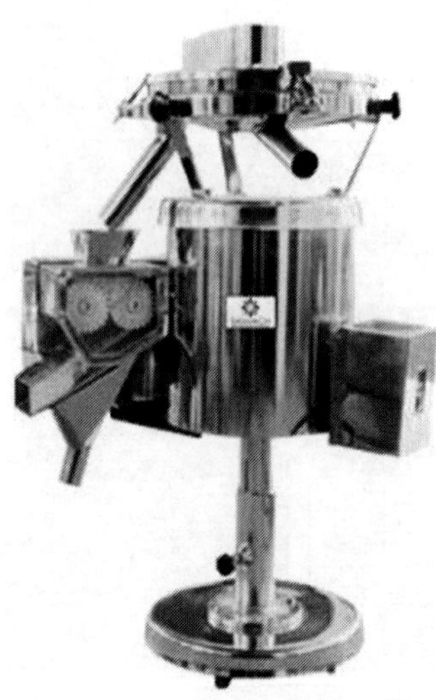

FIGURE 1.17: Tablet deduster

### iv. Fette machine

Fette machine is device that chills the compression components to allow the compression of low melting point substance such as waxes and thereby making it possible to compress products with low melting point.

## PACKAGING

Pharmaceutical manufacturers have to pack their medicines before they can be sent out for distribution. The type of packaging will depend on the formulation of the medicine.

'Blister packs' are a common form of packaging used for a wide variety of products. They are safe and easy to use and they allow the consumer to see the contents without opening the pack. Many pharmaceutical companies use a standard size of blister pack. This saves the cost of different tools and changes the production machinery between products. Sometimes, the pack may be perforated so that individual tablets can be detached. This means that the expiry date and the name of the product have to be printed on each part of the package. The blister pack itself must remain absolutely flat as it travels through the packaging processes, specially when it is inserted into a carton. This poses interesting problems for the designers.

## PROBLEMS IN TABLET MANUFACTURING

An ideal tablet should be free from any visual defect or functional defect. The advancements and innovations in tablet manufacture have not decreased the problems, often encountered in the production, instead have increased the problems, mainly because of the complexities of tablet presses; and/or the greater demands of quality.

An industrial pharmacist usually encounters number of problems during manufacturing. Majority of visual defects are due to inadequate fines or inadequate moisture in the granules ready for compression or due to faulty machine setting. Functional defects are due to faulty formulation. Solving many of the manufacturing problems requires an in-depth knowledge of granulation processing and tablet presses, and is acquired only through an exhaustive study and a rich experience.

Here, we will discuss the imperfections found in tablets along with their causes and related remedies. The imperfections are known as 'visual defects' and they are either related to imperfections in anyone or more of the following factors:

i. Tableting process
ii. Excipient
iii. Machine.

**The defects related to tableting process are as follows**:

- **Capping**: It is partial or complete separation of the top or bottom of tablet due to air entrapment in the granular material.
- **Lamination**: It is separation of tablet into two or more layers due to air entrapment in the granular material.
- **Cracking**: It is due to rapid expansion of tablets when deep concave punches are used.

**The defects related to excipient are as follows**:

- **Sticking**: It is the adhesion of granulation material to the die wall.
- **Picking**: It is the removal of material from the surface of tablet and its adherence to the face of punch.
- **Chipping**: Serious sticking causes chipping.

These problems are due to more amount of binder in the granules or wet granules.

**The defect related to more than one factor**:

**Mottling**: It is either due to anyone or more of these factors: due to a colored drug, which has different color than the rest of the granular material (excipient-related); improper mixing of granular material (process-related); dirt in the granular material or on punch faces; oil spots by using oily lubricant.

## The defect related to machine

**Double impression**: it is due to free rotation of the punches, which have some engraving on the punch faces.

### *a. Capping*

'Capping' is the term used, when the upper or lower segment of the tablet separates horizontally, either partially or completely from the main body of a tablet and comes off as a cap, during ejection from the tablet press, or during subsequent handling (Tables 1.15 and 1.16).

**Reason**: Capping is usually due to the air entrapment in a compact during compression, and subsequent expansion of tablet on ejection of a tablet from a die.

**Table 1.15**: Causes and remedies of capping related to formulation (granulation)

| *Causes* | *Remedies* |
|---|---|
| Large amount of fines in the granulation | - Remove some or all fines through 100–200 mesh screen |
| Too dry or very low moisture content (leading to loss of proper binding action) | - Moisten the granules suitably<br>- Add hygroscopic substance e.g. sorbitol, methylcellulose or PEG-4000 |
| Not thoroughly dried granules.<br>Insufficient amount of binder or improper binder | - Dry the granules properly<br>- Increasing the amount of binder or adding dry binder such as pre-gelatinized starch, gum acacia, powdered sorbitol, PVP, hydrophilic silica or powdered sugar |
| Insufficient or improper lubricant | - Increase the amount of lubricant or change the type of lubricant |
| Granular mass too cold to compress firm | - Compress at room temperature |

**Table 1.16**: Causes and remedies of capping related to machine (dies, punches and tablet press)

| *Causes* | *Remedies* |
|---|---|
| Poorly finished dies | - Polish dies properly<br>- Investigate other steels or other materials |
| Deep concave punches or beveled-edge faces of punches | - Use flat punches |
| Lower punch remains below the face of die during ejection | - Make proper setting of lower punch during ejection |
| Incorrect adjustment of sweep-off blade | - Adjust sweep-off blade correctly to facilitate proper ejection |
| High turret speed | - Reduce speed of turret (increase dwell time) |

### *b. Lamination/laminating*

Lamination is the separation of a tablet into two or more distinct horizontal layers (Tables 1.17 and 1.18).

**Reason**: Air entrapment during compression and subsequent release on ejection.

The condition is exaggerated by higher speed of turret.

**Table 1.17**: Causes and remedies of lamination related to formulation (granulation)

| *Causes* | *Remedies* |
|---|---|
| Oily or waxy materials in granules | - Modify mixing process<br>- Add adsorbent or absorbent |
| Too much of hydrophobic lubricant, e.g. Magnesium stearate | - Use a less amount of lubricant or change the type of lubricant |

**Table 1.18**: Causes and remedies of lamination related to machine (dies, punches and tablet press)

| *Causes* | *Remedies* |
|---|---|
| Rapid relaxation of the peripheral regions of a tablet, on ejection from a die | - Use tapered dies, i.e. upper part of the die bore has an outward taper of 3°–5° |
| Rapid decompression | - Use precompression step<br>- Reduce turret speed and reduce the final compression pressure |

### c. Cracking

Small, fine cracks observed on the upper and lower central surface of tablets, or very rarely on the sidewall are referred to as 'cracks' (Tables 1.19 and 1.20).

**Reason**: It is observed as a result of rapid expansion of tablets, specially when deep concave punches are used.

**Table 1.19**: Causes and remedies of cracking related to formulation (granulation)

| *Causes* | *Remedies* |
|---|---|
| Large size of granules | - Reduce granule size<br>- Add fines |
| Too dry granules | - Moisten the granules properly and add proper amount of binder |
| Tablets expand | - Improve granulation<br>- Add dry binders |
| Granulation too cold | - Compress at room temperature |

**Table 1.20**: Causes and remedies of cracking related to machine (dies, punches and tablet press)

| *Causes* | *Remedies* |
|---|---|
| Tablet expands on ejection due to air entrapment | - Use tapered die |
| Deep concavities cause cracking while removing tablets | - Use special take-off |

### e. Sticking / filming

Sticking refers to the tablet material adhering to the die wall.

Filming is a slow form of sticking and is largely due to excess moisture in the granulation (Tables 1.21 and 1.22).

**Reason**: Improperly dried or improperly lubricated granules.

### f. Picking

'Picking' is the term used when a small amount of material from a tablet is sticking to and being removed off from the tablet-surface by a punch face (Tables 1.23 and 1.24).

The problem is more prevalent on the upper punch faces than on the lower ones. The problem worsens, if tablets are repeatedly

**Table 1.21**: Causes and remedies of sticking related to formulation (granulation)

| *Causes* | *Remedies* |
|---|---|
| Granules not dried properly | - Dry the granules properly<br>- Make moisture analysis to determine limits |
| Too little or improper lubrication | - Increase or change lubricant |
| Too much binder | - Reduce the amount of binder or use a different type of binder |
| Hygroscopic granular material | - Modify granulation and compress under controlled humidity |
| Oily or way materials | - Modify mixing process<br>- Add an absorbent |
| Too soft or weak granules | - Optimize the amount of binder and granulation technique |

**Table 1.22**: Causes and remedies of sticking related to machine (dies, punches and tablet press)

| *Causes* | *Remedies* |
|---|---|
| Concavity too deep for granulation | - Reduce concavity to optimum |
| Too little pressure | - Increase pressure |
| Compressing too fast | - Reduce speed |

**Table 1.23**: Causes and remedies of picking related to formulation (granulation)

| *Causes* | *Remedies* |
|---|---|
| Excessive moisture in granules | - Dry properly the granules, determine optimum limit |
| Too little or improper lubrication | - Increase lubrication<br>- Use colloidal silica as a 'polishing agent', so that material does not cling to punch faces |
| Low melting point substances, may soften from the heat of compression and lead to picking | - Add high melting point materials<br>- Use high melting point lubricants |
| Low melting point medicament in high concentration | - Refrigerate granules and the entire tablet press |
| Too warm granules when compressing | - Compress at room temperature<br>- Cool sufficiently before compression |
| Too much amount of binder | - Reduce the amount of binder, change the type or use dry binders |

**Table 1.24:** Causes and remedies of picking related to machine (dies, punches and tablet press)

| Causes | Remedies |
|---|---|
| Rough or scratched punch faces | - Polish faces to high luster |
| Embossing or engraving letters on punch faces such as B, A, O, R, P, Q, G | - Design lettering as large as possible<br>- Plate the punch faces with chromium to produce a smooth and nonadherent face |
| Bevels or dividing lines too deep | - Reduce depths and sharpness |
| Pressure applied is not enough; too soft tablets | - Increase pressure to optimum |

manufactured in this station of tooling because of the more and more material getting added to the already stuck material on the punch face.

**Reason**: Picking is of particular concern when punch tips have engraving or embossing letters, as well as the granular material is improperly dried.

### *g. Chipping*

'Chipping' in the die, is the term used when the tablets adhere, seize or tear in the die. A film is formed in the die and ejection of tablet is hindered. With excessive chipping, the tablet sides are cracked and it may crumble apart (Tables 1.25 and 1.26).

**Table 1.25:** Causes and remedies of chipping related to formulation (granulation)

| Causes | Remedies |
|---|---|
| Too moist granules and extrudes around lower punch | - Dry the granules properly |
| Insufficient or improper lubricant | - Increase the amount of lubricant or<br>- Use a more effective lubricant |
| Too coarse granules | - Reduce granular size,<br>- Add more fines, and<br>- Increase the quantity of lubricant |
| Too hard granules for the lubricant to be effective | - Modify granulation<br>- Reduce granular size |
| Granular material very abrasive and cutting into dies | - If coarse granules, reduce its size<br>- Use wear-resistant dies |
| Granular material too warm, sticks to the die | - Reduce temperature<br>- Increase clearance if it is extruding |

**Table 1.26:** Causes and remedies of chipping related to machine (dies, punches and tablet press)

| *Causes* | *Remedies* |
|---|---|
| Poorly finished dies | - Polish the dies properly |
| Rough dies due to abrasion, corrosion | - Investigate other steels or other materials or modify granulation |
| Undersized dies. Too little clearance | - Rework to proper size or Increase clearance |
| Too much pressure in the tablet press | - Reduce pressure or Modify granulation |

**Reason:** Chipping is usually due to excessive amount of moisture in granules, lack of lubrication and/or use of worn dies.

### *h. Mottling*

'Mottling' is the term used to describe an unequal distribution of color on a tablet, with light or dark spots standing out in an otherwise uniform surface.

**Reason:** One cause of mottling may be a colored drug, whose color differs from the color of excipients used for granulation of a tablet.

**Table 1.27:** Causes and remedies of mottling

| *Causes* | *Remedies* |
|---|---|
| A colored drug used along with colorless or white-colored excipients | - Use appropriate colorants |
| A dye migrates to the surface of granulation while drying | - Change the solvent system<br>- Change the binder<br>- Reduce drying temperature and<br>- Use a smaller particle size |
| Improperly mixed dye, specially during 'direct compression' | - Mix properly and reduce size if it is of a larger size to prevent segregation |
| Improper mixing of a colored binder solution | Incorporate dry color additive during powder blending step, then add fine powdered adhesives such as acacia and tragacanth and mix well and finally add granulating liquid |

*i. Double impression*

Double impression involves only those punches, which have a monogram or other engraving on them (Table 1.28).

**Reason**: At the moment of compression, the tablet receives the imprint of the punch. Now, on some machines, the lower punch freely drops and travels uncontrolled for a short distance before riding up the ejection cam to push the tablet out of the die, now during this free travel, the punch rotates and at this point, the punch may make a new impression on the bottom of the tablet, resulting in double impression.

If the upper punch is uncontrolled, it can rotate during the short travel to the final compression stage and create a double impression.

**Table 1.28**: Causes and remedies of double impression

| *Causes* | *Remedies* |
|---|---|
| Free rotation of either upper punch or lower punch during ejection of a tablet | - Use keying in tooling, i.e. inset a key alongside of the punch, so that it fits the punch and prevents punch rotation<br>- Newer presses have antiturning devices, which prevent punch rotation |

## TABLET COATING

Coated tablets are defined as tablets covered with one or more layers of mixture of various substances such as natural or synthetic resins, gums, inactive and insoluble filler, sugar, plasticizer, polyhydric alcohol, waxes, coloring material and sometimes flavoring material.

Coating may also contain active ingredient. Substances used for coating are usually applied as solution or suspension under conditions where vehicle evaporates.

### Purpose of tablet coating

I. Therapy
   i. Avoid irritation of esophagus and stomach
   ii. Avoid bad taste
   iii. Avoid inactivation of drug in the stomach

iv. Improve drug effectiveness
v. Prolong dosing interval
vi. Improve dosing interval
vii. Improve patient compliance.

II. Technology
i. Reduce influence of moisture
ii. Avoid dust formation
iii. Reduce influence of atmosphere
iv. Improve drug stability
v. Prolong shelf life
vi. Improve product identity
vii. Improve appearance and acceptability.

## TYPES OF TABLET COATING PROCESS

Three types of tablet coating processes:
1. Sugar coating
2. Film coating
3. Press coating.

### 1. Sugar coating

Compressed tablets may be coated with colored or uncolored sugar layer. The coating is water soluble and quickly dissolves after swallowing. Sugar coat protects the enclosed drug from the environment and provides a barrier to objectionable taste or odor. The sugar coat also enhances the appearance of the compressed tablet and permit imprinting manufacturer's information. Sugar coating provides a combination of insulation, taste masking, smoothing the tablet core, coloring and modified release.

*Advantages*

1. It utilizes inexpensive and readily available raw materials.
2. Constituent raw materials are widely accepted—no regulatory problems.
3. Modern, simplified techniques have greatly reduced coating times over traditional sugar-coating methods.
4. No complex equipment or services are required.
5. The process is capable of being controlled and documented to meet modern GMP standards.
6. Simplicity of equipment and ready availability of raw materials make sugar coating an ideal coating method for developing countries.

7. The process is generally not as critical as film coating; recovering and reworking procedures are usually possible.
8. For high humidity climates, it generally offers a stability advantage over film-coated tablets.
9. Results are aesthetically pleasing and have wide consumer acceptability.

*Disadvantages*

The disadvantages of sugar coating are the time and expertise required in the coating process and thus increases size, weight and shipping costs.

## Processing steps (Fig. 1.18)

Sugar coating process involves five separate operations:

A. Sealing/water proofing: It provides a moisture barrier and harden the tablet surface.
B. Subcoating: It causes a rapid buildup to round off the tablet edges.
C. Grossing/smoothing: It smoothes out the subcoated surface and increases the tablet size to predetermined dimension.
D. Coloring: It gives the tablet its color and finished size.
E. Polishing: It produces the characteristics gloss.

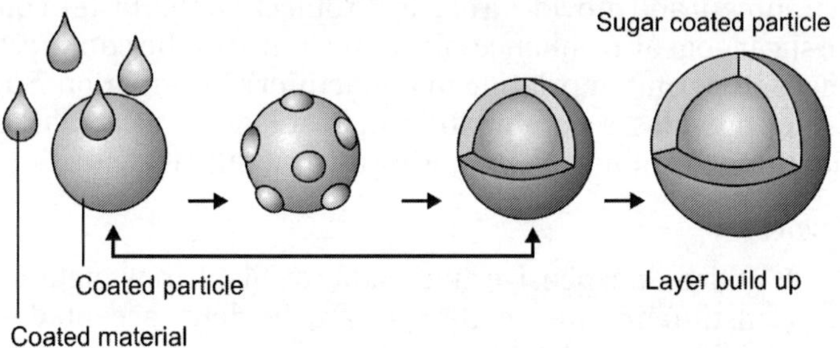


FIGURE 1.18: Simplified representation of sugar coating process

**Sugar coating technologies**: Three types of sugar coating technologies are used—

I. *Plain sugar coating* (*application of syrup at room temperature*): This coating technique includes three steps—application of coating formulation onto the core, distribution of formulation on the core surfaces, and drying to increase the strength of each coating layer. However, the time required for distribution and drying is critical to obtain a smooth even coating.

II. *Two components coating or lamination process* (*application of a syrup or binder solution first in a slight excess amount and then dusting with a powder to bind the excess solution*): Compared to the plain sugar coating technique the two component coating is a more complicated technique involving two steps of application of solution and powder. In order to obtain a high volume increase within a short period of time, adjustment must be made between powder and liquid quantities and performed by skillful operators.

III. *Hot sugar coating* (*application of heated syrup*): For the hot sugar coating technique, syrup is heated above room temperature to reduce the viscosity of the syrup. Therefore, a higher sugar content formulation can be used, with gelatin as a binder, and less water has to be removed during the drying process. However, the temperature used during this process must be controlled since the gelatin is prone to hydrolysis at temperatures above 60°C. Attempts to prevent sugar crystallization during processing may make this technique more complicated and more expensive since all equipment parts must be insulated and heated.

### *Steps involved in sugar coating process are:*

#### A. Sealing/water proofing

Prior to applying any sugar/water syrup, the tablet cores must be sealed, thoroughly dried and free of all residual solvents. The seal coat provides a moisture barrier and hardens the surface of the tablet in order to minimize attritional effects. Core tablets having very rapid disintegration rates conceivably could start the disintegration process during the initial phase of sugar coating.

The sealants are generally water-insoluble polymers/film formers applied from an organic solvent solution. The quantities of material applied as a sealing coat will depend primarily on the tablet porosity, since highly porous tablets will tend to soak up the first application of solution, thus preventing it from spreading uniformly across the surface of every tablet in the batch. Hence, one or more further application of resin solution may be required to ensure that the tablet cores are sealed effectively.

The common materials used as a sealant include shellac, zine, cellulose acetate phthalate (cap), polyvinylacetate phthalate, hydroxypropylmethylcellulose, etc.

### B. Subcoating

Subcoating is the actual start of the sugar coating process and provides the rapid build up necessary to round up the tablet edge. It also acts as the foundation for the smoothing and color coats.

Generally, two methods are used for subcoating:

i. The application of gum based solution followed by dusting with powder and then drying. This routine is repeated until the desired shape is achieved (Table 1.29).
ii. The application of a suspension of dry powder in gum/sucrose solution followed by drying (Table 1.30).

Thus, subcoating is a sandwich of alternate layer of gum and powder. It is necessary to remove the bulk of the water after each application of coating syrup.

**Table 1.29:** Typical binder solution formulation for subcoating

| | %w/w | %w/w |
|---|---|---|
| Gelatin | 6 | 3.3 |
| Gum acacia (powdered) | 8 | 8.7 |
| Sucrose (powdered) | 45 | 55.3 |
| Distilled water | upto 100 | upto 100 |

**Table 1.30:** Typical suspension subcoating formulation

| | %w/w |
|---|---|
| Sucrose | 40.0 |
| Calcium carbonate | 20.0 |
| Talc, asbestos free | 12.0 |
| Gum acacia (powdered) | 2.0 |
| Titanium dioxide | 1.0 |
| Distilled water | 25.0 |

### *C. Grossing/smoothing*

The grossing/smoothing process is specifically for smoothing and filing the irregularity on the surface generated during subcoating.

It also increases the tablet size to a predetermined dimension. If the subcoating is rough with high amount of irregularities then the use of grossing syrup containing suspended solids will provide more rapid build up and better filling qualities.

Smoothing usually can be accomplished by the application of a simple syrup solution (approximately 60%–70% sugar solid). This syrup generally contains pigments, starch, gelatin, acacia or opacifier if required. Small quantities of color suspension can be applied to impart a tint of the desired color when there are irregularities in coating.

### *D. Color coating*

This stage is often critical in the successful completion of a sugar coating process and involves the multiple application of syrup solution (60%–70% sugar solid) containing the requisite coloring matter. Mainly soluble dyes were used in the sugar coating to achieve the desired color, since the soluble dye will migrate to the surface during drying. But nowadays, the insoluble certified lakes have virtually replaced the soluble dyes in pharmaceutical tablet coating. The most efficient process for color coating involves the use of a predispersed opacified lake suspension.

#### Advantages of lakes over dyes

A pigment (lake) system is superior to a water-soluble dye for coloring sugar-coated tablets due to:

i. Maintenance of evenness of color because
   - The color is not water-soluble and thus is not prone to color migration problems.
   - The color is opaque, and thus is not affected by any minor unevenness in the subcoat layer.

ii. Maintenance of color uniformity from batch to batch, which results from the fact that, again because the colorant is opaque, the final color is not affected by small fluctuations in the quantity of color solution applied.

iii. Reduction in overall processing time.

iv. Reduction in the thickness of the color-coating layer.

### *E. Polishing*

After the color-coating process the tablets have a somewhat dull, matt appearance which requires a separate polishing step to give them the high degree of gloss.

Some examples of polishing methods which are currently in use include:

i. Application of an organic solvent solution/suspension of waxes, e.g. carnauba and beeswax. A recently available variant on this theme provides an emulsion of both waxes in an aqueous continuous phase stabilized by a food and pharmaceutically acceptable surfactant. The results obtained are equivalent to traditional methods utilizing organic solvent solutions but, of course, with the big bonus of aqueous processing.
ii. Use of wax-lined pan.
iii. Use of canvas-lined pan with wax solution/suspension.
iv. Finely powdered wax application.
v. Mineral oil application.

### *F. Printing*

Some regulatory authorities demand that tablets, be coated or uncoated, should possess some detailed identifying mark. Those authorities who do not actually require this actively encourage it as part of the overall GMP and product acceptability requirements. Unfortunately, unlike film-coated tablets, sugar-coated tablets cannot be monogrammed by engraving the punch tooling. Instead a printing process is used.

A typical edible pharmaceutical ink formulation is—shellac, alcohol, pigment, lecithin, antifoam and other organic solvents.

### Raw materials for sugar coating

A. **Coating formers**: They form the coating due to their mass and cohesion, typically consist of sugar, binders and fillers.

   i. **Sucrose, other sugars, and sugar alcohols**: Sucrose is used primarily as a coating material in concentrations ranging between 50%–60%, since syrups with a sugar content of less than 65% are stable at room temperature without crystallization occurring. Aqueous solubility of sucrose is increased by the use of heat.

   Due to major concerns in using the products in diabetic patients, and the fact that they cause dental caries, other sugars and sugar alcohols are used to replace sucrose. These include glucose, lactose, maltitol, mannitol, isomalt, sorbitol, xylitol, and sugar mixtures such as invert sugar and starch sugars.

ii. **Binders**: The commonly used binders are polyvinyl acetate, polyvinyl pyrrolidine, acacia gum, gelatin, agar-agar, sodium alginate, carboxymethyl starch, dextrin, cellulose ethers and starches.

iii. **Fillers**: Fillers builds up the structure adds mass to the coating. For example, kaolin, dextrin, precipitated calcium carbonate, powdered acacia, corn starch, talc and calcium sulfate.

B. **Colorants**: Colorants impart color to the coating and cover the imperfections. For example, pigments (titanium dioxide or other inorganic coloring agents), dyes and lakes.

C. **Flavors**: Flavors improve and enhance the acceptability and palatability of the dosage form. For example, cinnamon, fruit flavors.

D. **Lubricants, glidants, and antiadherents**: These materials reduce friction between the individual sugar-coated cores and prevent dust formation during the drying step. For example, talc and colloidal silicon dioxide.

E. **Smoothing agent**: For example, combination of syrup and acacia gum.

F. **Polishing agent**: For example, beeswax, carnauba wax.

G. **Suspension stabilizer**: They prevent phase separation or sedimentation of the coating suspensions. For example, it includes surface active agents (emulsifying agents, bentonite) or thickening agents.

2. Film coating

Film coating is deposition of a thin film of polymer surrounding the tablet core. Modern approach to coat tablets, capsules, or pellets is by surrounding them with a thin layer of polymeric material.

Comparison between film coating and sugar coating is shown in Table 1.31.

*Advantages*

i. Enhance the elegance and glossy appearance of the dosage form.
ii. Obtain legible logo and product identification after coating. Product information can be engraved on the tablet grove.
iii. Improve mechanical integrity and resistance of the dosage form upon handling and shipping from manufacturing site to patients.

**Table 1.31:** Comparison between film coating and sugar coating

| *Features* | *Film coating* | *Sugar coating* |
|---|---|---|
| Appearance | Retain contour of original core. Usually not as shiny as sugar coat type | Rounded with high degree of polish |
| Weight increase because of coating material | 2%–3% | 30%–50% |
| Logo or break lines | Possible | Not possible |
| Operator training required | Process tends itself to automation and easy training of operator | Considerable |
| Adaptability to GMP | High | Difficulty may arise |
| Process stages | Usually single stage | Multistage process |
| Functional coatings | Easily adaptable for controlled release | Not usually possible apart from enteric coating |

iv. Increase flexibility in types of formulations coated and processing equipment required.
v. Minimal weight increase (about 2%–3% of tablet core weight) compared to sizeable increase when using a sugar coating (doubling the weight of tablet core).
vi. Significant reduced processing in time, with increased process efficiency and output.
vii. Minimize dusting.

*Disadvantages*

There are environmental and safety implications of using organic solvents as well as their financial expense.

## Process description

Film coating is deposition of a thin film of polymer surrounding the tablet core. Conventional pan equipments may be used but nowaday more sophisticated equipments are employed to have a high degree of automation and coating time. The polymer is solubilized into solvent. Other additives like plasticizers and pigments are added. Resulting solution is sprayed onto a rotating tablet bed. The drying conditions cause removal of the solvent, giving thin deposition of coating material around each tablet core.

### Process details

Usually spray process is employed in preparation of film coated tablets. Accela Cota is the prototype of perforated cylindrical drum providing high drying air capacity. Fluidized bed equipment has made considerable impact where tablets are moving in a stream of air passing through the perforated bottom of a cylindrical column. With a smaller cylindrical insert, the stream of cores is rising in the center of the device together with a spray mist applied in the middle of the bottom. For fluidized bed coating, very hard tablets have to be used.

### Basic process requirements for film coating

The fundamental requirements are independent of the actual type of equipments being used and include adequate means of atomizing the spray liquid for application to the tablet core, adequate mixing and agitation of tablet bed, sufficient heat input in the form of drying air to provide the latent heat of evaporation of the solvent. This is particularly important with aqueous-based spraying and good exhaust facilities to remove dust and solvent laden air.

### Development of film coating formulations

If the following questions are answered concomitantly then one can go for film coating:

- Is it necessary to mask objectionable taste, color and odor?
- Is it necessary to control drug release?
- What tablets size, shape, or color constrains must be placed on the developmental work?

Color, shape and size of final coated tablet are important for marketing and these properties have a significant influence on the marketing strategies. An experienced formulator usually takes the pragmatic approach and develops a coating formulations modification of one that has performed well in the past. Spraying or casting films can preliminarily screen film formulations. Cast films cab is prepared by spreading the coating composition on teflon, glass or aluminum foil surface using a spreading bar to get a uniform film thickness. Sprayed films can be obtained by mounting a plastic-coated surface in a spray hood or coating pan.

## Materials used in film coating

i. Film formers, which may be enteric or nonenteric
ii. Solvents
iii. Plasticizers
iv. Colorants
v. Opaquant-extenders
vi. Miscellaneous coating solution components.

### *i. Film formers*

Materials used to coat pharmaceutical products are primarily based on acrylic and cellulosic polymers and the aqueous solubility characteristics of these compounds generally dictate their uses. Sustained release coatings are water-insoluble or swellable films through which the medicament slowly diffuses.

Common sustained release polymers commercially available include ethyl cellulose and water-insoluble polymethacrylates. In contrast, water-soluble polymers, including hydroxypropyl cellulose, hydroxypropyl methylcellulose, sodium carboxymethylcellulose, and polyvinyl pyrrolidone, are often used for rapidly disintegrating film-coated tablets. These materials have also been added to the water-insoluble polymers to accelerate drug release from sustained release films.

Enteric film coatings exhibit pH-dependent solubility and have been used to protect drugs from degradation in the stomach. In the low pH of the stomach, mixed acid and acid ester functional groups on the enteric polymers are unionized, and therefore, insoluble. As the pH increases in the intestinal tract, these functional groups ionize and the polymer becomes soluble. Thus, an enteric polymeric film allows the coated solid to pass through the stomach intact and release the medication in the small intestines. Common enteric polymers commercially available include cellulose acetate phthalate, hydroxypropyl methylcellulose phthalate, hydroxypropyl methylcellulose acetate succinate, polyvinyl acetate phthalate, and several methacrylic acid copolymers.

Ideal requirements of film coating materials are summarized below:

i. Solubility in solvent of choice for coating preparation.

ii. Solubility requirement for the intended use, e.g. free water-solubility, slow water-solubility, or pH-dependent solubility.
iii. Capacity to produce an elegant looking product.
iv. High stability against heat, light, moisture, air and the substrate being coated.
v. No inherent color, taste or odor
vi. High compatibility with other coating solution additives
vii. Nontoxic with no pharmacological activity
viii. High resistance to cracking
ix. Film former should not give bridging or filling of the debossed tablet
x. Compatible to printing procedure.

**Commonly used film formers are as follows:**

i. *Hydroxypropyl methylcellulose* (HPMC)
   - It is available in different viscosity grades.
   - It is a polymer of choice for air suspension and pan spray coating systems because of solubility characteristic in gastric fluid, organic and aqueous solvent system.

Advantages include:
– It does not affect tablet disintegration and drug availability.
– It is cheap, flexible.
– It is highly resistant to heat, light and moisture.
– It has no taste and odor.
– Color and other additives can be easily incorporated.

Disadvantages includes
– When it is used alone, the polymer has tendency to bridge or fill the debossed tablet surfaces. So mixture of HPMC and other polymers/plasticizers is used.

ii. *Methyl hydroxyethyl cellulose* (MHEC)
   - It is available in wide variety of viscosity grades.
   - It is not frequently used as HPMC because soluble in fewer organic solvents.

iii. *Ethyl cellulose* (EC)
   - Depending on the degree of ethoxy substitution, different viscosity grades are available.
   - It is completely insoluble in water and gastric fluids. Hence, it is used in combination with water-soluble additives like HPMC and not alone.

- Unplasticized ethylcellulose films are brittle and require film modifiers to obtain an acceptable film formulation.
- Aqua coat is aqueous polymeric dispersion utilizing ethyl cellulose. These pseudolatex systems contain high solids, low viscosity compositions that have coating properties quite different from regular ethylcellulose solution.

iv. *Hydroxypropyl cellulose* (HPC)
- It is soluble in water below 40°C (insoluble above 45°C), gastric fluid and many polar organic solvents.
- HPC is extremely tacky as it dries from solution system. It is used for subcoat and not for color or glass coat. It gives very flexible film.

v. *Povidone*
- Degree of polymerization decides molecular weight of material. It is available in four viscosity grades, i.e. K-15, K-30, K-60 and K-90.
- Average molecular weight of these grades is 10000, 40000, 160000 and 360000 respectively. K-30 is widely used as tablet binder and in tablet coating. It has excellent solubility in wide variety of organic solvents, water, gastric and intestinal fluids.
- Povidone can be cross-linked with other materials to produce films with enteric properties. It is used to improve dispersion of colorants in coating solution.

vi. *Sodium carboxy methyl cellulose* (NaCMC)
- It is available in medium, high and extra high viscosity grades.
- It is easily dispersed in water to form colloidal solutions but it is insoluble in most organic solvents and hence not a material of choice for coating solution based on organic solvents.
- Films prepared by it are brittle but adhere well to tablets. Partially dried films are tacky. So coating compositions must be modified with additives.

vii. *Acrylate polymers*
- It is marketed under the name of Eudragit.
- Eudragit E is cationic copolymer based on dimethyl aminoethyl methacrylate and other neutral methacrylic

acid esters. Only Eudragit E is freely soluble in gastric fluid up to pH 5, and expandable and permeable above pH 5.

- This material is available as organic solution (12.5% In isopropanol/acetone), solid material or 30% aqueous dispersion.
- Eudragit RL and RS are copolymers synthesized from acrylic and methacrylic acid esters with low content of quaternary ammonium groups. These are available only as organic solutions and solid materials. They produce films for delayed action (pH dependent).

### *ii. Solvents*

Solvents are used to dissolve or disperse the polymers and other additives and convey them to substrate surface.

Ideal requirement are summarized below:

i. It should be either dissolve/disperse polymer system.
ii. It should easily disperse other additives into solvent system.
iii. Small concentration of polymers (2%–10%) should not in an extremely viscous solution system creating processing problems.
iv. It should be colorless, tasteless, odorless, inexpensive, inert, nontoxic and nonflammable.
v. Rapid drying rate.
vi. No environmental pollution.

Mostly, solvents are used either alone or in combination with water, ethanol, methanol, isopropanol, chloroform, acetone, methylene chloride, etc. Water is more used because no environmental and economic considerations. For drugs that readily hydrolyze in presence of water, nonaqueous solvents are used.

### *iii. Plasticizers*

The quality of a film can be modified by the use of internal or external plasticizing techniques. Internal plasticizer causes chemical modification of the basic polymer that alters the physical properties of the polymer whereas, external plasticizer provides flexibility, tensile strength or adhesion properties of the resulting film. Combination of plasticizer may be used to get desired effect. Concentration of plasticizer is expressed in relation to the polymer being plasticized. Recommended levels of plasticizers range from 1%–50% by weight of the film former.

*Most commonly used plasticizers*

- Polyols: water miscible
  - Glycerol
  - Propylene glycol (PG)
  - Polyethylene glycol (PEG).
- Organic esters
  - Diethyl phthalate (DEP)—water-insoluble
  - Dibutyl phthalate (DBP)—water-insoluble
  - Dibutyl sebacate (DBS)—water-insoluble
  - Triethyl citrate (TEC)—water-miscible
  - Acetyl triethyl citrate (ATEC)—water-insoluble
  - Acetyl tributyl citrate (ATBC)—water-insoluble
  - Tributyl citrate (TBC)—water-insoluble
  - Triacetin (glyceryl triacetate; TA)—water-miscible.
- Oils/glycerides: water-insoluble
  - Castor oil
  - Acetylated monoglyceride (AMG)
  - Fractionated coconut oil.

For aqueous coating, PEG and PG are more used while castor oil and spans are primarily used for organic-solvent based coating solution. External plasticizer should be soluble in the solvent system used for dissolving the film former and plasticizer. The plasticizer and the film former must be at least partially soluble or miscible in each other. The plasticizer and the film former must be at least partially soluble or miscible in each other. To be effective, a plasticizer must partition from the solvent phase into the polymer phase and subsequently diffuse throughout the polymer to disrupt the intermolecular interactions. The rate and extent of this partitioning for an aqueous dispersion have been found to be dependent on the solubility of the plasticizer in water and its affinity for the polymer phase. The partitioning of water-soluble plasticizers in an aqueous dispersion occurs rapidly, whereas significantly longer equilibration times are required for water-insoluble plasticizing agents. For aqueous-based dispersed systems, water-insoluble plasticizers should be emulsified first and then added to the polymer. Sufficient time must be allowed for plasticizer uptake into the polymer phase prior to the initiation of coating. If insufficient time for plasticizer partitioning is given, the unincorporated plasticizer droplets, as well as the plasticized polymer particles, will be sprayed onto the substrates during the coating process, resulting in uneven plasticizer distribution within the film, which could potentially cause changes in the polymer properties of the film overtime. The effectiveness of a plasticizing agent is dependent, to a large extent, on the amount of plasticizer added to the film coating formulation and the extent of polymer-plasticizer interaction. Forces involved in polymer-plasticizer mixtures include hydrogen bonding, dipole-dipole, and dipole-induced dipole interactions, as well as dispersions forces.

*iv. Colorants*

Colorants can be used in solution form or in suspension form. To achieve proper distribution of suspended colorants in the coating solution requires the use of the powdered colorants (<10 μ).

Most common colorants in use are certified FD & C or D & C colorants. These are synthetic dyes or lakes. Lakes are choice for sugar or film coating as they give reproducible results. Concentration of colorants in the coating solutions depends on the color shade desired, the type of dye, and the concentration of opaquant-extenders. If very light shade is desired, concentration of less than 0.01% may be adequate, on the other hand if a dark color is desired a concentration of more than 2.0% may be required. The inorganic materials (e.g. iron oxide) and the natural coloring materials (e.g. anthocyanins, carotenoids, etc.) are also used to prepare coating solution. Magenta red dye is nonabsorbable in biologic system and resistant to degradation in the gastrointestinal tract.

The size, shape, surface chemistry, and concentration of the pigments have been shown to affect polymer properties. There is an inverse relationship between the particle size of the pigment and film–tablet adhesion. Larger particles disrupt the interfacial bonding between the polymer and the surface of the tablet to a greater extent than the smaller particles. Pigments with polar surfaces (such as titanium dioxide, iron oxide, and mica) produce films that are less permeable than when the hydrophobic talc is incorporated into the coating. Addition of titanium dioxide to acrylic and cellulosic films increases water vapor permeability and enhances polymer adhesion.

*v. Opaquant-extenders*

These are very fine inorganic powder used to provide more pastel colors and increase film coverage. These inorganic materials provide white coat or mask color of the tablet core. Colorants are very expensive and higher concentration is required. These inorganic materials are cheap. In presence of these inorganic materials, amount of colorants required decreases. Pigments were investigated in the production of opaque films and it was found that they have good hiding power.

Most commonly used materials are

- Titanium dioxide
- Silicate (talc and aluminum silicates)
- Carbonates (magnesium carbonates)
- Oxides (magnesium oxide)
- Hydroxides (aluminum hydroxides).

*vi. Miscellaneous coating solution component*

Flavors, sweeteners, surfactants, antioxidants, antimicrobials, etc. may be incorporated into the coating solution.

Enteric coating

The technique involved in enteric coating is protection of the tablet core from disintegration in the acidic environment of the stomach by employing pH sensitive polymer, which swell or solubilize in response to an increase in pH to release the drug. This type of coating is used to protect tablet core from disintegration in the acid environment of the stomach for one or more of the following reasons:

i. To prevent degradation of acid sensitive API.
ii. To prevent irritation of stomach by certain drugs like sodium salicylate.
iii. Delivery of API into intestine.
iv. To provide a delayed release component for repeat action tablet.

*The pH status of enteric coated polymers in the stomach:*

The polymers used for enteric coatings remain unionize at low pH, and therefore remain insoluble. As the pH increases in the gastrointestinal tract the acidic functional groups are capable of ionization, and the polymer swells or becomes soluble in the intestinal fluid.

Thus, an enteric polymeric film coating allows the coated solid to pass intact through the stomach to the small intestine, where the drug is then released for absorption through the intestinal mucosa into the human body where it can exert its pharmacologic effects.

*Ideal properties of enteric coating material are summarized as below:*

i. Resistance to gastric fluids.
ii. Susceptible/permeable to intestinal fluid.
iii. Compatibility with most coating solution components and the drug substrate.
iv. Formation of continuous film.
v. Nontoxic, cheap and ease of application.
vi. Ability to be readily printed.

*Commonly used enteric film formers are as follows:*

A. Cellulose acetate phthalate (CAP)
   - It is widely used in industry.
   - It dissolves above pH 6 only, delays absorption of drugs.
   - It is hygroscopic and permeable to moisture in comparison with other enteric polymer.
   - It is susceptible to hydrolytic removal of phthalic and acetic acid changing film properties.
   - Cap films are brittle and usually used with other hydrophobic film forming materials.

B. Acrylate polymers
   - Eudragit L and Eudragit S are two forms of commercially available enteric acrylic resins. Both of them produce films resistant to gastric fluid.
   - Eudragit L and S are soluble in intestinal fluid at pH 6 and 7 respectively.
   - Eudragit L is available as an organic solution (isopropanol), solid or aqueous dispersion. Eudragit S is available only as an organic solution (isopropanol) and solid.

C. Hydroxypropyl methylcellulose phthalate (HPMCP)
   - HPMCP 50, 55 and 55-S (also called HP-50, HP-55 and HP-55-S) is widely used.

- HP-55 is recommended for general enteric preparation while HP-50 and HP-55-S for special cases.
- These polymers dissolve at a pH 5-5.5.

D. Polyvinyl acetate phthalate (PVAP)
- It is similar to HP-55 in stability and pH dependent solubility.

**3. Press coating (Fig. 1.19)**

Press coating process involves compaction of coating material around a preformed core. The technique differs from sugar and film coating process.

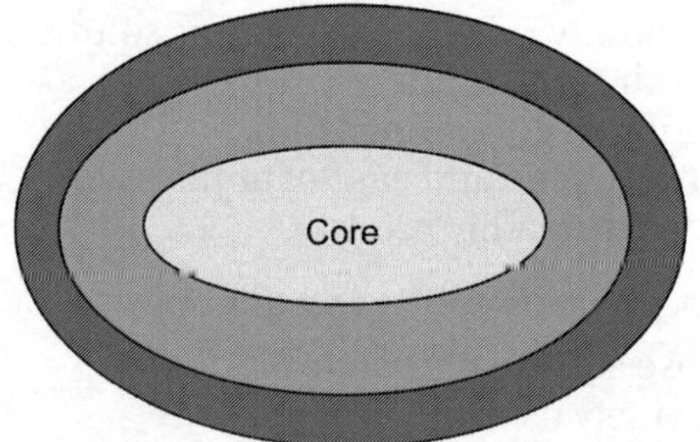


FIGURE 1.19: Press coated tablet

*Advantages*

This coating process enables incompatible materials to be formulated together, such that one chemical or more is placed in the core and the other(s) in the coating material.

*Disadvantages*

Formulation and processing of the coating layer requires some care and relative complexities of the mechanism used in the compressing equipment.

## SPECIALIZED COATING

### A. Compressed coating

This type of coating requires a specialization tablet machine. Compression coating is not widely used but it has advantages in some cases in which the tablet core cannot tolerate organic solvent or water and yet needs to be coated for taste masking or to provide delayed or enteric properties to the finished product and also to avoid incompatibility by separating incompatible ingredients.

### B. Electrostatic coating

Electrostatic coating is an efficient method of applying coating to conductive substrates. A strong electrostatic charge is applied to the substrate. The coating material containing conductive ionic species of opposite charge is sprayed onto the charged substrate. Complete and uniform coating of corners and adaptability of this method to such relatively nonconductive substrate as pharmaceutical is limited.

### C. Dip coating

Coating is applied to the tablet cores by dipping them into the coating liquid. The wet tablets are dried in a conventional manner in coating pan. Alternative dipping and drying steps may be repeated several times to obtain the desired coating. This process lacks the speed, versatility, and reliability of spray-coating techniques. Specialized equipment has been developed to dip-coat tablets, but no commercial pharmaceutical application has been obtained.

### D. Vacuum film coating

Vacuum film coating is a new coating procedure that employs a specially designed baffled pan. The pan is hot water jacketed, and it can be sealed to achieve a vacuum system. The tablets are placed in the sealed pan, and the air in the pan is displaced by nitrogen before the desired vacuum level is obtained. The coating solution is then applied with airless spray system. The evaporation is caused by the heated pan, and the vapor is removed by the vacuum system. Because there is no high-velocity heated air, the energy requirement is low and coating efficiency is high. Organic solvent can be effectively used with this coating system with minimum environmental or safety concerns.

## TABLET COATING EQUIPMENTS

Most coating processes use one of three general types of equipment:

- Standard coating pan

- Perforated coating pan
- Fluidized bed coater

a. **Standard coating pan**: The standard coating pan system consists of a circular metal pan mounted angularly on a stand. The pan is 8–60 inches in diameter and is rotated on its horizontal axis by a motor. Heated air is directed into the pan and onto the tablet bed surface and is exhausted by means of duct positioned through the front of the pan. Coating solutions are applied to the tablets by ladling or spraying the material onto the rotating tablet bed (Fig. 1.20).

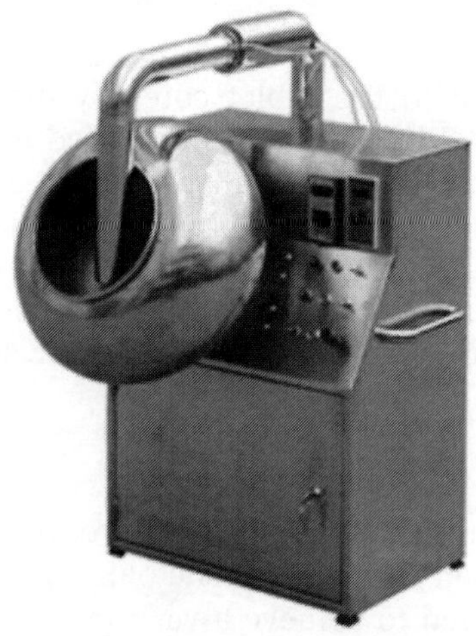

FIGURE 1.20: Standard coating pan

A significant landmark in the performance of standard coating pan systems has been introduced with the development of Pellegrini pan, immersion sword and immersion tube systems as in these systems coating solutions are applied by an atomized spray system directed to the surface of the rotating tablet bed.

Pellegrini system has a baffled pan and diffuser that distributes the drying air uniformly over the tablet bed surface. With the immersion sword system, drying air is introduced through a perforated metal sword device that is immersed in the tablet bed. Drying air flows upward from the sword through the tablet bed. With the immersion tube system, a tube is immersed in the tablet. The tube delivers the heated air and a spray nozzle is built in the tip of the tube. During the operation, coating solution is applied simultaneously with the heated air from the immersed tube. The drying air flows upward through the tablet bed and is exhausted by a conventional duct.

**Advantages**

Simple design, inexpensive, easy to clean and adaptable to sugar coating, film coating, etc.

**Major drawbacks**

- Relatively ineffective drying by pulsed hot air at the substrate surface.
- Extensive dust formation if extraction system not appropriate.

b. **Perforated coating pan system**: All the equipment of this type consists of a perforated or partially perforated drum that is rotated on its horizontal axis in an enclosed housing. These housings enables to control: airflow, air temperature, air pressure and coating application. Tablet coating takes place in a controlled atmosphere inside the rotating drum.

In perforated pan systems several air flow configurations are possible. In Accela Cota (Fig. 1.21) and hi-coater systems, drying air is directed into the drum, is passed through the tablet bed and is exhausted through perforations in the drum. The driacoater introduces drying air through hollow perforated ribs located on the inside periphery of the drum. As the coating pan rotates, the

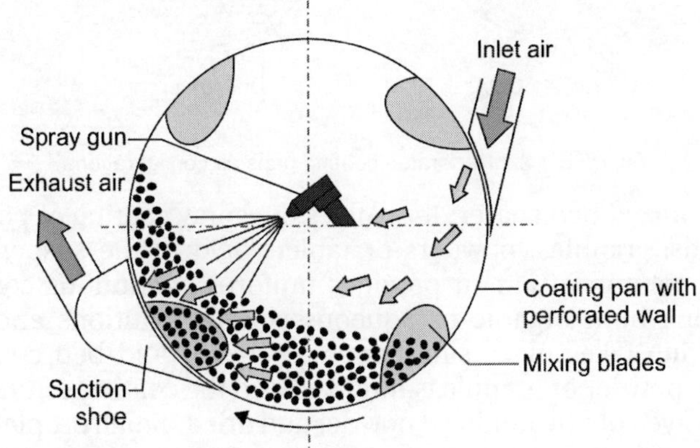


FIGURE 1.21: Simplified diagram of Accela-Cota system

ribs dip into the tablet bed and drying air passes through and fluidizes the tablet bed. Exhaust is from the back of the pan. In the Glatt coater, drying air can be directed from inside the drum through the tablet bed and out an exhaust duct.

In all four of these perforated pan systems, the coating solution is applied to the surface of the rotating bed of tablets through spraying nozzles that are positioned inside the drum (Fig. 1.22).

## Advantages

- Efficient drying with high coating capacity.
- Completely automated for both sugar coating and film coating processes.

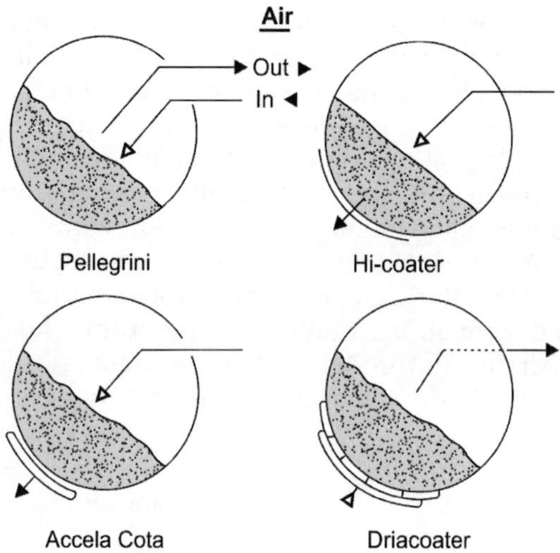


FIGURE 1.22: Perforated coating pans air configurations

c. **Fluidized bed coater**: It involves the spray coating of pellets, beds, granules, powders or tablets held in the suspension by column of air. It provides uniform continuous coating using both organic or aqueous coating solutions and the drying takes place simultaneously. With fluid bed coating, the powder or granule is fluidized and the coating solution is sprayed on the fluidized powder and dried. Small droplet and low viscosity of the coating solution ensure uniform coating with capability for controlled coat thickness.

The equipment developed commercially has provision for three types of coating system—top spray coating, bottom spray coating and tangential spray coating (Fig. 1.23).

i. **Top spray coating**: Top spray coating is recommended for taste masking, coating of enteric release and barrier films on particles or tablets. The method is of special significance when coatings are being applied from aqueous solutions, latexes or hot melts. Here the spray liquid is sprayed on to the fluidized powder against the air flow, from the nozzle provided at the top. Drying takes place as the coated particles continue to move upwards in the air flow.

ii. **Bottom spray coating (Wurster coating)**: Bottom spray coating is recommended for sustained release and enteric release products in which fluidization of the tablet mass is achieved in a columnar chamber by the upward flow of drying air.

The air flow is controlled, so that more air enters the center of the column, causing the tablets to rise in the center. The movement of tablets is upward through the center of the chamber. They then fall towards the chamber wall and move downward to re-enter the air stream at the bottom of the chamber. Coating solution applied continuously from spray nozzle located at the bottom of the chamber.

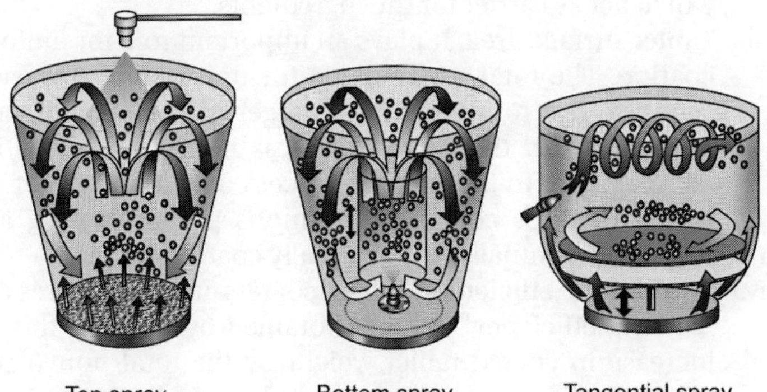


FIGURE 1.23: Spray pattern in fluidized bed coater

iii. **Tangential spray coating**: The tangential spray technique is recommended for layering coatings and also for sustained release and enteric release products. Here the product is set into a spiral motion by means of a rotating base plate, which has air fed into the powder bed at its edge. The spray nozzle is fitted tangentially to the rotating base plate, which spray coat solution on the fluidized powder bed.

### Application

The fluid bed processing equipment is multifunctional and may be used in preparing tablet granulation as well.

### Limitation

Tablet cores that are friable and prone to chipping and edge abrasion are not coated in fluidized bed coater.

## PROCESS PARAMETERS

Some generally used process parameters are:

i. **Air capacity**: This value represents the quantity of water or solvent that can be removed during the coating process which depends on the quantity of air flowing through the tablet bed, temperature of the air and quantity of water that the inlet air contains.
ii. **Coating composition**: The coating contains the ingredients that are to be applied on the tablet surface and solvents which act as carrier for the ingredients.
iii. **Tablet surface area**: It plays an important role for uniform coating. The total surface area for unit weight decreases significantly from smaller to larger tablets. Application of a film with the same thickness requires less coating composition. In the coating process only a portion of the total surface is coated. Continuous partial coating and recycling eventually results in fully coated tablets.
iv. **Equipment efficiency**: Tablet coaters use the expression "coating efficiency" a value obtained by dividing the net increase in coated tablet weight by the total nonvolatile coating weight applied to the tablet. Ideally 90%–95% of the applied film coating should be on the tablet surface. Coating efficiency for conventional sugar coating is much

less and 60% would be acceptable. The significant difference in coating efficiency between film and sugar coating relates to the quantity of coating material that collects on the wall.

## PROBLEMS AND REMEDIES FOR TABLET COATING

Variations in formulation and processing conditions may result in unacceptable quality defects in the film coating.

The sources of these defects and some of their probable causes are:

a. **Blistering:** It is local detachment of film from the substrate forming blister (Table 1.32).
*Reason*: Entrapment of gases in or underneath the film due to overheating either during spraying or at the end of the coating run.

**Table 1.32**: Causes and remedies of blistering

| *Causes* | *Remedies* |
|---|---|
| Effect of temperature on the strength, elasticity and adhesion of the film | - Use mild drying condition |

b. **Chipping:** It is the defect where the film becomes chipped and dented, usually at the edges of the tablet (Table 1.33 and Fig. 1.24).
*Reason*: Decrease in fluidizing air or speed of rotation of the drum in pan coating.

**Table 1.33**: Causes and remedies of chipping

| *Causes* | *Remedies* |
|---|---|
| High degree of attrition associated with the coating process | - Increase hardness of the film by increasing the molecular weight of polymer |

c. **Cratering:** It is a defect of film coating whereby volcanic-like craters appears exposing the tablet surface (Table 1.34).

**Table 1.34**: Causes and remedies of cratering

| *Causes* | *Remedies* |
|---|---|
| Inefficient drying | - Use efficient and optimum drying conditions |
| Higher rate of application of coating solution | - Increase viscosity of coating solution to decrease spray application rate |

*Reason*: The coating solution penetrates the surface of the tablet, often at the crown where the surface is more porous, causing localized disintegration of the core and disruption of the coating.

d. **Picking**: It is the defect where isolated areas of film are pulled away from the surface when the tablet sticks together and then part (Table 1.35 and Fig. 1.24).

*Reason*: Conditions similar to cratering that produces an overly wet tablet bed where adjacent tablets can stick together and then break apart.

**Table 1.35**: Causes and remedies of picking

| *Causes* | *Remedies* |
|---|---|
| Inefficient drying | - Use optimum and efficient drying conditions or<br>- Increase the inlet air temperature |
| Higher rate of application of coating solution | - Decrease the rate of application of coating solution by increasing viscosity of coating solution |

e. **Pitting/roughness**: It is the defect whereby pits occur in the surface of a tablet core without any visible disruption of the film coating (Table 1.36 and Fig. 1.24).

*Reason*: Temperature of the tablet core is greater than the melting point of the materials used in the tablet formulation.

**Table 1.36**: Causes and remedies of pitting/roughness

| *Causes* | *Remedies* |
|---|---|
| Inappropriate drying (inlet air) temperature | - Dispensing with preheating procedures at the initiation of coating and modifying the drying (inlet air) temperature such that the temperature of the tablet core is not greater than the melting point of the batch of additives used. |

f. **Blooming**: It is the defect where coating becomes dull immediately or after prolonged storage at high temperatures (Table 1.37).

*Reason*: It is due to collection on the surface of low molecular weight ingredients included in the coating formulation. In most circumstances, the ingredient will be plasticizer.

**Table 1.37:** Causes and remedies of blooming

| *Causes* | *Remedies* |
|---|---|
| High concentration and low molecular weight of plasticizer | - Decrease plasticizer concentration and increase molecular weight of plasticizer |

g. **Blushing**: It is the defect best described as whitish specks or haziness in the film (Table 1.38).

*Reason*: It is thought to be due to precipitated polymer exacerbated by the use of high coating temperature at or above the thermal gelation temperature of the polymers.

**Table 1.38:** Causes and remedies of blushing

| *Causes* | *Remedies* |
|---|---|
| High coating temperature | - Decrease the drying air temperature |
| Use of sorbitol in formulation which causes largest fall in the thermal gelation temperature of the hydroxypropyl cellulose, hydroxypropyl methylcellulose, methylcellulose and Cellulose ethers | - Avoid use of sorbitol with hydroxypropyl cellulose, hydroxypropyl methylcellulose, methylcellulose and Cellulose ethers |

h. **Color variation**: A defect which involves variation in color of the film (Table 1.39).

*Reason*: Alteration of the frequency and duration of appearance of tablets in the spray zone or the size/shape of the spray zone.

**Table 1.39:** Causes and remedies of color variation

| *Causes* | *Remedies* |
|---|---|
| Improper mixing, uneven spray pattern, insufficient coating, migration of soluble dyes-plasticizers and other additives during drying | - Go for geometric mixing, reformulation with different plasticizers and additives or use mild drying conditions |

i. **Infilling**: It is a defect that renders the intagliations indistinctly.

*Reason*: Inability of foam, formed by air spraying of a polymer solution, to break. The foam droplets on the surface of the tablet breakdown readily due to attrition but the intagliations form a protected area allowing the foam to accumulate and set. Once the foam has accumulated to a level approaching the outer contour of the tablet surface, normal attrition can occur allowing the structure to be covered with a continuous film.

**Table 1.40:** Causes and remedies of infilling

| *Causes* | *Remedies* |
|---|---|
| Bubble or foam formation because of air spraying of a polymer solution | - Add alcohol or use spray nozzle capable of finer atomization |

j. **Orange peel/roughness**: It is surface defect resulting in the film being rough and nonglossy. Appearance is similar to that of an orange.

*Reason*: Inadequate spreading of the coating solution before drying.

**Table 1.41:** Causes and remedies of orange peel/roughness

| *Causes* | *Remedies* |
|---|---|
| Rapid drying | - Use mild drying conditions |
| High solution viscosity | - Use additional solvents to decrease viscosity of solution |

k. **Cracking/splitting**: It is defect in which the film either cracks across the crown of the tablet (cracking) or splits around the edges of the tablet (splitting).

*Reason*: Internal stress in the film exceeds tensile strength of the film.

**Table 1.42:** Causes and remedies of cracking/splitting

| *Causes* | *Remedies* |
|---|---|
| Use of higher molecular weight polymers or polymeric blends | - Use lower molecular weight polymers or polymeric blends<br>- Adjust plasticizer type and concentration |

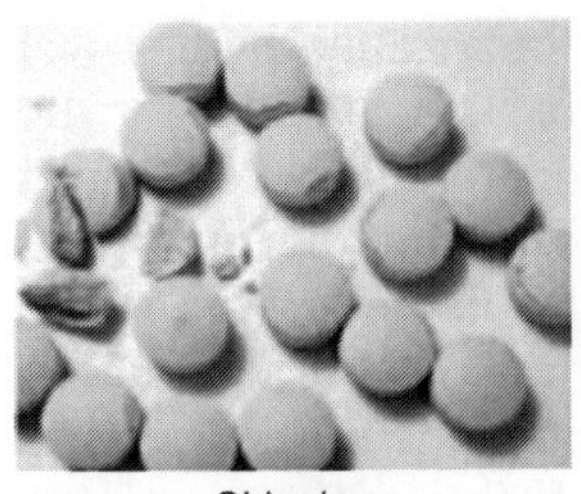

Chipping

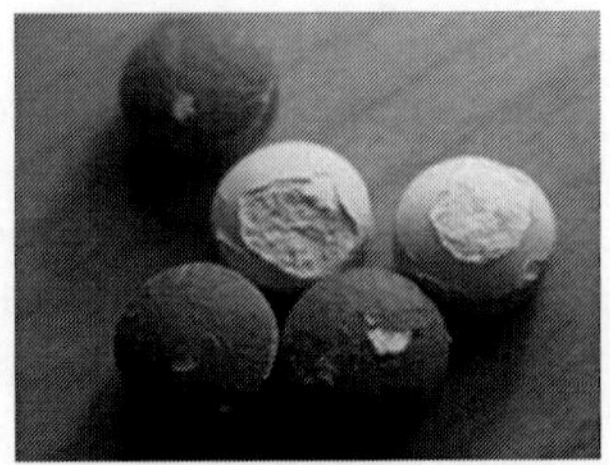

Picking

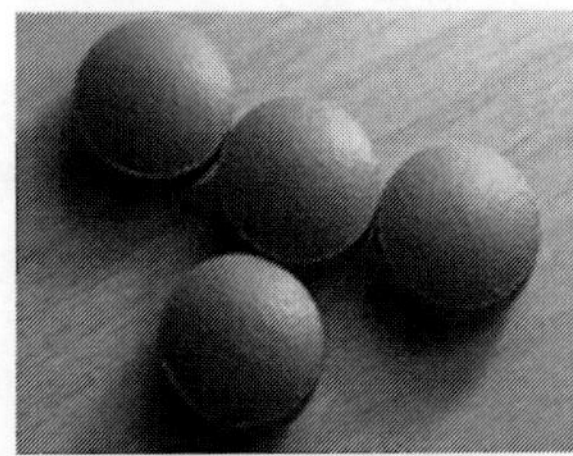

Pitting/roughness

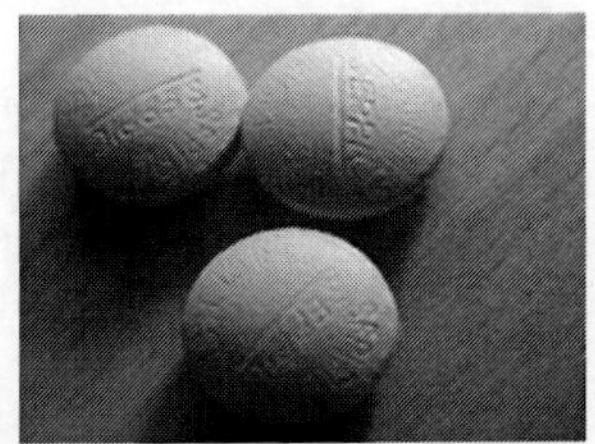

Filling

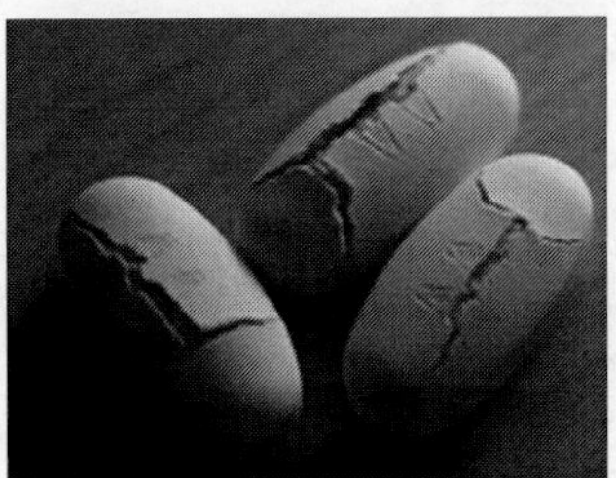

Film cracking

FIGURE 1.24: Film coating defects

## IN PROCESS QUALITY CONTROL (IPQC) TESTS FOR TABLETS

The quantitative evaluation and assessment of a tablet's chemical, physical and bioavailability properties are important in the design of tablets and to monitor product quality. These properties are important since chemical breakdown or interactions between tablet components may alter the physical tablet properties, and greatly affect the bioavailability of the tablet system. There are various standards that have been set in the various pharmacopoeias regarding the quality of pharmaceutical tablets. These include the diameter, size, shape, thickness, weight, hardness, disintegration and dissolution characters. The diameters and shape depends on the die and punches selected for the compression of tablets. The remaining specifications assure that tablets do not vary from one production lot to another.

## Classifications

Quality control tests are classified in two categories. These are:

A. Official or compendial tests
   - Weight variation test
   - Content uniformity test
   - Friability test
   - Disintegration time
   - Dissolution test.

B. Nonofficial or noncompendial tests
   - General appearance
   - Hardness test.

### *i. General appearance*

The general appearance of tablets, its visual identity and overall elegance is essential for consumer acceptance, control of batch-to-batch uniformity and general tablet-to-tablet uniformity and for monitoring the production process. The control of general appearance involves measurement of attributes such as a tablet's size, shape, color, presence or absence of odor, taste, surface textures, and quality of identification markings.

#### a. Tablets size and shape

The shape and dimensions of compressed tablets are determined by the type of tooling during the compression process. At a constant compressive load, tablets thickness varies with changes in die fill, particle size distribution and packing of the powder mix being compressed and with tablet weight, while with a constant die fill, thickness varies with variation in compressive load. Tablet thickness is consistent from batch-to-batch or within a batch only if the tablet granulation or powder blend is adequately consistent in particle size and particle size distribution, if the punch tooling is of consistent length, and if the tablet press is clean and in good working condition.

The thickness of individual tablets may be measured with a micrometer or vernier caliper, (Fig. 1.25) which permits accurate measurements and provides information of the variation between tablets. Tablet thickness should be controlled within a ±5% variation of a standard value.

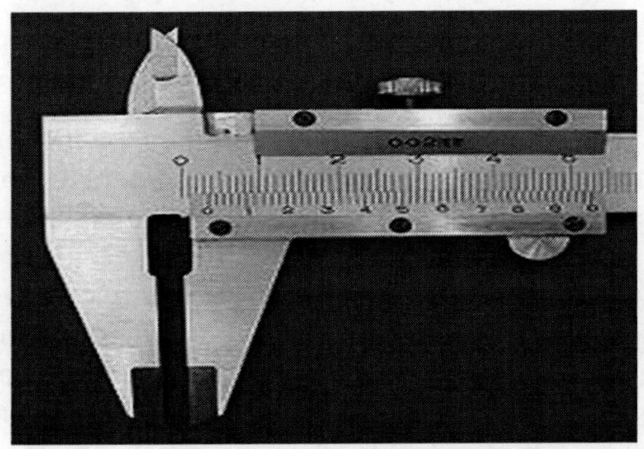

FIGURE 1.25: Vernier caliper

b. Organoleptic properties

Color is a vital means of identification for many pharmaceutical tablets and is also usually important for consumer acceptance. The color of the product must be uniform within a single tablet, from tablet-to-tablet and from batch-to-batch. Nonuniformity of coloring not only lack esthetic appeal but could be associated by the consumer with nonuniformity of content and general poor product quality. Nonuniformity of coloring is usually referred to as mottling. Reflectance spectrophotometry measurements and microreflectance photometer have been used to measure color uniformity and gloss on a tablet surface.

Odor may also be important for consumer acceptance of tablets and can provide an indication of the quality of tablets as the presence of an odor in a batch of tablets could indicate a stability problem, such as the characteristic odor of acetic acid in degrading aspirin tablets. However, the presence of an odor may be characteristic of the drug (e.g. vitamins), added ingredients (e.g. flavoring agent) or the dosage form (e.g. filmcoated tablets).

Taste is also important for consumer acceptance of certain tablets (e.g. chewable tablets) and many companies utilize taste panels to judge the preference of different flavors and flavor levels in the development of a product. Taste preference is, however, subjective and the control of taste in the production of chewable tablets is usually based on the presence or absence of a specified taste.

### *ii. Weight variation test*

The physical dimensions of the tablet along with the density of the material in the tablet formulation and their proportions, determine the weight of the tablet. The size and shape of the tablet can also influence the choice of tablet machine to use, the best particle size for granulation, production lot size that can be made, the best type of tableting processing that can be used, packaging operations, and the cost of production. The USP has provided limits for the average weight of uncoated compressed tablets. These are applicable when the tablet contains 50 mg or more of the drug substance or when the latter comprises 50% or more, by weight of the dosage form.

**Procedure**: Twenty tablets are weighed individually and the average weight is calculated. The individual tablet weights are then compared to the average weight. Not more than two of the tablets must differ from the average weight by the percentages stated in Tables 1.43 and 1.44. No tablet must differ by more than double the relevant percentage. Tablets that are coated are exempted from these requirements but must conform to the test for content uniformity if applicable.

**Table 1.43**: Weight variation requirements as per USP

| *Average wt. of tablet (mg)* | *Maximum % difference allowed* |
|---|---|
| 130 or less | 10% |
| 130–324 | 7.5% |
| More than 324 | 5% |

Table 1.44: Weight variation requirements as per IP

| *Average wt. of tablet (mg)* | *Maximum % difference allowed* |
|---|---|
| 84 or less | 10% |
| 84–250 | 7.5% |
| More than 250 | 5% |

### *iii. Content uniformity test*

The content uniformity test is used to ensure the uniform potency, for tablets of low dose drugs. USP defines content uniformity test for tablets containing 50 mg or less of drug substance in case of uncoated tablets and for all sugar coated tablets regardless to the drug content.

Procedure

- Representative samples of 30 tablets are selected randomly and 10 are assayed individually for their content (according to the method described in the individual monograph).
- Requirements are met if amount of drug in each tablet lies within the range of 85%–115% of the labeled claim.
- If the above conditions are not met, the results should be as follows in order to pass the test.
- Remaining 20 tablets are assayed. Out of 30 tablets, 1 tablet can be outside 85%–115% of the labeled claim and not even one should be above 75%–125% of the labeled claim.

* Content uniformity test ensures that every dosage form contains equal amount of drug substance, i.e. Active pharmaceutical ingredient within a batch.

### *iv. Hardness test*

The resistance of tablets to capping, abrasion or breakage under conditions of storage, transportation and handling before usage depends on its hardness. Hardness, which is now more appropriately called crushing strength determinations are made during tablet production to determine the need for pressure adjustment on tablet machine. If the tablet is too hard, it may not disintegrate in the required period of time to meet the dissolution specifications; if it is too soft, it may not be able to withstand the handling during subsequent processing such as coating or packaging and shipping operations.

Hardness or crushing strength of tablets is measured by hardness or crushing strength testers. They measure the force required to break the tablet. The force measured in kilograms and a crushing strength of 4 kg is usually considered to be the minimum for satisfactory tablets. Oral tablets normally have a hardness of 4–10 kg, however, hypodermic and chewable tablets are usually much softer (3 kg) and some sustained release tablets are much harder (10–20 kg). Tablet hardness has been associated with other tablet properties such as density and porosity. Hardness generally increases with normal storage of tablets and depends on the shape, chemical properties, binding agent and pressure applied during compression.

*Hardness or crushing strength testers*: The small and portable hardness tester was manufactured and introduced by Monsanto in the Mid 1930s. It is now designated as either the Monsanto or Stokes hardness tester. The instrument measures the force required to break the tablet when the force generated by a coil spring is applied diametrically to the tablet. The Strong-Cobb, Erweka Pfizer and Schleuniger apparatus which were later introduced measures the diametrically applied force required to break the tablet (Fig. 1.26).

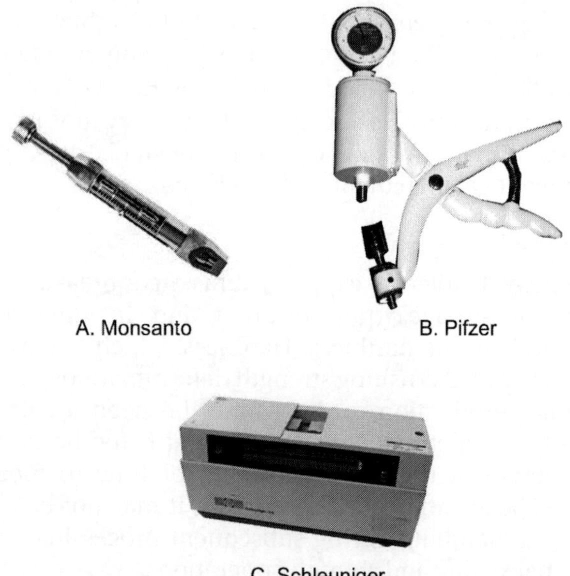

A. Monsanto B. Pifzer

C. Schleuniger

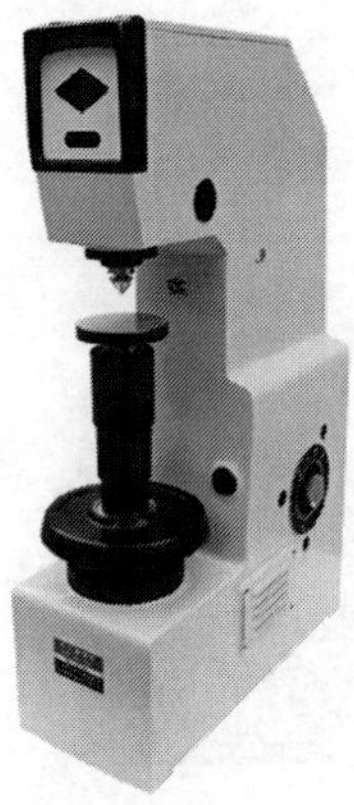

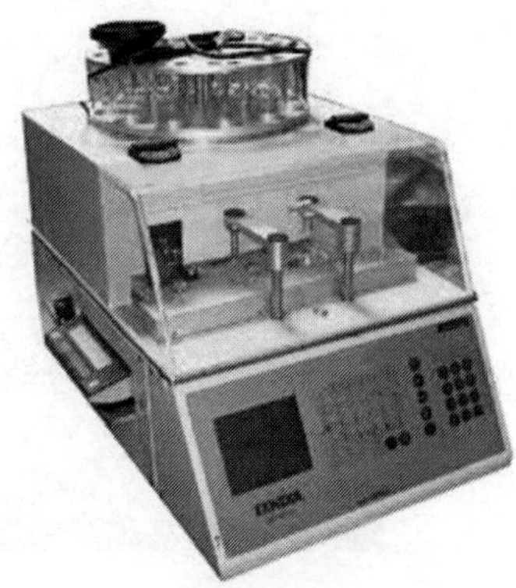

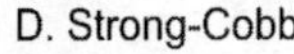

D. Strong-Cobb E. Erweka

FIGURES 1.26A to E: Hardness testers

## v. *Friability test*

Measuring the hardness of a tablet is not a reliable indicator for tablet strength as some formulations when compressed into very hard tablets tend to 'cap' or lose their crown portions on attrition. Such tablets tend to powder, chip and fragment. They not only lack elegance and consumer acceptance but also spoil the areas of manufacturing such as coating and packaging. Friction and shocks are the forces that most often cause tablets to chip, cap or break. The friability test is closely related to tablet hardness and is designed to evaluate the ability of the tablet to withstand abrasion in packaging, handling and shipping.

*Friability test apparatus*: The friability test is carried out in an instrument called a friabilator (commonly used friabilator in laboratories is the Roche friabilator). A friability testing apparatus should stimulate the conditions that the product will be exposed to during the process of production. This test is a method to determine physical strength of uncoated tablets upon exposure to mechanical shock and attrition.

This instrument consists of a plastic chamber for placing the tablets which are attached to a horizontal axis. The drum has an inside diameter of 287 mm and is about 38 mm in depth, made of a transparent synthetic polymer with polished internal surface. The plastic chamber revolves at 25 rpm, dropping the tablets a distance of 6 inches with each revolution (Fig. 1.27).

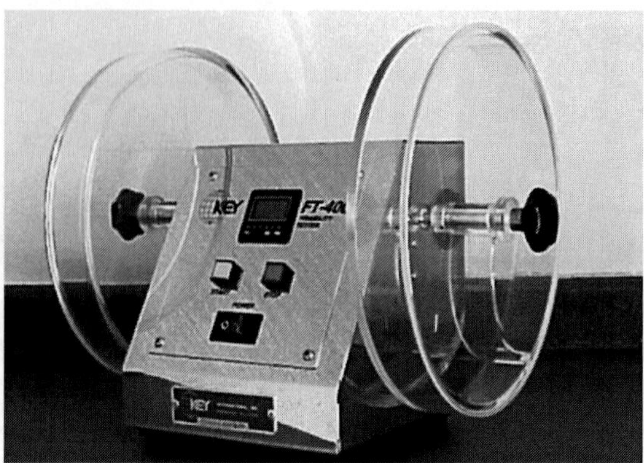


FIGURE 1.27: Friability test apparatus

*Procedure*: 10 tablets are weighed and placed in the apparatus where they are exposed to rolling and repeated shocks as they fall 6 inches in each turn within the apparatus. After four minutes of this treatment or 100 revolutions, the tablets are weighed and the weight compared with the initial weight. The loss due to abrasion is a measure of the tablet friability. The value is expressed as a percentage. A maximum weight loss of 0.5%–1% is considered acceptable. Normally, when capping occurs, friability values are not calculated. A thick tablet may have less tendency to cap whereas thin tablets of large diameter often show extensive capping, thus indicating that tablets with greater thickness have reduced internal stress.

Most effervescent tablets and some chewable tablets undergo high friability weight loss which is an indication for the special stack packing that is required for these types of tablets. In case of hygroscopic tablets a humidity-controlled environment (relative humidity less than 40%) is required for testing. Tablets prone to capping during the test are considered unfit for commercial use.

Friability is affected by various external and internal factors like:

1. Punches that are in poor condition or worn at their surface edges, resulting in 'whiskering' at the tablet edge and show higher than normal friability values.
2. Friability test is influenced by internal factors like the moisture content of tablet granules and finished tablets. Moisture at low and acceptable level acts as a binder.

*vi. Disintegration time*

For a drug to be absorbed from a solid dosage form after oral administration, it must first be in solution, and the first important step toward this condition is usually the break-up of the tablet; a process known as disintegration. The disintegration test is a measure of the time required under a given set of conditions for a group of tablets to disintegrate into particles which will pass through a 10 mesh screen. Generally, the test is useful as a quality assurance tool for conventional dosage forms.

*Disintegration test apparatus*: The disintegration test is carried out using the USP disintegration test apparatus, which consists of a basket rack assembly holding 6 glass tubes that are 3 inches long, open at the top, and held against a 10 mesh screen at the bottom end of the basket rack assembly (Figs 1.28 and 1.29).

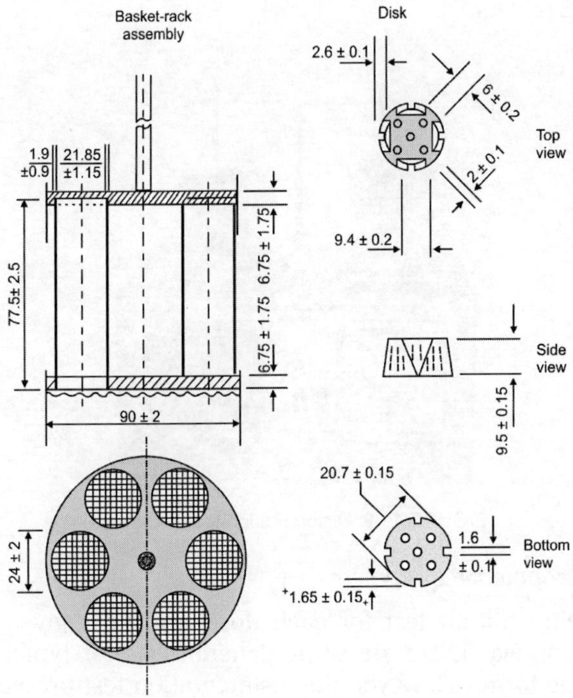


FIGURE 1.28: Disintegration test apparatus assembly

To test for the disintegration time, a single tablet is placed in each tube, and the basket rack is positioned in a 1-L beaker containing water or simulated gastric fluid, or stimulated intestinal fluid. The temperature of the system is maintained at 37± 2°C. A standard motor-driven device is used to move the basket assembly containing the tablets up and down through a distance of 5–6 cm at a frequency of 28–32 cycles per minute. During the movement of basket rack assembly, the tablets remain 2.5 cm below the surface of the liquid on their upward movement and descend not closer than 2.5 cm from the bottom of the beaker. Perforated plastic disks may also be used in the test. These disks are placed on top of the tablets. The disks are useful for preventing the tablets from coming out of the assembly. If the tablets are to be declared as USP compliant, they must disintegrate and all particles must pass through the 10 mesh screen in the specified time. If one or two tablets fail to disintegrate, the test is repeated using 12 tablets.

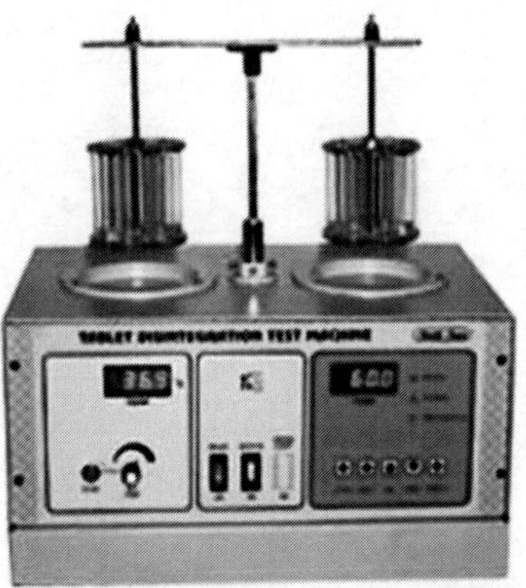

FIGURE 1.29: Disintegration test apparatus

*Pharmacopoieal requirements*

The disintegration test for each dosage form is given in the pharmacopeia. There are some general tests for typical types of dosage forms. However, the disintegration test prescribed in the individual monograph of a product is to be followed. If the monograph does not specify any specific test, the general test for the specific dosage form may be employed. Some of the types of dosage forms and their disintegration tests are (Table 1.45).

**Table 1.45:** Disintegration testing conditions and interpretation

| *Type of tablets* | *Medium* | Temperature | Time limit |
|---|---|---|---|
| Compressed uncoated | | 37 ± 2°C | 15 minutes or as per individual monograph |
| Sugar coated if 1 or 2 tablets fail | Water, 0.1 N HCl | 37 ± 2°C | 60 minutes or as per individual monograph |
| Film coated | Water | 37 ± 2°C | 30 minutes or as per individual monograph |
| Enteric coated | 0.1 N HCl and phosphate buffer pH 6.8 | 37 ± 2°C | 1 hour or as per individual monograph |
| Dispersible/ Effervescent | Water | 37 ± 2°C | LST < 3 minutes or as per individual monograph |
| Buccal | 37 ± 2°C | | 4 hours or as per individual monograph |

1. *Uncoated tablets*—Tested using distilled water as medium at 37+/-2°C at 29–32 cycles per minute; test is completed after 15 minutes. It is acceptable when there is no palpable core at the end of the cycle (for at least 5 tablets or capsules) and if the mass does not stick to the immersion disk.
2. *Coated tablets*—The same test procedure is adapted but the time of operation is 30 minutes.
3. *Enteric coated/gastric resistant tablets*—The test is carried out first in distilled water (at room temperature for 5 min; USP and no distilled water per BP and IP), then it is tested in 0.1 M HCl (upto 2 hours; BP) or stimulated gastric fluid (1 hour; USP) followed by phosphate buffer, pH 6.8 (1 hour; BP) or stimulated intestinal fluid without enzymes (1 hour; USP).
4. Chewable tablets—Exempted from disintegration test (BP and IP), 4 hours (USP).

### *vii. Dissolution test*

Dissolution is the process by which a solid solute enters a solution. In the pharmaceutical industry, it may be defined as the amount of drug substance that goes into solution per unit time under standardized conditions of liquid/solid interface, temperature and solvent composition. Dissolution is considered one of the most important quality control tests performed on pharmaceutical dosage forms and is now developing into a tool for predicting bioavailability, and in some cases, replacing clinical studies to determine bioequivalence. Dissolution behavior of drugs has a significant effect on their pharmacological activity. In fact, a direct relationship between in vitro dissolution rate of many drugs and their bioavailability has been demonstrated and is generally referred to as in vitro-in vivo correlation (IVIVC).

Dissolution test measures the availability of drug into systemic circulation. It is widely used in the pharmaceutical industry for optimization of formulation and quality control of different dosage forms.

**– What is the definition of dissolution?**

Dissolution is pharmaceutically defined as the rate of mass transfer from a solid surface into the dissolution medium or solvent under standardized conditions of liquid/solid interface, temperature and solvent composition. It is a dynamic property that changes with time and explains the process by which a homogenous mixture of a solid or a liquid can be obtained in a solvent. It happens to chemically occur by the crystal break down into individual ions, atoms or molecules and their transport into the solvent.

**– Why dissolution testing is used for pharmaceuticals?**

Dissolution testing is a critical preformulation solubility analysis research tool in the process of drug discovery that entails measuring the stability of the investigational product, achieving uniformity in production lots and determining its in vivo availability. Thus, this dissolution testing is an essential requirement for the development, establishment of in vitro dissolution and in vivo performance (IVIVR), registration and quality control of different dosage forms.

**– What are the applications of dissolution testing?**

Dissolution testing is widely used in the pharmaceutical industry for optimization of formulation and quality control.

*Dissolution test apparatus*: The dissolution test is carried out using the USP dissolution test apparatus, generally for tablets two types of apparatus is used (Fig. 1.30):

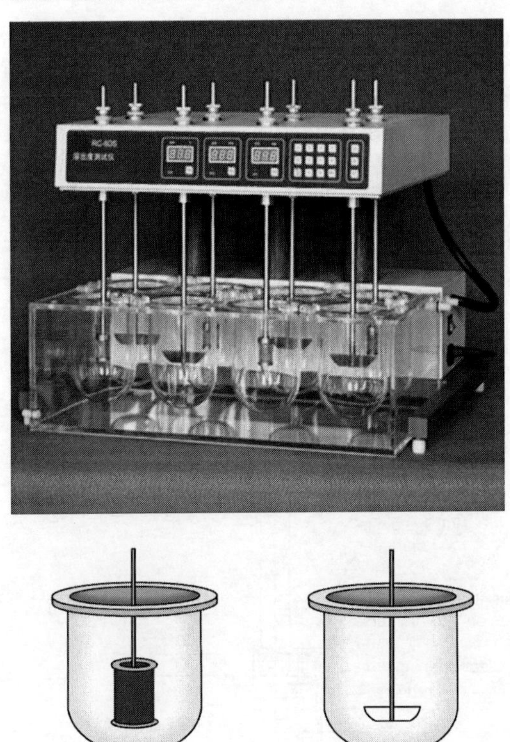

(a) Apparatus 1 (b) Apparatus 2

FIGURE 1.30: USP dissolution test apparatus

1. **Rotating basket apparatus**: It is also called USP type I apparatus; the basket of 22 mesh screen fastened to the bottom of the shaft. Basket is immersed in the dissolution medium contained in a 1-L flask. Flask is cylindrical with a hemispherical bottom maintained at 37°C ± 0.5°C by a constant temperature bath. Basket is placed at a distance of 2.5 cm from the bottom of the vessel, is centered within 2 mm of the centerline of the vessel. For the determination of dissolution rate single tablet is placed into basket and samples of fluid are withdrawn at intervals to determine the amount of drug in solution (Fig. 1.31).

2. **Rotating paddle apparatus**: It is also called USP type II apparatus; here basket is replaced by paddle, formed from a blade and a shaft as stirring element. The dosage form is allowed to sink to the bottom of the flask before stirring (Fig. 1.32).

   * Dissolution test medium, volume, which apparatus is to be used, speed (rpm), time limit of the tests and assay procedure is specified in USP/NF monographs.

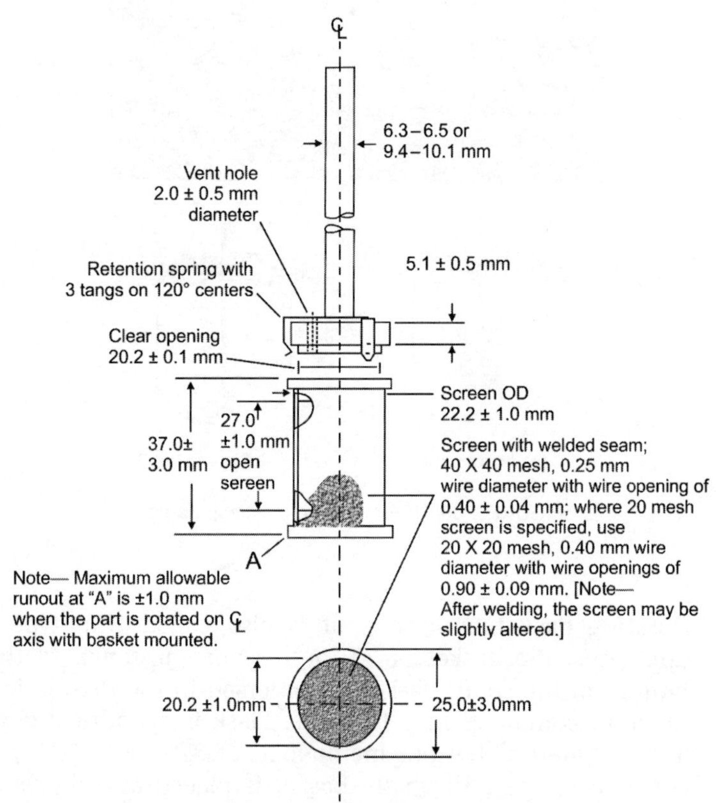


FIGURE 1.31: USP specification for type I (rotating basket) dissolution apparatus

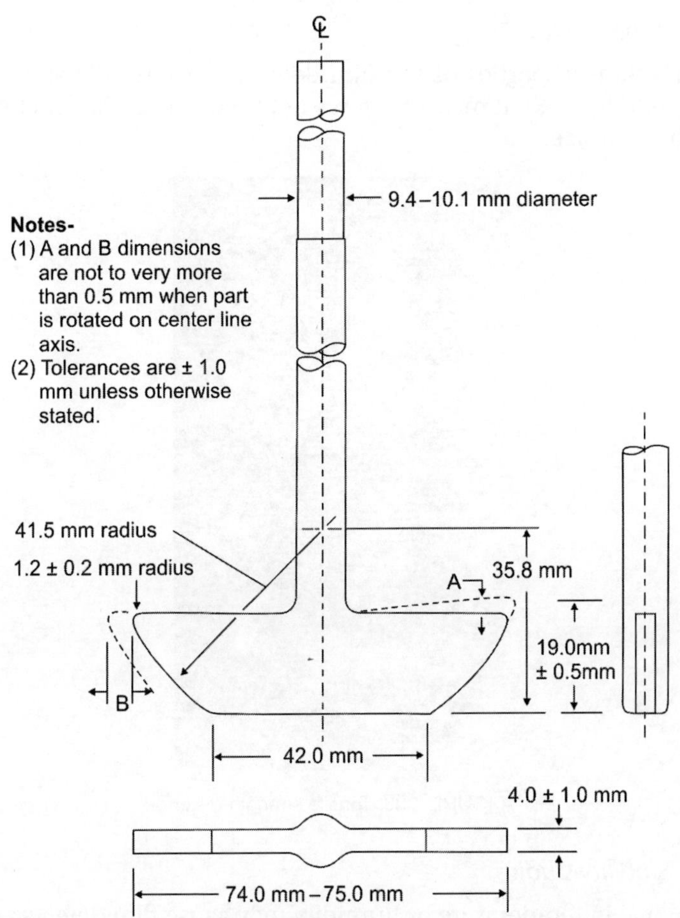


FIGURE 1.32: USP specification for type II (rotating paddle) dissolution apparatus

There are certain tests that are conducted on coated tablets to evaluate the suitability of film with respect to adhesion, tensile strength, etc.

*viii. Crushing strength of coated tablet*

For the determination of crushing strength of coated tablets, hardness testers are used. This test gives information on the relative increase in crushing strength provided by the film and contribution made by changes in the film composition.

*ix. Adhesion test*

Adhesion properties of the film determine by tensile strength tester (Fig. 1.33). It measures force required to peel the film from tablet surface.

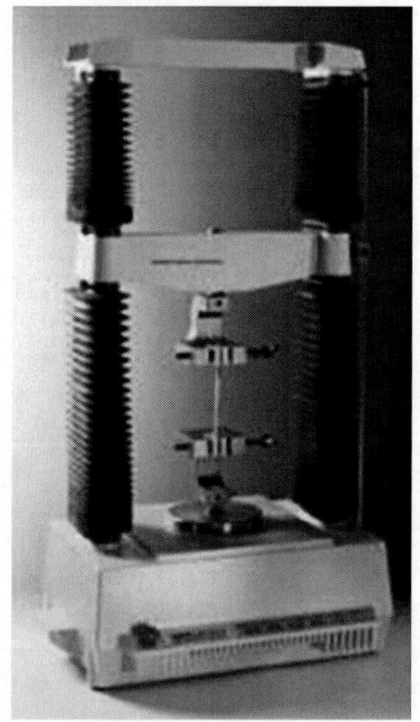

FIGURE 1.33: Tensile strength tester

*x. Stability studies*

Change in temperature or humidity may cause film defects and hence, studies are to be carried out in this respect also. Exposure of coated tablet to elevated humidity and measurement of tablet weight gain provide relative information on the protection provided by the film.

# Chapter 2

# Capsules

## INTRODUCTION

Capsule is the most versatile of all dosage forms. Capsules are solid dosage forms in which unit doses of powders, semi-solid or liquid drugs are enclosed in either a hard or soft envelop or shell. The shells are generally made of gelatin.

There are two types of capsules, "hard" and "soft". The hard gelatin capsule is also called as "two piece" as it consists of two pieces, smaller wider part of the capsule is "cap" and larger narrower part of the capsule is "body". The soft gelatin capsule is also called as "one piece". Although capsules are made from gelatin predominate, nongelatin capsules are also available in the market. Hard shell capsule made from starch were developed by "Capsugel". Shells made from hydroxypropyl methylcellulose (HPMC) are also available. HPMC capsules have been developed for both pharmaceutical products and dietary supplements. Qualicaps, is the first HPMC capsule developed for eventual use in pharmaceutical products. Capsules are available in many sizes to provide dosing flexibility. Unpleasant drug tastes and odors can be masked by the tasteless gelatin shell. The administration of liquid and solid drugs enclosed in hard gelatin capsules is one of the most frequently utilized dosage forms.

Capsules equal the tablets in their popularity and usage. They are convenient means of dispensing a variety of solids, semi-solids and liquids. All capsules basically consist of soluble shells of a material like gelatin. The solid substances are dispensed in hard capsules while for dispensation of liquids and semisolids soft capsules are preferred. Capsules are generally employed for enclosing materials meant for oral administration and are swallowed as a whole. Nowadays some capsules are administered through rectum or vagina and are useful substitutes for the more conventional types of suppositories based on oleaginous or water soluble bases. Soft capsules can also be employed for enclosing single application of eye ointments. Here the capsules have to be pricked with needle and the contained ointment transferred to ophthalmic cavity by application of slight pressure.

## HARD GELATIN CAPSULES (HGC) (FIG. 2.1)

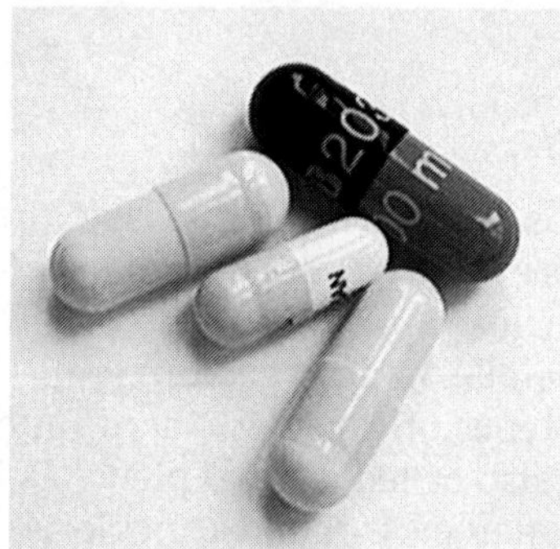

FIGURE 2.1: Hard gelatin capsules

These are solid dosage form of medicaments, in which drug is enclosed within the shells made up of gelatin. HGC are produced empty and are then filled in a separate operation. HGC are usually filled with powders, granules, pellets or small tablets containing the drug. Some semisolids (thixotropic mixtures and pastes) can also be filled in HGC. After ingestion, the gelatin shell softens swells and begins to dissolve in the gastrointestinal tract.

### Advantages of HGC

i. Beneficial for drugs having unpleasant taste or odor.
ii. They are attractive in appearance.
iii. They are slippery when moist and, hence, easy to swallow with a draught of water.
iv. As compared to tablets fewer adjuncts are required.
v. Possibility of filling diverse systems in HGC including beads, granules, small tablets and powders.
vi. The shells are physiologically inert and easily and quickly digested in the gastrointestinal tract.

vii. They have better bioavailability than tablets.
viii. They are economical.
ix. They are easy to handle and carry.
x. The shells can be opacified (with titanium dioxide) or colored, to give protection from light.

## Disadvantages of HGC

i. HGC should not be used for highly effervescent or deliquescent materials. Effervescent materials tends capsule to soften and deliquescent materials dry the capsules to excessive brittleness.
ii. Highly soluble salts such as iodides, bromides and chlorides generally should not be dispensed in HGC. Since, sudden release of such compounds in the stomach could result in irritating concentrations.
iii. Relatively costlier than tablets.

## Size and Shapes of HGC (Table 2.1)

**Table 2.1**: Standard sizes of hard gelatin capsules and their filling capacities

| *Capsule no.* | *Volume in ml* | *Size in mm* |
|---|---|---|
| 000 | 1.37 | 26.3 |
| 00 | 0.95 | 23.7 |
| 0 | 0.68 | 21.8 |
| 1 | 0.50 | 19.2 |
| 2 | 0.37 | 18.3 |
| 3 | 0.30 | 15.3 |
| 4 | 0.21 | 14.7 |
| 5 | 0.15 | 11.9 |

For human use empty gelatin capsules are manufactured in eight sizes ranging from 000 (largest) to 5 (smallest) (Fig. 2.2). Approximate filling capacity of capsule ranges from 1400 to 30 mg depending upon the types and bulk densities of powdered drug materials. Normally, the shell manufacturers give a guidance of the approximate quantities of selected drugs that can be contained in different sizes. For veterinary use larger capsules No. 10, 11 and 12 approximating to capacities of 30 gm, 15 gm and 7.5 gm are also marketed.

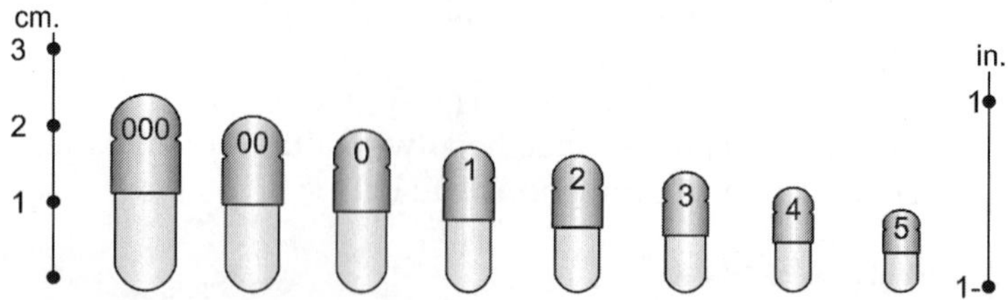


– The largest size of the capsule is No: 000.
– The smallest size is No: 5.
– The standard shape of capsules is traditional, symmetrical bullet shape.

FIGURE 2.2: Standard sizes of hard gelatin capsules

## Composition of HGC

The shell of hard gelatin capsules basically consists of gelatin, plasticizers and water. Modern day shells may, in addition, consist of preservatives, colors, opacifying agents, flavors, sugars, acids, enteric materials, etc.

1. *Gelatin*: Gelatin is the major component of the capsules shell and has been the material from which they have traditionally been made. Gelatin is a translucent brittle solid substance, colorless or slightly yellow, nearly tasteless and odorless, which is created by prolonged boiling of animal skin connective tissue or bones.

Gelatin has been the raw material of choice because of the ability of a solution of gel to form a solid at a temperature just above ambient temperate conditions, which enables a homogeneous film to be formed rapidly on a mould pin.

The reason for this is that gelatin possesses the following basic properties:

- It is nontoxic, widely used in foodstuffs and acceptable for use worldwide.
- It is readily soluble in biological fluids at body temperature.
- It is good film-forming material, producing a strong flexible film.
- The gelatin films are homogeneous in structure, which gives them strength.

**Some of the disadvantages with using gelatin for hard capsules include**—It has a high moisture content, which is essential because this is the plasticizer for the film and, under

International Conference on Harmonization of Technical Requirements for Registration of Pharmaceuticals for Human Use (ICH) conditions for accelerated storage testing, gelatin undergoes a cross-linking reaction that reduces its solubility.

**Production of gelatin**: Gelatin is prepared by the hydrolysis of collagen obtained from animal connective tissues, bones and skin. On hydrolysis, this long polypeptide chain yields 18 amino acids, of which most prevalent is glycine and alanine.

Gelatin can vary in its chemical and physical properties depending on the source of the collagen and the manner of extraction (Fig. 2.3). There are basic two types of gelatin: Type A and Type B. Characteristics of these two types of gelatin discussed in Table 2.2. Average molecular weight of gelatin varies between 20,000 and 200,000. Pharmagel A and Pharmagel B are the most popular grades, which are derived from an acid and alkali treated precursor respectively. Capsules may be made from either type of gelatin, but combination of both types of gelatin is often used to optimize shell characteristics. Difference in the physical properties of finished capsules as a function of the type of gelatin used is slight.

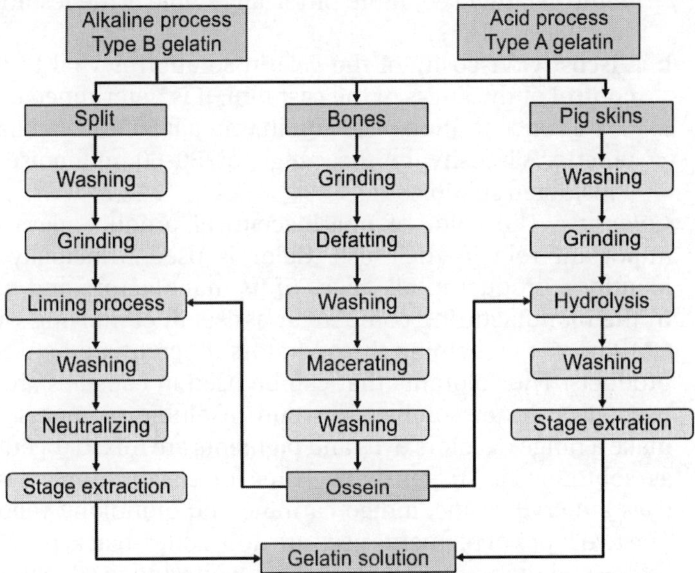


FIGURE 2.3: Gelatin production process

Table 2.2: Characteristics of Type A and Type B gelatin

| *Type A* | *Type B* |
|---|---|
| Produced by acid hydrolysis | Produced by alkaline hydrolysis |
| Manufactured from pork skin | Manufactured from animal bones |
| Exhibit isoelectric point in the region of pH 7.0–9.0 | Exhibit isoelectric point in the region of pH 4.8–5.0 |
| Gelatin is obtained from pork skin contributes plasticity and clarity | Gelatin is obtained from bone gelatin contribute firmness |

*Physiochemical properties of gelatin*

a. **Bloom or gel strength of gelatin**: It is a measure of cohesive strength of the cross-linking that occurs between gelatin molecules and is proportional to the molecular weight of the gelatin. It is determined by measuring the weight in gm required to move a plastic plunger to a fixed distance into the surface of a $6^{2/3}$% w/w gelatin gel that has been held at 10°C for 17 hours.

   Bloom strength in the range of 150–280 gm is considered suitable for capsule. The higher the bloom strength of the gelatin used, more physically stable is the resulting capsule shell.

b. **Viscosity**: Viscosity of the gelatin solution is vital to the control of thickness of the cast film. It is determined on a $6^{2/3}$% concentration of gelatin in water at 60°C in capillary pipette. Viscosity in the range of 30–60 millipoise is considered suitable.

2. *Colorants*: The color of pharmaceutical product plays an important role in their use. Color is used principally to identify a product in all stages of its manufacture and use. In the manufacturing company it assists in complying with GMP norms by helping the operators differentiate between products. The colorants that can be used in capsules are of two types: water soluble dyes and insoluble pigments. To make a range of colors dyes and pigments are mixed together as solutions or suspensions. Three most commonly used dyes are erythrosine, indigo carmine and quinolone yellow. The two types of pigments used are iron oxides-black, red and yellow and titanium dioxide which is white and used to make the capsule opaque. Capsules are colored by the addition of

colorants to the gelatin solution during the manufacturing stage.

3. *Process aids*: Preservatives and surfactants are added to the gelatin solution during capsule manufacture to aid in processing. Gelatin solution is an ideal medium for bacterial growth at temperatures below 55°C. Preservatives are added to the gelatin and colorant solutions to reduce the growth of micro-organisms. Preservatives generally used are sodium sulfite, sodium metabisulfite, methyl paraben, propyl paraben, benzoic and propanoic acids.

Some hard gelatin capsules may contain 0.15% w/w of sodium lauryl sulfate which functions as wetting agent, to ensure that the lubricated metal moulds are uniformly covered when dipped into the gelatin solution. Capsules are available in many different sizes and shapes and can be used for the administration of powders, semisolids and liquids. Unpleasant tastes and odors of drugs are effectively masked by the practically tasteless capsule shell which dissolves or is digested in the stomach after about 10–20 minutes.

4. *Water*: Hot and dimineralized water is used in the preparation of gelatin solution.

## Method of production of empty hard gelatin shells

The capsule shells are nowadays produced on mass scale by sophisticated machinery. Some of the major suppliers of empty gelatin capsules are: Eli Lilly and Company, Warner Lambert's Capsugel (formerly Park Davis) and RP Scherer Corporation. The metal moulds at room temperature are dipped into a hot gelatin solution, which gels to form a film. This is dried, cut to length, removed from the moulds and the two parts are joined together, these processes are carried out as a continuous process in large machines.

*Steps involved in making empty gelatin capsules are (Fig. 2.4):*

i. Preparation of dipping solution: In the capsule manufacturing process firstly 30%–40% w/w solution of gelatin is prepared in large stainless steel tanks. Vacuum may be applied to assist in the removal of entrapped air from the viscous preparation. Portion of this stock solution are removed and mixed with any other ingredients as required, to prepare the dipping solution. At this point, the viscosity of the dipping solution is measured and adjusted. The viscosity of the dipping solution is critical to the control of the thickness of the capsule wall.

ii. Dipping: Pairs of stainless steel pins, lubricated with a mold releasing agent, are dipped into dipping solution to simultaneously form the cap and bodies. During dipping the pins are at ambient temperature (about 22°C), whereas the dipping solution is maintained at a temperature of about 50°C in a heated, jacketed dipping pan.

    The length of time to cast the film has been reported to be about 12 second, with larger capsule requiring longer dipping times.

iii. Rotation or spinning: After dipping, the pins are withdrawn from the dipping solution and as they are done so, they are elevated and rotated to distribute the gelatin over the pins uniformly and to avoid the formation of a bead at the capsule ends. After rotation, they are given a stream of cool air to set the film.

iv. Drying: The rack of gelatin coated pins then passes through the upper and lower kilns of capsule machine drying system. Here gently moving air which is precisely controlled for volume, temperature, and humidity, removes the exact amount of moisture from the capsule halves. Precision controls constantly monitor humidity, temperature and gelatin viscosity throughout the production process.

v. Stripping: Once drying is complete, a series of bronze jaws strip the cap and body portions of the capsules from the pins.

vi. Trimming: The stripped cap and body portions are delivered to collets in which they are firmly held. As the collets rotate, knives are brought against the shell to trim them to the required length.

vii. Joining: After trimming to the right length, the cap and body portions are aligned concentrically in channels, and the two portions are slowly pushed together. The cap and body portion are joined and ejected from the machine.

    The entire cycle takes about 45 minutes, about 2/3 of which is required for the drying step alone.

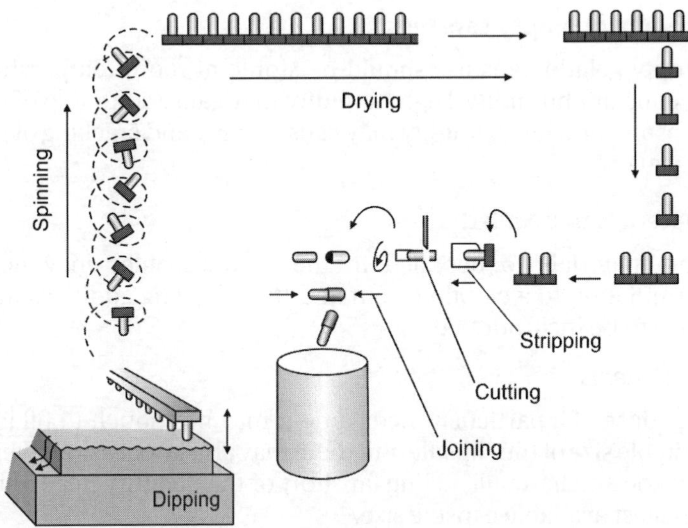


FIGURE 2.4: Steps involved in hard gelatin shells manufacturing

## Properties of empty capsule

Empty capsules contain a significant amount of water that acts as a plasticizer for the gelatin film and is essential for their function. The standard moisture content specification for hard gelatin capsules is between 13% w/w and 16% w/w. This value can vary depending upon the conditions to which they are exposed that is at low humidity they will lose moisture and become brittle, and at high humidity they will gain moisture and soften. The moisture content can be maintained within the correct specification by storing them in sealed containers at an even temperature.

Capsules are readily soluble in water at 37°C. When the temperature falls below, their rate of solubility decreases. At below about 30°C they are insoluble and simply absorb water, swell and distort. This is an important factor to take into account during disintegration and dissolution testing. Because of this most pharmacopoeias have set a limit of 37°C ± 1°C for the media for carrying out these tests.

## Storage of empty capsules

Empty gelatin capsules should be stored at room temperature at constant humidity. High humidity may cause softening of the capsules and low humidity may cause drying and cracking of the capsules.

## Materials to be filled

The materials to be filled in the hard capsules may need formulation to a certain extent and the following additives may have to be incorporated:

### *1. Diluents*

The dose of a particular medicament may be enough to fill in a suitable size of the capsule. But there may also be occasions when it is too small in bulk falling far short of the quantity needed for smallest available capsule size.

In such instances, one or the other diluents has to be added to bring the medicament up to a desired bulk. The usual diluents selected are lactose, mannitol, sorbitol, starch, etc. The quantities of diluents are related to the dose of the medicament and the capsule size.

### *2. Protective sorbents*

In some cases, inclusion of inert materials may be called for to physically separate incompatible or eutectic substances. Sometimes, some inert materials are included to prevent absorption of moisture by hygroscopic substances. Materials like oxides and carbonates of magnesium or calcium are suitable for these purposes.

### *3. Glidants*

Glidants become essential when the powders are filled by automated machinery requiring their regular flow into the capsule bodies. Many materials by themselves lack the desired degree of flow and hence glidants like talcum, stearates, etc. are included in suitable amounts.

### *4. Antidusting compounds*

In large scale filling operations dust is a real problem and if allowed to go unchecked, can pose serious health hazards for the workers. Presence of potent drugs in the dust can cause its continuous inhalation. Hence, material to be filled in the capsules should include some antidusting components like inert edible oils. The quantities of oils have to be carefully worked out, since excessive amounts can cause the particles to cohese together.

## Capsule Filling

Capsules are generally filled with powder blend containing drug and other inactive ingredients. However, in exceptional cases hard gelatin capsules are also filled with other forms of materials like mini tablets, granules, pellets and semisolids. Such cases are mostly to prevent incompatibility, provide extraordinary performance like desired dissolution profile, sustained release or to overcome certain specific technical problems. Hand operated machines are developed for small scale operation. On large-scale manufacturing various types of semiautomatic and automatic machines are used. They operate on the same principle as manual filling, namely the caps are removed, powder filled in the bodies, caps replaced and filled capsules are ejected out (Fig. 2.5). With automatic capsule filling machines powders or granulated products can be filled into hard gelatin capsules.

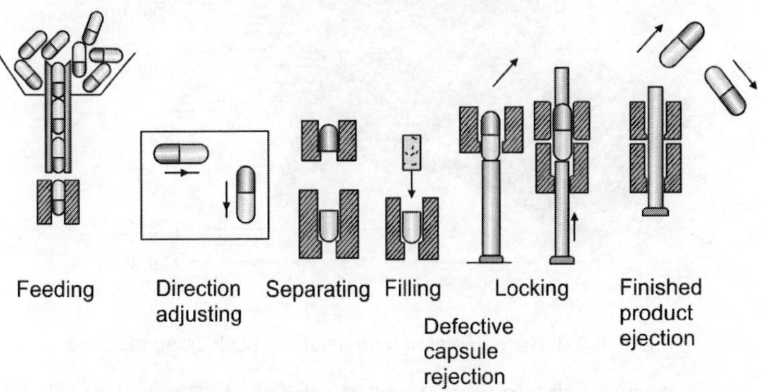


FIGURE 2.5: Operation sequences of capsule filling

### *a. Hand operated hard gelatin capsule filling machines*

Hand operated and electrically operated machines are in practice for filling the capsules but for small and quick dispensing hand operated machines are quite economical.

A hand operated gelatin capsule filling machine consists of the following parts and is shown in Figure 2.6.

– A filler unit with 200–300 holes
– A capsule loading tray
– A powder tray
– A pin plate having 200 or 300 pins corresponding to the number of holes in the filler unit and capsule loading tray.
– A lever
– A handle
– A plate fitted with rubber top.

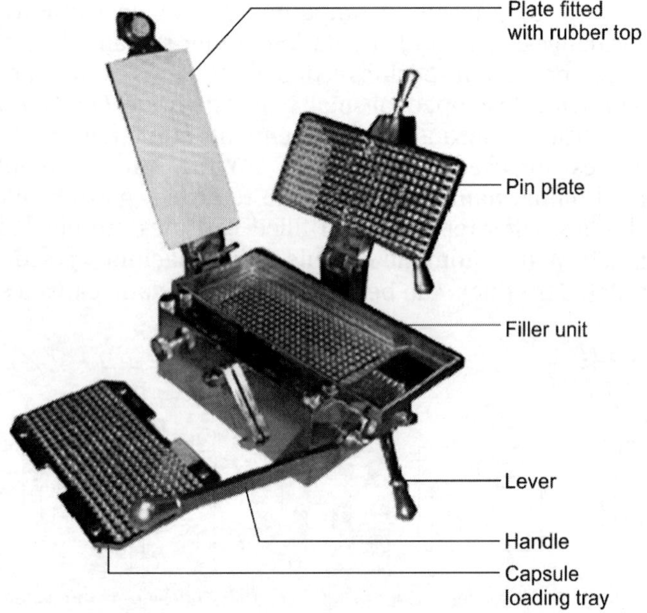


FIGURE 2.6: Hand operated hard gelatin capsule filling machine

All parts of the machine are made up of stainless steel. The machines are generally supplied with additional loading trays, filler units, and pin plates with various diameters of holes so as to fill the desired size of the capsules. These machines are very simple to operate, can be easily dismantled and reassembled.

*Working*: The empty capsules are loaded into the loading tray which is then placed over the filler unit. By opening the handle, the bodies of the capsules are locked and caps separated in the loading tray itself which is then removed by operating the liver. The weighed amount of the drug to be filled in the capsules is placed in powder tray already kept in position over the filler unit. Spread the powder with the help of a powder spreader so as to fill the bodies of the capsules uniformly. Collect excess of the powder on the platform of the powder tray. Lower the pin plate and move it downward so as to press the powder in the bodies. Remove the powder tray and place the caps holding tray in position. Press the caps with the help of plate with rubber top and operate the lever to unlock the cap and body of the capsules. Remove the loading tray and collect the filled capsules in a tray. With 200 hole machine about 5000 capsules can be filled per hour and with 300 hole machine 7500 capsules can be filled per hour.

*b. Semiautomatic capsule filling machine (Fig. 2.7)*

Semiautomatic capsule filling machines are designed with functions quite similar to the hand operating machine. These machines perform filling operation in 4 steps (Figs 2.8A to D):

i. First step includes feeding, aligning and insertion of capsules into holes of two piece filling ring. Empty capsules are oriented so that all points are in same direction, i.e. body end downward. As the ring is rotated, vacuum is applied on its underside to seats the bodies into lower half of the ring while caps are retained in the upper portion.
ii. After separation, cap containing portion is kept aside and body containing portion is placed on turntable and rotated under powder hopper.
iii. After one complete cycle of the ring, the powder hopper is removed and the two segments of ring are rejoined. Intact ring is placed in front of peg ring and the closing plate is pivoted to 180° position. Pneumatic pressure is applied to the ring which forces the capsule body into the cap and the closing plate held the capsules in place.
iv. For ejection of capsules, pressure is released and closing plate is restored to original position. Capsules are expelled through upper portions of ring.

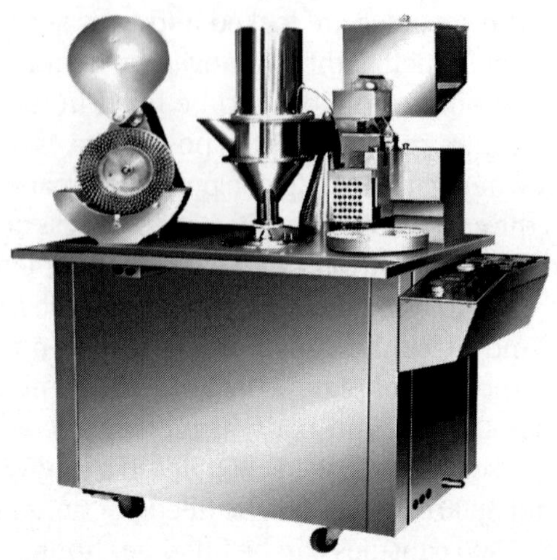

FIGURE 2.7: Semiautomatic capsule filling machine

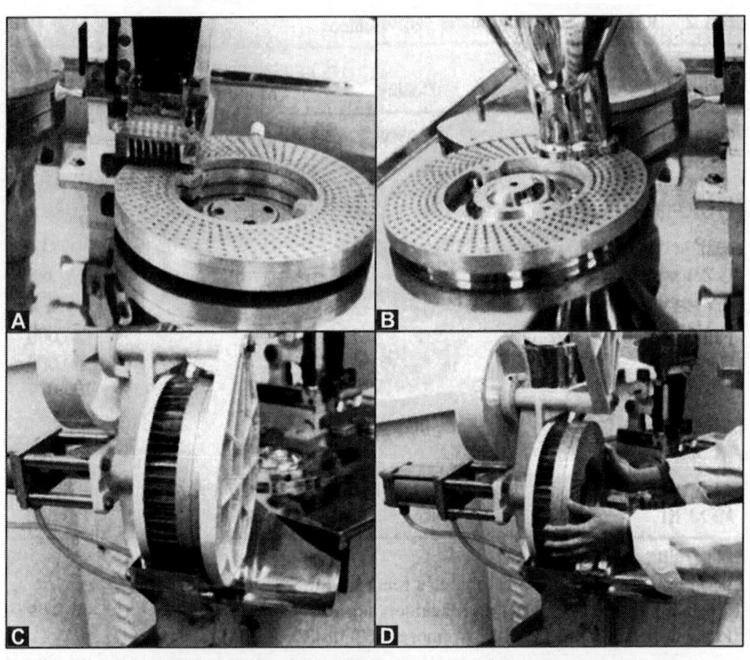

FIGURES 2.8A to D: Stages in semiautomatic capsule filling machine: A. Orientation and separation of capsule, B. Filling of powder, C. Joining of cap and body portion, D. Ejection of filled capsule

### c. *Automatic capsule filling machine (Fig. 2.9)*

It is a continuous operating machine where the cycle of operations continues in sequential manner. The major operational sequences include rectification, pre-fill powder compression and finally filling in capsules. The machines have capabilities to give an output of 40,000 capsules per hour with high filling accuracy and uniformity in dosing.

Automatic machines can be either continuous in motion, like a rotary tablet press, or intermittent, where the machine stops to perform a function and then indexes round to the next position to repeat the operation on a further set of capsules. High speed automatic capsule filling machines are suitable for filling powders and pellets. These are versatile machines with several outstanding features both functional and mechanical. Most machines conform to the GMP guidelines with various safety features for maximum operator protection. Here, fillers generate minimum dust with lowest level of product loss. Non-separated, double loaded capsules and improperly inserted capsules are automatically rejected by machines to maintain the consistency in the quality of product. Most capsule fillers are characterized with fast changeover time to accommodate a variety of capsules in terms of shapes and size. High quality capsule filling machine requires minimal maintenance and easy to clean. Another important feature is the installation of speed adjusting equipment and automatic counters ensuring the right quantity of capsules being filled and packed. ROTOFIL is a high speed, automatic, continuous – motion machine, is available from Eli Lilly and Company. This machine is specially designed to fill pellets.

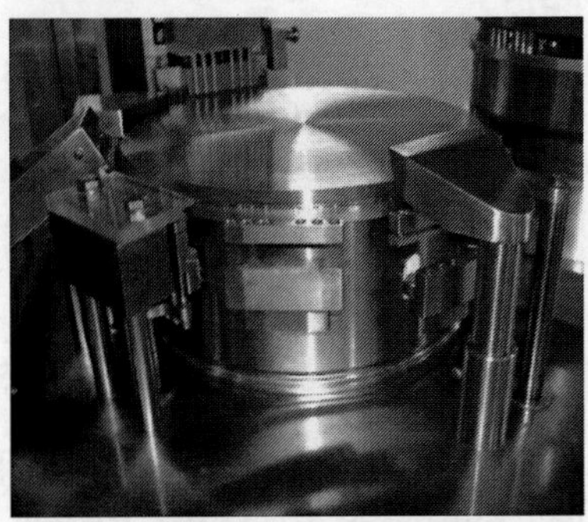

Figure 2.9: Automatic capsule filling machine

## Finishing

The filled and sealed capsules necessitate a finishing operation before inspection, bottling or packing in strips/blisters and labeling. The following steps are involved in the finishing process:

- **Salt polishing**: In salt polishing, the capsules are rotated in an Accela Cota pan along with sodium chloride granules. Later the capsules and granules are separated by screening on a suitable device. Such a polishing removes adhering materials from the surfaces of capsules. However, salt polishing should be done before imprinting, if any, since imprinting may be affected by salt.
- **Cloth dusting**: In this process individual capsules are rubbed with cloth which may or may not contain inert oil. This removes some remaining materials and also imparts improved gloss.
- **Brushing**: In brushing, capsules are projected under soft a rotating brush which removes all remaining dust. This operation must be supplemented by exposure of capsules to regulated vacuum.

## Sorting

This process is desirable to pick up imperfect and damaged capsules manually or with automated inspecting systems. ROTOSORT is a new filled capsule-sorting machine sold by Eli Lilly and Company. It is a mechanical sorting device that removes loose powder, unfilled joined capsules, filled or unfilled bodies and loose caps. It can handle upto 150,000 capsules per hour, and it can run directly off a filling machine or be used separately.

## Sealing and locking

Sealing and locking devices invented by various manufacturers as their novelties are basically guards against separation of the caps from the bodies during handling, transport, etc.

Sealing of the caps onto bodies is possible by moistening the upper part of the body and slipping the cap on. However, many manufacturers seal capsules by means of a colored band of gelatin placed at the junction of the body and the cap. More recently, some configurations have been developed in the bodies and caps which enable their mechanical locking. For instance, Snap Fit capsules, marketed by Parke Davis, have matching interlocking rings on the body and in the cap. Another method suggested is to bring a hot needle-like structure against the cap where it overlies the body to form a sort of spot weld.

### Storage of filled capsules

The capsules shells should be stored under controlled conditions of temperature and humidity. The normal moisture content of shell is 10%–15%. Under conditions of low humidity, they may soften and grow tacky. Ideally, humidity range of storage room is 30%–45%.

## SOFT GELATIN CAPSULES (SGC)

A soft gel (a soft gelatin capsule) is a solid capsule (outer shell) surrounding a liquid or semisolid center (inner fill), as shown in Figure 2.10. An active ingredient can be incorporated into the outer shell, the inner fill, or both.

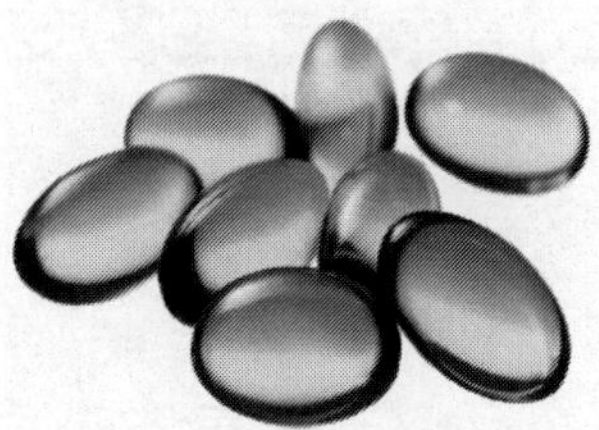

FIGURE 2.10: Soft gel capsule in the form of cod liver oil capsules

### Advantages of soft gel capsules

i. Ease of use-easy to swallow, no taste, unit dose delivery, tamper proof.
ii. Versatile
  - Accommodates a wide variety of compounds filled as a semisolid, liquid, gel or paste.
  - Wide variety of colors, shapes and sizes.
iii. Immediate or delayed drug delivery—It can be used to improve bioavailability by delivering drug in solution or other absorption enhancing media.
iv. Improved bioavailability, as the drug is presented in a solubilised form.
v. Enhanced drug stability.
vi. Consumer preference regarding ease of swallowing, convenience, and taste can improve compliance.

vii. Offer opportunities for product differentiation via color, shape and size and product line extension.
viii. The soft gels can be enteric coated for delayed release.
ix. They are popular for pharmaceuticals, cosmetics and nutritional products.

## Disadvantages of soft gel capsules

i. It requires special manufacturing equipment.
ii. Stability concerns with highly water-soluble compounds, and compounds susceptible to hydrolysis.
iii. There is more intimate contact between the shell and its liquid contents than exists with dry filled hard gelatin capsules which increase the possibility of interactions.
iv. Limited choices of excipients / carriers compatible with the gelatin.

**Table 2.3:** Shapes of soft gelatin capsule and their filling capacities

| *Shape* | *Volume in ml* |
|---|---|
| Spherical | 0.05–5 |
| Ovoid | 0.05–7 |
| Cylindrical | 0.15–25 |
| Tubes | 0.5–0 |
| Pear-shaped | 0.3–5 |

## Shape of capsule

SGC are available in variety of shapes and sizes as shown in Figure 2.11.

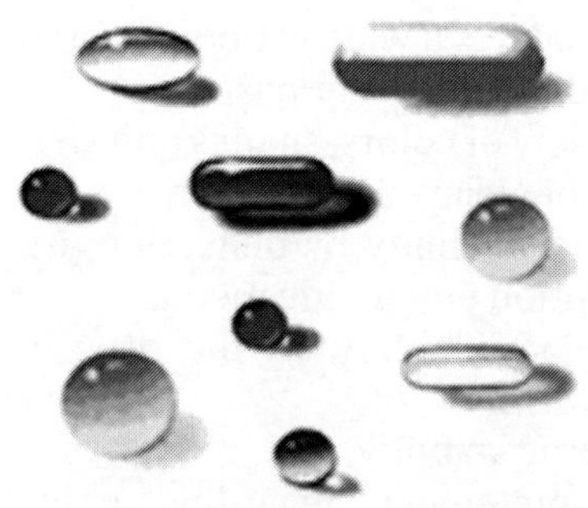

FIGURE 2.11: Different shapes of soft gel capsules

They are most suitable for liquids and semisolids and are widely used, in spherical and ovoid forms for vitamin preparations such as cod liver oil, vitamins A and D and multiple vitamins.

## Composition of soft gelatin capsules

Soft gels are made up of gelatin, plasticizer, and water. It may contain additional ingredients such as preservatives, coloring agents, opacifying agents, acids and medicaments to achieve desired.

a. *Gelatin*: Gelatin's chemical, physical and physiological properties make it ideal substance for the capsulation of pharmaceutical products.
b. *Plasticizers*: These are used to make the soft gel shell elastic and pliable. They usually account for 20%–30%. The most common plasticizers used in soft gels is glycerol, although sorbitol and propylene glycol are used frequently often in combination with glycerol. The amount and choice of the plasticizer contribute to the hardness of the final product and may even affect its dissolution or disintegration characteristics, as well as its physical and chemical stability. Plasticizers are selected on the basis of their compatibility with the fill formulation, ease of processing and the desired properties of the final soft gel, including hardness, appearance, handling characteristics and physical stability. One of the most important aspects of soft gel formulation is to ensure that there is minimum interaction or migration between the liquid fill matrix and the soft gel shell. The choice of plasticizer type and concentration is important in ensuring optimum compatibility of the shell with the liquid fill matrix.
c. *Water*: The other essential component of the soft gel shell is water. Water usually accounts for 30%–40% of the wet gel formulation and its presence is important to ensure proper processing during gel preparation and soft gel encapsulation. Following encapsulation, excess water is removed from the soft gels through controlled drying. In dry gels the equilibrium water content is typically in the range 5%–8% w/w, which represents the proportion of water that is bound to the gelatin in the soft gel shell. This level of water is important for good physical stability, because in harsh storage conditions soft gels will become either too soft and fuse together, or too hard and embrittled.

d. *Colorants/opacifiers*: Colorants (soluble dyes, or insoluble pigments or lakes) and opacifiers are typically used in the wet gel formulation. Colorants can be either synthetic or natural, and are used to impart the desired shell color for product identification. An opacifier, usually titanium dioxide may be added to produce an opaque shell when the fill formulation is a suspension, or to prevent photo degradation of light-sensitive fill ingredients. Titanium dioxide can either be used alone to produce a white opaque shell or in combination with pigments to produce a colored opaque shell.
e. *Preservatives*: Preservatives are added to the gelatin solution to reduce the growth of micro-organisms. Preservatives generally used are methyl paraben, propyl paraben, sodium sulfite, etc.
f. *Acidifiers*: Acidifiers aids solubility and reduces aldehydric tanning of gelatin.

## Materials to be filled

Content of a soft gel capsule is a liquid, or a combination of miscible liquids, a solution of a solid(s) in a liquid(s) or a suspension of a solid(s) in a liquid(s).

**Liquids**: Liquids are an essential part of the soft gel capsule content.

*Limitations*

- Only those liquids that are both water miscible and volatile cannot be included as major constituents of the capsule content since they can migrate into the hydrophilic gelatin shell and volatilize from its surface. Water, ethyl alcohol and emulsions fall into this category.
- Gelatin plasticizers such as glycerin and propylene glycol cannot be the major constituents of the capsule content, owing to their softening effect on the gelatin shell, which makes the capsule more susceptible to the effects of heat and humidity. As minor constituent (upto about 5% of the capsule content), water and alcohol can be used as cosolvent to aid in the preparation of solution for capsulation.

The types of liquids used in soft gelatin capsule fall into two main categories:

a. **Water immiscible, volatile or more likely nonvolatile liquids** such as vegetable oils, aromatic and aliphatic hydrocarbons (mineral oil), medium chain trigycerides and acetylated glycerides.

b. **Water miscible, nonvolatile liquids** such as low molecular weight polyethylene glycol (PEG-400 and PEG-600). Such liquids mixed with water readily and accelerate dissolution of dissolved or suspended drugs.

All liquids used for filling should be homogeneous and air free. Liquids should be flow by gravity at room temperature, but not at temperature exceeding 35°C at the point of capsulation, since the sealing temperature of the gelatin films is usually in the range of 37–40°C. Also, preparations for encapsulation should have a pH between 2.5 and 7.5, since preparations that are more acidic can cause hydrolysis and leakage of the gelatin shell and preparations that are more alkaline (>7.5) decreases shell solubility by tanning the gelatin.

**Solids**: Solids that are not sufficiently soluble in liquids or in combinations of liquids are capsulated as suspensions. Most organic and inorganic solids or compounds may be capsulated. Such materials must be 80 mesh or finer in particle size, owing to certain close tolerances of the capsulation equipment and for the maximum homogeneity of the suspension. The soft gelatin capsules these days are being increasingly used for encapsulation of suspensions of solids in suitable bases. The important requirement that a suspension should necessarily meet is that it must have flow properties similar to liquids and the suspended solids remain uniformly suspended during the filling operation to ensure homogeneity of the encapsulated mix. To achieve this liquid bases should be carefully chosen. The common materials cited in literature for this purpose are admixtures of vegetable oils and nonionic surfactants, carbowax 400, etc. These bases could be used for oral as well as topical dosage forms. The formulation of suspensions for soft gelatin capsules involves the consideration of "base adsorption" of the solid(s) to be suspended.

**Base adsorption**—Base adsorption is expressed as the number of grams of liquid base required to produce a capsulatable mixture when mixed with 1 gm of solid(s). The base adsorption of a solid is influenced by factors such as the solids particle size and shape, its physical state (fibrous, amorphous, or crystalline), its density, its moisture content, and its oleophilic or hydrophilic nature.

In the determination of base adsorption, the solid(s) must be completely wetted by the liquid base. For glycol and nonionic type bases, the addition of a wetting agent is seldom required, but for vegetable oil bases, complete wetting of the solid(s) is not achieved without an additive. Soy lecithin, at a concentration of 2%–3% by weight of the oil, serves excellently for this purpose, and being a natural product, is universally accepted for good drug use. Increasing the concentration above 3% appears to have no added advantage.

A practical procedure for determining base adsorption and for judging the adequate fluidity of a mixture is as follows: Weigh a definite amount of the solid (40 gm is convenient) into a 150 ml tared beaker. In a separate 150 ml beaker tared beaker, place about 100 gm of the solid base. Add small increments of the liquid base to the solid, and using a spatula, stir the base into the solid after each addition until the solid is thoroughly wetted and uniformly coated with the base. This should produce a mixture that has a soft ointment like consistency. Continue to add liquid and stir until the mixture flows steadily from the spatula blade when held at a 45° angle above the mixture.

The base adsorption is obtained by means of the following formula—

$$\text{Weight of the base} / \text{Weight of the solid} = \text{Base adsorption}$$

Base adsorption is used to determine the "minim per gram" factor (M/g) of the solid(s). The minim per gram factor is the volume in minims that is occupied by one gram (S) of the solid plus the weight of the liquid base (BA) required making a capsulatable mixture. The minim per gram factor is calculated by dividing the weight of the base plus the gram of solid base (BA+ S) by the weight of the mixture (W) per cubic centimeter or 16.23 minims (V).

A convenient formula is—

$$(BA + S) \times V / W = M/g$$

Thus, lower the base adsorption of the solid(s) and higher the density of the mixture, the smaller the capsule will be. This also indicates the importance of establishing specifications for the control of those physical properties of a solid mentioned previously that can affect its base adsorption.

The final formulation of a suspension invariably requires a suspending agent to prevent the settling of the solids and to maintain homogeneity prior to, during and after capsulation. The nature and the concentration of the suspending agent vary. In all instances, the suspending agent used is melted in a suitable portion of the liquid base, and the hot melt is added slowly, with stirring, into the bulk portion of the base, which has been pre-heated to 40°C prior to the addition of any solids. The solids are then added, one by one, with sufficient mixing between additions to ensure complete wetting. Incompatible solids are added as far as possible in the mixing order to prevent interaction prior to complete wetting by the base.

**Examples of suspension fills include drug suspended in the following carriers**:

1. Oily mixtures:
   - Soybean oil with beeswax (4%–10% w/w) and lecithin (2%–4% w/w). The lecithin improves material flow, and imparts some lubrication during filling. Add enough beeswax to get a good suspension, but avoid creating a non-dispersible plug.
   - Gelified oil (e.g. Geloil® SC), a ready to use system composed of soybean oil, a suspending agent and a wetting agent.
2. Polyethylene glycol:
   - PEG 800–1000 for semisolid fills.
   - PEG 10,000–100,000 for solid fills.
   - Or mixtures of the above (heat upto 35°C to make fluid enough for filling).
3. Optional ingredients that can be added in the suspension fill:
   - Surfactant: Sorbitan derivatives such as polysorbate 80 or lecithin.
   - For hydrophobic drugs dissolved or dispersed in an oily matrix, a surfactant of HLB 10 will increase the dispersibility of the product in aqueous fluids and also may improve bioavailability.

## Manufacture of soft gelatin capsules

Soft gelatin capsules is manufactured by four methods:

i. Plate process
ii. Rotary die process
iii. Accogel machine
iv. Bubble method.

a. *Plate process*: It is an oldest commercial process. It is a batch process requiring two or three operators for each machine. This process involves:
   - Placing the upper half of a gelatin sheet over a die plate containing numerous die pockets.
   - Application of vacuum to draw the sheet into the die pockets.
   - Filling the pockets with liquid or paste.
   - Folding lower half of the gelatin sheet back over the filled pockets.
   - Inserting the "Sandwich" under a die press where the capsules are formed and cut out.

b. *Rotary die process (Fig. 2.12)*: In this process die cavities are machined into the outer surfaces of two rollers, (i.e. die rolls).

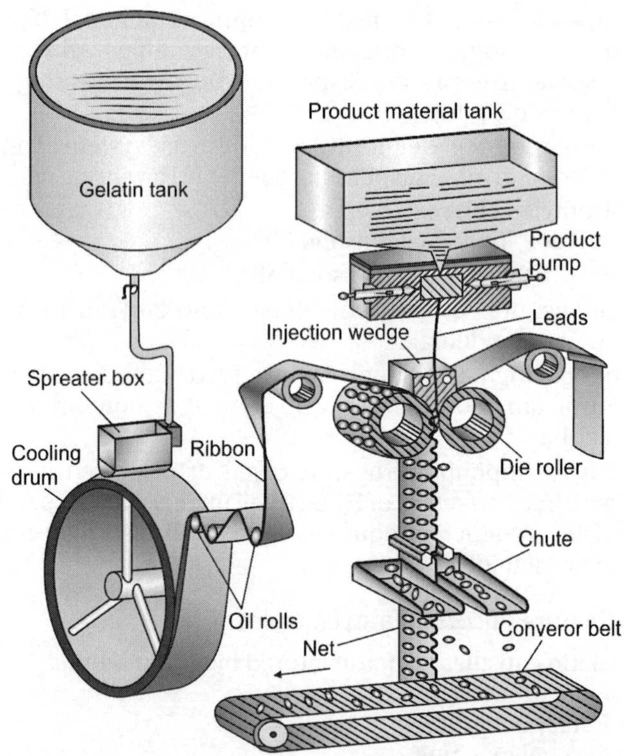


FIGURE 2.12: Schematic drawing of rotary die process

The die pockets on the left hand roller form left side of the capsule and the die pockets on the right hand roller form right side of the capsule. The die pockets on the two rollers matches as the rollers rotate. Two plasticized gelatin ribbons prepared in the machine are continuously and simultaneously fed with the liquid or paste fill between the rollers of the rotary die mechanism. The material to be capsulated flows by gravity into a positive displacement pump. The pump accurately meters the material through the lead and wedges and into the gelatin ribbons between the die rolls. The bottom of the wedge contains small orifice lined up with the die pockets of the die rolls. The capsule is about half sealed when the pressure of the pumped material forces the gelatin into the die pockets, where the capsules are simultaneously filled, shaped, hermatically sealed and cut from the gelatin ribbon. The sealing of capsule is achieved by mechanical pressure on the die rolls and the heating (37–40°C) of the ribbons by the wedges (Fig. 2.12).

From the capsulating machines, the soft, moist capsules are transferred to drying drums or the chambers for rapid drying. The extent of moisture to be removed during drying depends upon the size of the capsule, the number of capsules and the period of time over which this moisture can be removed. Typically the environment to be maintained for effective and rapid drying corresponds to forced air conditions of 20%–30% relative humidity at 21°–24°C.

The following are typical design conditions:

| Temperature | Humidity |
|---|---|
| 25°C | 15% RH |
| 20°C | 20% RH |

In order to achieve the controlled air requirement listed above, refrigeration equipment alone becomes uneconomical, impractical and cumbersome to design, operate and maintain. On the other hand, desiccant type dehumidifiers combined with refrigeration can offer a simple and economical solution to controlling both temperature and humidity levels as low as necessary.

c. ***Bubble method***: This is an alternative technology to manufacture round seamless capsules (pearls) using the physical properties of surface tension. This method of making soft capsules takes advantage of the phenomenon of drop formation. The essential part of the apparatus consists of two concentric tubes. Through the inner tube flows the medicament and through the surrounding outer tube, the gelatin solution. The medicament, therefore, issues from the tube surrounded by gelatin and forming a spherical drop. This is ensured by allowing the drop to form in liquid paraffin in which the gelatin is insoluble. Regular induced pulsations cause drops of the correct size to be formed, and a temperature of 4°C ensures that the gelatin shell is rapidly congealed. The capsules are subsequently degreased and dried.
d. ***Accogel machine***: It is a continuous process specially designed for filling of powdered dry solids into soft gelatin capsules.

## QUALITY CONTROL TESTS FOR CAPSULES

Whether capsules are produced on a small scale or large scale all of them are required to pass not only the disintegration test, weight variation test and percentage of medicament test but a visual inspection must be made as they roll off the capsule machine onto a conveyor belt regarding uniformity in shape, size, color and filling. As the capsules moves in front of the inspectors the visibly defective or suspected of being less than the perfect are picked out.

The hard and soft gelatin capsules should be subjected to following tests for their standardization.

i. Shape and size
ii. Color
iii. Thickness of capsule shell
iv. Leaking test for semisolid and liquid ingredients from soft capsules
v. Disintegration tests
vi. Weight variation test
vii. Percentage of medicament test.

*In official books the following quality control tests are recommended for capsules*:

### i. Disintegration test

For performing disintegration test on capsules the tablet disintegration test apparatus is used but the guiding disk may not be used except that the capsules float on top of the water. One capsule is placed in each tube which is then suspended in the beakers to move up and down for 30 minutes, unless otherwise stated in the monograph. The capsules pass the test if no residue of drug or other than fragments of shell remains on No. 10 mesh screen of the tubes.

### ii. Weight variation test

Twenty capsules are taken at random and weighed. Their average weight is calculated, then each capsule is weighed individually and their weight noted. The capsule passes the test if the weight of individual capsule falls within 90%–110% of the average weight. If this requirement is not met, then the weight of the contents for each individual capsule is determined and compared with the average weight of the contents. The contents from the shells can be removed just by emptying or with the help of small brush. From soft gelatin capsules the contents are removed by squeezing the shells which has been carefully cut. The remainder contents are removed by washing with a suitable solvent. After drying the shells, they are weighed and the content weights of the individual capsules are calculated. The requirements are met if (1) not more than 2 of the differences are greater than 10% of the average net content and (2) in no case the difference is greater than 25%.

### iii. Content uniformity test

This test is applicable to all capsules which are meant for oral administration. For this test a sample of the contents is assayed as described in individual monographs and the values calculated which must comply with the prescribed standards.

### iv. Dissolution test

For performing the dissolution test on capsules, the USP dissolution test apparatus is used. Dissolution test medium, volume, which apparatus is to be used, speed (RPM), time limit of the tests and assay procedeere is specified in USP/NF monographs.

### v. Capsule stability

Unprotected soft capsules (i.e. capsules that can breathe) rapidly reach equilibrium with the atmospheric conditions under which they are stored. This inherent characteristic warrants a brief discussion of the effects of temperature and humidity on these products, and points to the necessity of proper storage and packaging conditions and to the necessity of choosing an appropriate retail package. The variety of materials capsulated, which may have an effect on the gelatin shell, together with the many gelatin formulations that can be used, makes it imperative that physical standards are established for each product.

General statements relative to the effects of temperature and humidity on soft gelatin capsules must be confined to a control capsule that contains mineral oil, with a gelatin shell having a dry glycerin to dry gelatin ratio of about 0.5:1 and a water to dry gelatin ratio of 1:1, and that is dried to equilibrium with 20%–30% RH at 21–24°C, the physical stability of soft gelatin capsules is associated primarily with the pick-up or loss of water by the capsule shell. If these are prevented by proper packaging, the above control capsule should have satisfactory physical stability at temperature ranging from just above freezing to as high as 60°C, for the unprotected control capsule, low humidities (less than 20% RH), low temperature (less than 2°C) and high temperatures (greater than 38°C) or combinations of these conditions have only transient effects. The capsule returns to normal when returned to optimum storage conditions. As the humidity is increased, within a reasonable temperature range, the shell of the unprotected control capsule should pick up moisture in proportion to its glycerin and gelatin content.

The total moisture content of the capsule shell, at equilibrium with any given relative humidity within a reasonable temperature range, should closely approximate the sum of the moisture content of the glycerin and the gelatin when held separately at the stated conditions.

The effect of temperature and humidity on capsule shell has been illustrated in Table 2.4.

Capsules containing water-soluble or miscible liquid bases may be affected to a greater extent than oil-based capsules, owing to the residual moisture in the capsule content and to the dynamic relationship existing between capsule shell and capsule fill during the drying process.

**Table 2.4:** Effect of temperature and humidity on capsule shell

| *Temperature* | *Humidity* | *Effect on capsule shell* |
|---|---|---|
| 21–24°C | 60% | Capsules become softer, tackier and bloated |
| Greater than 24°C | Greater than 45% | More rapid and pronounced effects—unprotected capsules melt and fuse together |

The capsule manufacturers routinely conduct accelerated physical stability tests on all new capsule products as an integral part of the product development program. The following tests have proved adequate for determining the effect of the capsule shell content on the gelatin shell. The tests are strictly relevant to the integrity of the gelatin shell and should not be confused as stability tests for the active ingredients in the capsule content. The results of such tests are used as a guide for the reformulation of the capsule content or the capsule shell, or for the selection of the proper retail package. The test conditions for such accelerated physical stability tests are shown in Table 2.5.

**Table 2.5:** Test conditions for accelerated physical stability tests for capsule dosage forms

| *Test conditions* | *Observation* |
|---|---|
| 80% RH at room temperature in an open container | Capsules are observed periodically for 2 weeks; both gross and subtle effects of the storage conditions are noted and recorded |
| 40°C in an open container | The control capsule should not be affected |
| 40°C in a closed container (glass bottle with tight screw-cap) | Except at the 80% RH station |

The capsules at these stations are observed periodically for 2 weeks. Both gross and subtle effects of the storage conditions on the capsule shell are noted and recorded. The control capsule should not be affected except at the 80% RH station, where the capsule would react as described under the effects of high humidity.

## SPECIAL TYPES OF HARD GELATIN AND SOFT GELATIN CAPSULES

### a. Altered release

The rate of release of capsule contents can be varied according to the nature of the drug and the capsule excipients. If the drug is water-soluble and a fast release is desired, the excipients should be hydrophilic and neutral. If a slow release of water-soluble drug is desired, hydrophobic excipients will reduce the rate of drug dissolution. If the drug is insoluble in water, hydrophilic excipients will provide a faster release; hydrophobic and neutral excipients will slow its release. A very rapid release of the capsule contents can be obtained by piercing holes in the capsule to allow faster penetration by fluids in the gastrointestinal tract, or by adding a small quantity of sodium bicarbonate and citric acid to assist in opening the capsule by the evolution of carbon dioxide.

About 0.1%–1% of sodium lauryl sulfate may be added to enhance the penetration of water into the capsule and speed dissolution. If slower release of the active drug is desired, it can be mixed with various excipients, such as cellulose polymers (methylcellulose) or sodium alginate. In general, the rate of release is delayed as the proportion of polymer or alginate is increased relative to water-soluble ingredients, such as lactose. It should be mentioned that it is difficult to predict the exact release profile for a drug and to obtain consistent results from batch-to-batch. Further, reliable, consistent blood levels and duration of action can only be proved with controlled bioequivalence studies. In addition, many medications exhibit narrow therapeutic indices as the toxic and therapeutic doses are very close. Therefore, extemporaneous attempts to alter release rates to this extent should be avoided.

### b. Coating capsules

Coatings have been applied extemporaneously to enhance appearance and conceal taste, as well as to prevent release of the medication in the stomach (enteric coated products). Most coating of capsules requires considerable formulation skill and quality control equipment found in manufacturing facilities. Capsules can be coated to delay the release of the active drug until it reaches a selected portion of the gastrointestinal tract. Materials found suitable for coating of capsules include stearic acid, shellac, casein, cellulose acetate phthalate and natural and synthetic waxes; the basis of their use is their acid insolubility but alkaline solubility. Many of the newer coating materials are time: erosion-dependent rather than acid: base-dependent, i.e. they erode over time on exposure to gastrointestinal contents rather than over a pH gradient. There are, in addition, a number of newer materials with predictable pH solubility profiles.

*Enteric-coated capsules*: Enteric-coated capsules resist disintegration in the stomach but break up in the intestine. They have largely been superseded by enteric-coated tablets. Types of coating used commercially include cellulose acetate phthalate and mixtures of waxes and fatty acids and/or their esters. Enteric coating may be given to following categories of drugs—

- For substances that irritate the gastric mucosa or are destroyed by the gastric juice, and for medicaments, such as amoebicides and anthelmintics that are intended to act in the intestine.
- Which interfere with digestion, e.g. tannins, silver nitrate and other salts of heavy metals.
- Which are required to produce delayed action of the drug.

In general, the application of a coating requires skill and additional equipment. A general coating can be applied but should probably only be used in medications that would not be of a critical nature. In many cases, experience must be developed for specific formulations depending upon the requests of the physicians and the needs of the individual patients.

## PACKAGING

Capsules are normally packaged in glass or plastic containers, sometimes containing packets of a desiccant like silica gel or anhydrous calcium chloride to prevent the absorption of excessive moisture by the capsule. These type of containers have advantage over cardboard boxes that they are more convenient to handle and transport and protect the capsules from moisture and dust. Soft gel capsules should be kept at cool and dry place. Capsules can also be strip or blister packaged, which have obvious advantages.

# Chapter 3

# Microencapsulation

## INTRODUCTION

Microencapsulation is the process of applying relatively thin coatings to small particles of solids or droplets of liquids and dispersions. Microencapsulation provides the means for converting liquids to solids, for altering colloidal and surface properties, for providing environmental protection and for controlling the release characteristics or availability of coated materials. Microencapsulation is receiving considerable attention fundamentally, developmentally and commercially. The term microcapsule is defined as a spherical particle with size varying from 50 nm to 2 μm, containing a core substance. Microspheres are, in strict sense, spherical empty particles. However, the terms microcapsule and microsphere are often used synonymously. Over the last 25 years, numerous patents have been taken out by pharmaceutical companies for microencapsulated drugs.

### Dimensions

At present, there is no universally accepted size range that particles must have in order to be classified as microcapsules. However, many workers classify capsules as follows in Table 3.1:

**Table 3.1**: Types of capsules and their size range

| *Diameter* | *Type of capsule* |
|---|---|
| Less than 1 micron | Nanocapsule |
| 3–800 micron | Microcapsule |
| Larger than 1000 micron | Macrocapsule |

### Reasons for microencapsulation

i. The primary reason for microencapsulation is found to be either for sustained or prolonged drug release.
ii. This technique has been widely used for masking taste and odor of many drugs to improve patient compliance.
iii. This technique can be used for converting liquid drugs in a free-flowing powder.
iv. The drugs, which are sensitive to oxygen, moisture or light, can be stabilized by microencapsulation.
v. Incompatibility among the drugs can be prevented by microencapsulation.
vi. Vaporization of many volatile drugs, e.g. methyl salicylate and peppermint oil can be prevented by microencapsulation.
vii. Many drugs have been microencapsulated to reduce toxicity and GI irritation including ferrous sulfate and potassium chloride.
viii. Alteration in site of absorption can also be achieved by microencapsulation.
ix. Toxic chemicals such as insecticides may be microencapsulated to reduce the possibility of sensitization of factorial person.

Microencapsulation process involves the basic understanding of the general properties of microcapsules such as the nature of core and coating materials, the stability and release characteristics of the coated materials and the microencapsulation methods.

## CORE MATERIAL

The core material is the material over which coating has to be applied to serve the specific purpose. Core material may be in form of solids or droplets of liquids and dispersions. The composition of core material can vary and thus furnish definite flexibility and allow effectual design and development of the desired microcapsule properties. A substance may be microencapsulated for a number of reasons. Examples may include protection of reactive material from their environment, safe and convenient handling of the materials which are otherwise toxic or noxious, taste masking, means for controlled or modified release properties means of handling liquids as solids, preparation of free flow powders and in modification of physical properties of the drug.

### Liquid core materials

Perfumes, solvents, vegetable oils, pesticides, dyes, catalysts, bleaches, cosmetics, insecticides, sugars, salts, acids, pigments, fungicides, nutrients.

### Solid core materials

Dextrins, bases, herbicides, pharmaceuticals, biocides, minerals.

## COATING MATERIAL

A wide variety of coating materials are available for microencapsulation. However, many traditional coating materials are satisfactory for the use in the gastrointestinal tract. They include inert polymers such as ethyl cellulose and pH sensitive ones, such as carboxylate and amino derivatives, which swell or dissolve according to the degree of cross-linking. Depending upon the method of microencapsulation employed and properties of final product needed, coatings solution may contain different additive such as film formers, plasticizers and fillers and may be applied through different solvent system.

### Ideal characteristics of coating material

1. It should be capable of forming a film that is cohesive with the core material.
2. It should be chemically compatible and nonreactive with the core material.
3. It should provide desired coating properties such as strength, flexibility, impermeability, optical properties and stability.
   *Examples of coating materials*:
   a. Water-soluble resins—Gelatin, gum arabic, starch, methyl cellulose, hydroxylpropyl methylcellulose (HPMC), PVP and polyvinyl acetate.
   b. Water-insoluble resins—Ethyl cellulose, polyethylene, cellulose nitrate and silicones.
   c. Waxes and lipids—Paraffin, carnauba wax, beeswax, stearic acid and stearyl alcohol.
   d. Enteric resins—Shellac, cellulose acetate phthalate, zein, etc.

## TECHNIQUES OF MICROENCAPSULATION

Various processes that have been adopted for preparing microcapsules include:

1. Air suspension process
2. Coacervation—Phase separation process
3. Pan coating
4. Solvent evaporation
5. Spray drying and spray congealing
6. Interfacial polymerization
7. Multiorifice centrifugal process.

### 1. Air suspension process

Air suspension process is also known as Wurster process. It consists of dispersing of solid, particulate core materials in a supporting air stream and the spray coating of the air suspended

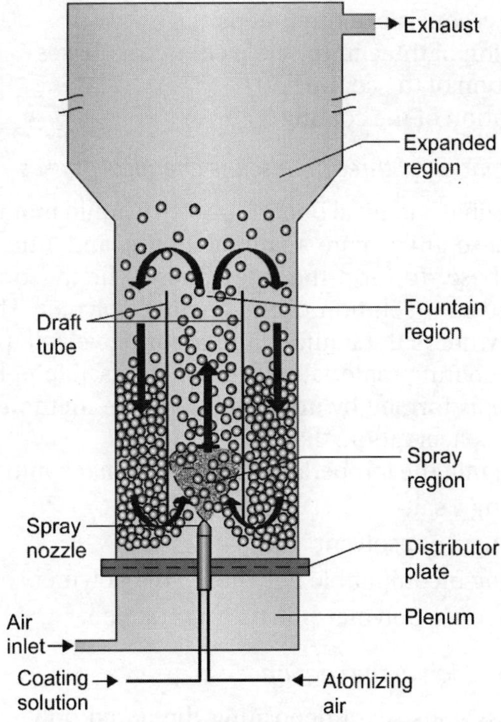


FIGURE 3.1: Air suspension coater

particles. Within the coating chamber, particles are suspended on an upward moving air stream. Particles are recirculated through coating zone portion of the chamber, where coating material, usually a polymer solution is spray applied to the moving particles. During each pass through the coating zone, the core material receives an increment of coating material (Fig. 3.1).

The cyclic process is repeated several hundred times during processing, depending on the purpose of microencapsulation and the coating thickness desired or whether the core material particles are thoroughly encapsulated. The supporting air stream also serves to dry the product while it is being encapsulated. Drying rates are directly related to the volume temperature of the supporting air stream. This process is applicable only for the encapsulation of solid core material.

### 2. Coacervation—Phase separation process

This process consists of three steps:

a. Formation of three immiscible chemical phases
b. Deposition of the coating
c. Rigidization of the coating

#### *Step I: Formation of three immiscible chemical phases*

The immiscible chemical phases are—(i) a liquid manufacturing vehicle phase (ii) a core material phase and (iii) a coating material phase. To form the three phases, firstly core material is dispersed in a solution of the coating polymer. The solvent for the polymer is the liquid manufacturing vehicle phase (Fig. 3.2A). The coating material phase, an immiscible polymer in a liquid state, is formed by utilizing one of the methods of phase separation coacervation, that is:

- By changing the temperature of the polymer solution
- By adding a salt
- By adding a nonsolvent
- By adding incompatible polymer to the polymer solution
- By inducing a polymer-polymer interaction.

#### *Step II: Deposition of the coating*

This process consists of depositing the liquid polymer coating upon the core material. This is accomplished by controlled physical mixing of the coating material and the core material in the manufacturing vehicle. Deposition of the liquid polymer coating around the core material occours if the polymer is adsorbed at the interface formed between the core material and the liquid vehicle phase. This adsorption phenomenon results in effective coating (Fig. 3.2B).

*Step III: Rigidization of the coating*

Rigidization of coating is done by thermal, cross-linking or desolvation techniques to form self-sustaining microcapsules (Fig. 3.2C).

Coacervation—Phase separation process applicable for solids and liquids.

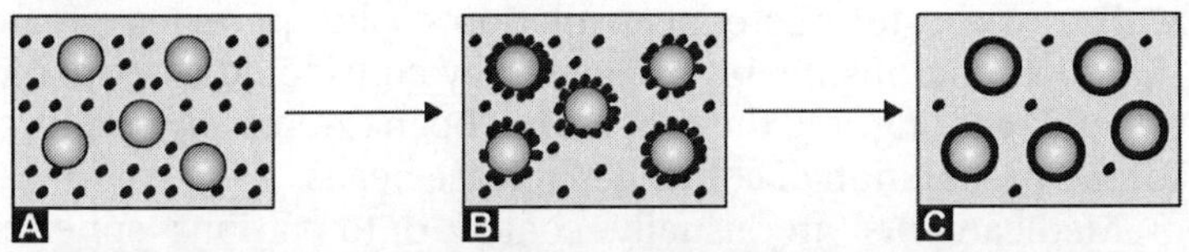


FIGURE 3.2A to C: Coacervation–Phase separation process (a) Formation of three immiscible chemical phases, (b) Deposition of the coating, and (c) Rigidization of the coating

## Methods for phase—Separation

i. **Temperature change**: It involves the change in temperature, which results in separation of phases. With decrease in temperature, one phase become polymer poor (microencapsulation vehicle phase) and second phase (coating material phase) become polymer rich. Phase separation of the dissolved polymer occurs in the form of immiscible droplets.

   Under proper polymer concentration, temperature and agitation condition, liquid polymer droplets coalesce around the dispersed core material particle, this result in formation of embryonic microcapsule.

ii. **Incompatible polymer addition**: Liquid phase separation of a polymeric coating material and microencapsulation can be accomplished by utilizing the incompatibility of dissimilar polymer existing in a common solvent.

iii. **Nonsolvent addition**: This method involves the addition of a liquid that is a nonsolvent for a given polymer to a solution of the polymer, to induce phase separation.

iv. **Salt addition**: It involves the addition of soluble inorganic salts to aqueous solution of certain water-soluble polymers to cause phase separation.

v. **Polymer-polymer interaction**: It involves the interaction of oppositively charged polyelectrolyte, which results in formation of a complex having such reduced solubility that causes phase separation.

## 3. Pan coating

The pan coating process, widely used in the pharmaceutical industry, is among the oldest industrial procedures for forming small, coated particles or tablets. The particles are tumbled in a pan or other device while the coating material is applied slowly with respect to microencapsulation, solid particles greater than 600 microns in size are generally considered essential for effective coating, and the process has been extensively employed for the preparation of controlled release beads.

Medicaments are usually coated onto various spherical substrates such as nonpareil sugar seeds, and then coated with protective layers of various polymers. In practice, the coating is applied as a solution, or as an atomized spray, to the desired solid core material in the coating pans. Usually, to remove the coating solvent, warm air is passed over the coated materials as the coatings are being applied in the coating pans. In some cases, final solvent removal is accomplished in a drying oven (Fig. 3.3).

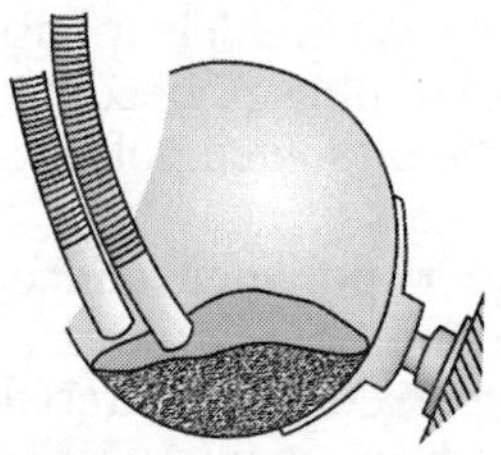

FIGURE 3.3: Pan coating

## 4. Solvent evaporation

Solvent evaporation techniques are carried out in a liquid manufacturing vehicle (O/W emulsion) which is prepared by agitation of two immiscible liquids. The process involves dissolving microcapsule coating (polymer) in a volatile solvent which is immiscible with the liquid manufacturing vehicle phase. A core material (drug) to be microencapsulated is dissolved or dispersed in the coating polymer solution. With agitation, the core-coating material mixture is dispersed in the liquid manufacturing vehicle phase to obtain appropriate size microcapsules. Agitation of system is continued until the solvent partitions into the aqueous phase and is removed by evaporation (Fig. 3.4). This process results in hardened microspheres which contain the active moiety. Several methods can be used to achieve dispersion of the oil phase in the continuous phase. The most common method is the use of a propeller style blade attached to a variable speed motor.

Various process variables include methods of forming dispersions, evaporation rate of the solvent for the coating polymer, temperature cycles and agitation rates. Important factors that must be considered when preparing microcapsules by solvent evaporation techniques include choice of vehicle phase and solvent for the polymer coating, as these choices greatly influence microcapsule properties as well as the choice of solvent recovery techniques.

The solvent evaporation technique to produce microcapsules is applicable to a wide variety of liquid and solid core materials. The core materials may be either water-soluble or water-insoluble materials. A variety of film forming polymers can be used as coatings.

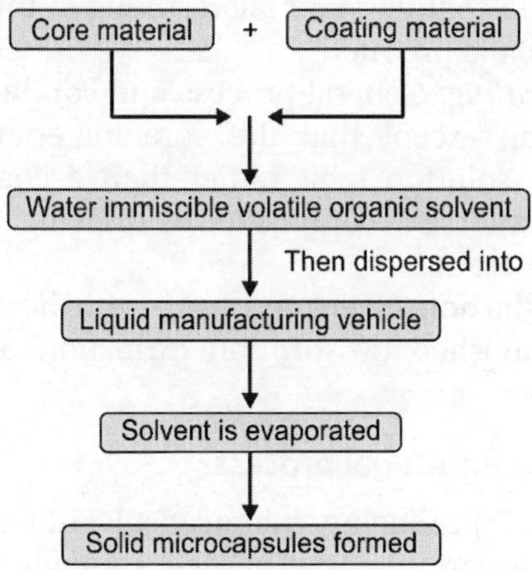


FIGURE 3.4: Solvent evaporation process

### 5. Interfacial polymerization

This process involves the dispersion of organic phase containing core material into the liquid manufacturing vehicle containing monomers, whereby the monomers react at a liquid-liquid interface to form a coating. A cross- linking agent may be added to the continuous phase to effect polymerization at interface. This method is suitable for low melting point solids or poorly soluble organic liquids.

### 6. Spray drying and spray congealing

Spray drying and spray congealing methods have been used for many years as microencapsulation techniques. Because of certain similarities of the two processes, they are discussed together. Spray drying and spray congealing processes are similar, both involves the dispersion of core material in a liquefied coating substance and spraying or introducing the core-coating mixture into some environmental condition, whereby relatively rapid solidification of the coating is affected. Both processes are applicable for encapsulation of solids and liquids.

*Spray drying (Fig. 3.5)*: This method involves the dispersion of core material into coating solution (core material must be insoluble in coating solution), then spraying the mixture as atomized spray into air stream. The air is usually heated, which provides the latent heat of vaporization required to remove the solvent from the coating material, resulting in the formation of microencapsulated product.

*Spray congealing*: General process and conditions are same as spray drying except that the core material is dispersed into a coating solution melt rather than a coating solution. Microencapsulation is accomplished by spraying the hot mixture into a cool air stream.

Removal of the nonsolvent or solvent from the coated product is then accomplished by sorption extraction or evaporation techniques.

### 7. Multiorifice centrifugal process

This method of producing microcapsule utilizes centrifugal forces to hurl a core material particle through an enveloping microencapsulation membrane, which result in formation of

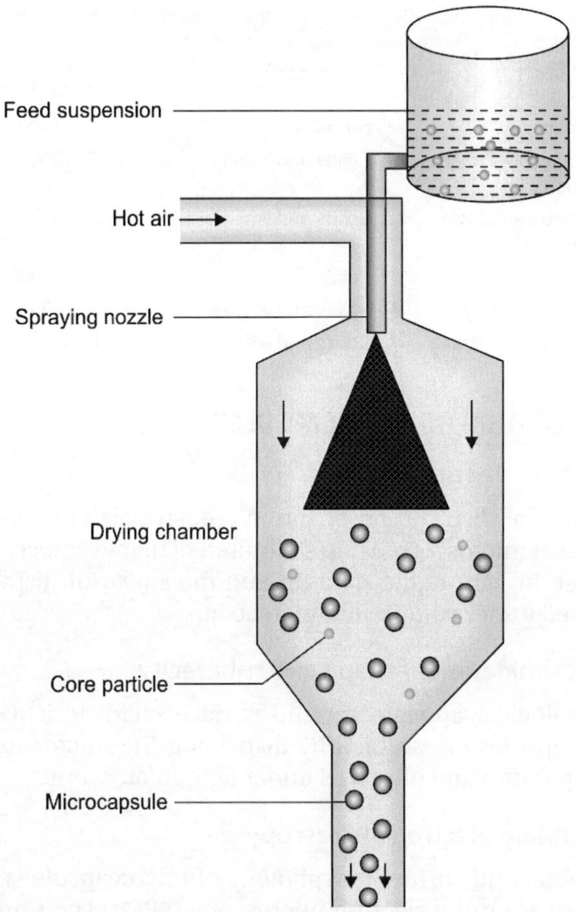


FIGURE 3.5: Schematic diagram of a spray dryer

microcapsules. Processing variables include the rotational speed of the cylinder, the flow rate of the core and coating materials, the concentration and viscosity and surface tension of the core material. The multiorifice centrifugal process is capable for microencapsulating liquids and solids of varied size ranges, with diverse coating materials. The encapsulated product can be supplied as slurry in the hardening media or as a dry powder. Production rates of 50–75 pounds per hour have been achieved with the process.

**Table 3.2:** Microencapsulation processes and their applicability

| *Microencapsulation process* | *Applicable core material* | *Approximate particle size (μm)* |
|---|---|---|
| Air suspension | Solids | 35–5000 |
| Coacervation—Phase separation | Solids and liquids | 2–5000 |
| Multiorifice centrifugal process | Solids and liquids | 1–5000 |
| Pan coating | Solids | 600–5000 |
| Solvent evaporation | Solids and liquids | 5–5000 |
| Spray drying and spray congealing | Solids and liquids | 600 |

## EVALUATION OF MICROCAPSULES

### 1. Particle size analysis

Particle size distribution of the microcapsules are determined by optical microscopy using calibrated ocular eyepiece. Product disperse in light liquid paraffin and the smear of dispersion is observed under compound microscope.

### 2. Determination of shape and spherecity

Morphological appearance and surface characteristics of the microcapsules are studied by dispersing the microcapsules in liquid paraffin and observed under light microscope.

### 3. Scanning electron microscopy

The shape and surface morphology of microcapsule is studied by using scanning electron microscopy (SEM). The samples for SEM study is prepared by lightly sprinkling the microcapsules on a double-adhesive tape stuck to an aluminum stub. The stubs are then coated with gold to a thickness of ~300 Å under an argon atmosphere using a gold sputter module in a high-vacuum evaporator. The coated samples are then randomly scanned and photomicrographs are taken with a scanning electron microscope.

### 4. Percentage yield

Percentage practical yield is calculated to know about percentage yield or efficiency of any method, thus it helps in selection of appropriate method of production. Practical yield is calculated as the weight of microcapsules recovered from each batch in relation to the sum of starting material. The percentage yield of prepared microcapsules is determined by using the formula.

$$\text{Percentage yield} = \frac{\text{Total wt. of microcapsules}}{\text{Total wt. of drug and polymer}} \times 100$$

## 5. Drug entrapment efficiency

The amount of drug present in the microcapsule is determined by extracting the drug into solvent under magnetic stirring for a period of approximately 2 hours. The solution is filtered through filter paper. Sample is suitably diluted and estimated for drug content spectrophotometrically.

The incorporation efficiency was calculated by the following formula:

$$\text{Drug entrapment efficiency(\%)} = \frac{\text{Experimental drug content (mg)}}{\text{Theoretical drug content (mg)}} \times 100$$

Theoretical drug content was determined by calculation assuming that the entire drug present in the polymer solution used gets entrapped in microcapsules and no loss occurs at any stage of preparation of microcapsules.

## 6. Flow properties of microcapsules

Flowability of microcapsules is investigated by determining angle of repose, bulk density, tapped density, Carr's index and Hausner's ratio. The angle of repose is determined by fixed funnel method. The microcapsules are tapped using bulk density apparatus for 1000 taps in a cylinder and the change in volume is measured. Carr's index and Hausner's ratio are calculated by the formula,

Carr's index = (Tapped density – Bulk density/Tapped density) × 100

Hausner's ratio = Tapped density/Bulk density

## 7. Determination of swelling properties

Microcapsules of known weight are placed in dissolution media for 6 hours and the swollen microcapsules are collected by the centrifugation. The net weight of the swollen microcapsules was determined by first blotting the particles with filter paper to remove absorbed water on surface and then weighing immediately on an electronic balance. The percentage of swelling of microcapsules in the dissolution media is then calculated by using equation,

$$Sw = [(Wt - Wo)/Wo] \times 100,$$

Where, Sw = Percentage of swelling of microcapsules,
Wt = Weight of the microcapsules at time t,
Wo = Initial weight of the microcapsules.

### 8. In vitro drug release study

In vitro drug release study is carried out in USP type I (Basket type) dissolution apparatus. Microcapsules are placed in the basket and immersed in the dissolution medium maintained at 37 ± 5°C and stirred for specified period. Samples are withdrawn from the dissolution medium at various time intervals using a pipette fitted with a microfilter (0.45-μm). The rate of drug release is analyzed using UV spectrophotometer.

# Chapter 4

# Parenteral Products

## INTRODUCTION

Parenteral (Gk, para—beside and enteron—the intestine) dosage forms differ from all other drug dosage forms, because they are injected directly into body tissue through the primary protective systems of the human body, the skin, and mucous membranes. They must be exceptionally pure and free from physical, chemical and biological contaminants. These requirements place a heavy responsibility on the pharmaceutical industry to practice current good manufacturing practices (cGMPs) in the manufacture of parenteral dosage forms and on pharmacists and other health care professionals to practice good aseptic practices (GAPs) in dispensing parenteral dosage forms for administration to patients.

Certain pharmaceutical agents, particularly peptides, proteins and many chemotherapeutic agents, can only be given parenterally, because they are inactivated in the gastrointestinal tract when given by mouth. Parenterally administered drugs are relatively unstable and generally highly potent drugs that require strict control of administration to the patient. Due to the advent of biotechnology, parenteral products have grown in number and usage around the world.

### Advantages

1. Parenterals are unique among dosage forms of drugs because they are injected through the skin or mucous membranes into internal body compartments. Parenterals are useful for patients who cannot take drug orally and in emergency situation.

2. Drugs may be injected into the specialized area of the body, including joints (intra-articular), joint fluid area (intrasynovial), spinal column (intraspinal), spinal fluid (intrathecal), arteries (intra-arterial) and in emergency, even the heart (intracardiac).
3. Parenterals possess better and faster onset of action and bioavailability than other dosage forms (solid and liquid orals, etc.). Biologic products viz peptide hormones, vaccines, toxoids and antitoxins are best suited for parenteral route of administration.
4. Useful for delivering fluids, electrolytes or nutrients (total parenteral nutrition) to patients.
5. Useful for drugs that are inactivated in the GIT or susceptible first pass metabolism by liver.
6. Parenteral products could be administered as sterile solution during an irrigation procedure as these solutions can enter the blood stream directly through open blood vessels of wounds or abraded mucous membranes.
7. Sterile parenteral products could be administered even as solid pellets/tablets for tissue implantation and useful for providing sustained drug delivery (depot injection).
8. Parenterals as a dosage form scores better over other conventional dosage forms (solid/liquid orals) for administration of special categories of drugs like anticancer agents, immunosuppressants, hormones and peptides, radiopaque and diagnostic agents, etc.

### Disadvantages

1. More expensive and costly to produce as compared to other formulations.
2. Potential for infection at the site of injection, thrombophlebitis, extravasation, fluid overload and air embolism.
3. Risk of needle stick injuries and exposure to blood borne pathogens by health care workers.
4. Disposal of needles, syringes and other infusion devices requires special consideration.
5. Improper injection procedures could cause damage to the patient's nerves, tissue, veins and other blood vessels.
6. The presence of traces of physical/chemical contaminants cause irritation to body tissues and also leads to degradation

of product due to chemical change when thermal sterilization is employed.

Example: Minute traces of copper increases the rate of oxidation of ascorbic acid in solution. The contamination arises from water or chemical components or even the container.

## Routes of administration

*Intravenous route (IV)* – IV injection of drugs provide rapid action compared with other routes of administration and because drug absorption is not a factor, optimum blood levels may be achieved with accuracy which is not possible by other routes.

In emergencies, IV administration of a drug may be life-saving because of placement of drug directly into the circulation and on the negative side, once a drug is administered intravenously, it cannot be retrieved.

Both small and large volumes of drug solutions may be administered intravenously. IV drugs must be in aqueous solution, they must mix with the circulating blood and not precipitate from solution.

*Intramuscular route (IM)*—IM injections of drugs provide effects that are less rapid but generally longer lasting than those obtained from IV administration. Aqueous or oleaginous solutions or suspensions of drug substances may be administered intramuscularly. IM injections are performed deep into skeletal muscles.

*Subcutaneous route (SC)*—This route may be used for injection of small amounts of medication. Injection of a drug beneath the skin is usually made in the loose interstitial tissue of the outer upper arm, the anterior thigh, or the lower abdomen. Prior to injection, the skin at injection site should be thoroughly cleansed. Irrigating drugs and those in thick suspension may produce induration, sloughing or abscess and may be painful. Such preparations are not suitable for SC injections.

*Intradermal route*—A number of substances may be effectively injected into the corium, the more vascular layer of skin just beneath the epidermis. These substances includes various agents for diagnostic detections, desensitization or immunization. The usual site for intradermal injection is the anterior forearm.

## FORMULATION REQUIREMENTS

Parenteral drugs are formulated as solutions, suspensions, emulsions and powders to be reconstituted as solutions. In general, there are two important aspects concerned with the development of these formulations:

- Vehicles and solvents for parenteral products
- Solutes.

### 1. Vehicles and solvents for parenteral products

The vehicle refers to a carrier or inert medium invariably being employed as a solvent (or diluents) in which a medicinally active ingredient is formulated and/or administered.

Some vehicles which are official in USP as follows:

- Aqueous vehicles
- Aqueous isotonic vehicles
- Nonaqueous vehicles.

#### *a. Aqueous vehicles*

Most commonly used vehicle for parenteral products is water, as it is the vehicle for all natural body fluids.

Types of water used in parenteral products:

- Water for injection, USP
  - Most frequently used for parenteral formulation.
  - Purified water underwent distillation or reverse osmosis.
  - Total dissolved solids not more than 1mg in 100 ml.
  - No added substances.
  - May not sterile.
  - Pyrogen free.
  - Used for manufacture of parenteral products to be sterilized after preparation.
  - Must store in tight container at suitable temperature.
  - Must be used within 24 hours.
  - Collected in sterile and pyrogen free container (glass or glass lined).
- Sterile water for injection
  - Water for injection which has been sterilized and packed in container of 1 L or less.

– Pyrogen free.
– No antimicrobial preservation or added substances.
– Due to sterilization may contain slightly more solid content.
– Intended to be used to reconstitute sterile solids and dilute sterile solution.
– Must be added ascetically.

- Bacteriostatic water for injection
  – Sterile water for injection with suitable antimicrobial agent(s).
  – Filled in vials/syringe in volume not more than 30 ml.
  – Name and concentration of preservative must be stated.
  – Intended for small volume injectables (multidose vials).
  – Not to be used with large volume parenterals (usually with 5 ml or less).
- Sterile water for irrigation USP
  – Available as sterilized and packaged in a single dose container.
  – No added substances.
  – Packaged in container 1 L or larger.
  – Not intended for parenteral uses.
  – Labeled as "For Irrigation Only".

*b. Aqueous isotonic vehicles*

Isotonic relates to a solution which essentially has the same number of dissolved particles as the body fluids (e.g. blood, nasal secretions, tears). In general, the aqueous isotonic vehicles are employed quite often in parenteral products particularly.

Few typical examples are as follows:

- Sodium chloride injection, USP
  – Sterile, isotonic solution of sodium chloride in water for injection.
  – No antimicrobial agent.
  – Used as vehicle in preparing solutions/suspension for parenteral administration.
- Bacteriostatic sodium chloride injection, USP
  – Sterile, isotonic solution of sodium chloride in water for injection.

  - Contain one or more antimicrobial agents (specify in label).
  - Volume not more than 30 ml (5 ml preferred).
- Miscellaneous
- Ringer's injection
  - Sterile solution of sodium chloride, potassium chloride and calcium chloride in water for injection.
  - Concentration as physiological concentrations.
  - Can be used as vehicle or electrolyte replenisher or fluid extender.
- Lactate Ringer's injection, USP
  - Sterile solution of sodium chloride, potassium chloride, calcium chloride and sodium lactate.
  - Intended to be used as fluid and electrolyte replenisher and systematic alkalyzer.

*c. Nonaqueous vehicles*

In formulation of sterile products, it is sometimes necessary to eliminate water entirely or in part from the vehicle, primarily because of solubility factors or hydrolytic reactions.

Nonaqueous solvents selected with great care:

- Must be nontoxic.
- Must be nonirritant.
- Must be nonsensitizing.
- Must not exert an adverse effect on ingredients of the formulation.

So that solvents are evaluated for its physical properties such as density, viscosity, miscibility, polarity, stability, solvent activity and toxicity.

i. **Solvents that are miscible with water and that are usually used in combination with water as vehicle**—Dioxalanes, butylenes glycol, polyethylene glycol 400 and 600, dimethylacetamide, propylene glycol, glycerine and ethyl alcohol.
ii. **Water immiscible solvents**—They include fixed oils (corn oil, cottonseed oil, peanut oil, and sesame oil), ethyl oleate, isopropyl myristate and benzyl benzoate.

Fixed oils are used as vehicles for certain hormone (e.g. progesterone, testosterone, deoxycorticosterone) and vitamin (e.g. Vitamin K, Vitamin E) preparations. The label of these preparations must state the name of the vehicle, so the user may beware in case of known sensitivity or other reactions to it.

## 2. Solutes

Solute represents a substance which is dissolved by a solvent. In other words, the solute designate the chemicals dissolved in vehicles, which must be best quality, because the presence of even small traces of contaminants may be detrimental to products. Obviously the solute may be the active ingredients (or drugs) which exerts a therapeutic effect.

**Added substances or excipients**: Apart from active ingredients, added substances are also added in the product (Table 4.1). They are added to enhance stability of the product. Such substances include:

- Buffers
- Tonicity contributors
- Antimicrobial agents
- Antioxidants
- Wetting, suspending and emulsifying agents
- Solublizers
- Stabilizers.

*Desired characteristics*

- It must be nontoxic in the quantity administered to the patients.
- They should not interfere with the therapeutic efficacy nor with the assay of the active therapeutic compound.
  a. **Buffers**: Buffers are added to maintain required pH of the product. Ideal pH for parenteral product is 7.4, the pH of blood. Extreme deviation can cause complications. Above pH 9, tissue necrosis often occur. If pH below 3, then extreme pain is experienced at the site of injection. Thus, the acceptable pH range is 3–10.5. For IV preparation pH is wider (pH 4–9) than the acceptable range for others. Buffers should not be used in intracardiac and intraocular injections. Acetate, phosphate, citrate and glutamate are most commonly used buffers.
  b. **Tonicity contributors**: These are the compounds contributing to the isotonicity of a product and reduces the pain of injection in the area with nerve endings. Injections

should be made isotonic with blood by the addition of sodium chloride or dextrose. Buffers also acts as tonicity contributors.

c. **Antimicrobial agents**: Antimicrobial agents are included in multidose packaging, to prevent multiplication of any accidently introduced microbes in the products during the withdrawal of dosages. Some commonly used antimicrobial agents are: Benzyl alcohol, benzalkonium chloride, methylparaben, propylparaben, thiomersal, phenylmercuric nitrate.
d. **Antioxidants**: Antioxidants are included in formulation to protect therapeutic agents susceptible to oxidation, particularly under the accelerated conditions of thermal sterilization. Antioxidants acts by various ways, on the basis they are classified as:
   i. *Reducing agents*: These agents preferentially oxidized and gradually used up.
   *For example*: Ascorbic acid, sodium bisulfate, sodium metabisulfite, thiourea.
   ii. *Blocking agents*: They block oxidative chain reaction in which they are not usually consumed.
   *For example*: Ascorbic acid esters, BHT, tocopherol.
   iii. *Synergistic agents*: These compounds acts as synergists. They increases the effectiveness of antioxidants those block oxidative reactions.
   *For examples*: Ascorbic acid, citric acid, tartaric acid, phosphoric acid.
   iv. *Chelating agents*: These compounds forms complex with catalysts that otherwise accelerate the oxidative reaction.
   *For example*: EDTA salts.
e. **Wetting agents**: Wetting agent used in preparation of parenteral suspension to maintain particle size and to counteract caking. For examples: Tween 80, sorbitan trioleate.
f. **Suspending agents**: The improper formulation of suspension not only affects the dose uniformity but determines syringeability and injectability. The sedimentation of insoluble drugs makes it difficult to take accurate dose in the syringe (syringeability) and to inject in even row without clogging under given

pressure (injectability). Sodium carboxymethylcellulose, methylcellulose, acacia, gelatin, polyvinylprollidone (PVP) may be used to prevent sedimentation of suspended particles.

g. **Emulsifying agents**: Emulsifying agents are used to prevent coalescence of dispersed globules and hence stabilizes the parenteral emulsion. For example: Lecithin.

h. **Stabilizers**: Drug in the solution form liable to undergo degradation through oxidation and hydrolysis. stabilizers are added to ensure the stability of drug compound in the preparation. For examples: Glycine, creatinine, sodium saccharin, sodium caprylate.

   i. *Solubilizing agents*: To enhance the solubility of drugs, parenteral formulation contains cosolvents such as alcohol, polyethylene glycol (PEG), nonionic surfactants. They are used to solubilize drugs such as vitamins, hormones and volatile oils.

**Table 4.1**: Common excipients used in parenterals

| *Excipients* | *Concentration range (%)* |
|---|---|
| Antimicrobial preservatives | |
| a. Benzyl alcohol | 0.5–10.0 |
| b. Phenylmercuric nitrate | 0.001 |
| c. Thimerosal | 0.001–0.02 |
| d. Propylparaben | 0.005–0.035 |
| Solubilizers, wetting agents/emulsifiers | |
| a. Dimethylacetamide | 0.01 |
| b. Ethanol | 0.61–49.0 |
| c. Glycerol | 14.6–25.0 |
| d. PEG 300 | 0.01–50.0 |
| Buffers | |
| a. Acetic acid | 0.22 |
| b. Citric acid | 0.5 |
| c. Maleic acid | 1.6 |
| d. Lactic acid | 0.1 |
| Tonicity modifiers | |
| a. Lactose | 0.14–5.0 |
| b. Mannitol | 0.4–2.5 |
| c. Sorbitol | 2.0 |
| d. NaCl | varies |

*Contd...*

*Contd...*

| *Excipients* | *Concentration range (%)* |
|---|---|
| Suspending agents | |
| a. Gelatin | 2.0 |
| b. Pectin | 0.2 |
| c. PEG 4000 | 2.7–3.0 |
| Antioxidants | |
| a. Ascorbic acid | 0.02–0.1 |
| b. Thiourea | 0.005 |
| c. BHT | 0.005–0.002 |
| Stabilizers | |
| a. Niacin | 1.25–2.5 |
| b. Sodium caprylate | 0.4 |
| c. Glycine | 1.5–2.25 |

## GENERAL MANUFACTURING PROCESS

The preparation of a parenteral product may encompass four general areas:

1. Procurement and accumulation of all components in a warehouse area, until released to manufacturing.
2. Processing the dosage form in appropriately designed and operated facilities.
3. Packaging and labeling in a quarantine area, to ensure integrity and completion of the product.
4. Controlling the quality of the product throughout the process.

Procurement encompasses selecting and testing according to specifications of the raw-material ingredients and the containers and closures for the primary and secondary packages. Microbiological purity, in the form of bioburden and endotoxin levels, has become standard requirements for raw materials.

Processing includes cleaning containers and equipment to validated specifications, compounding the solution (or other dosage form), filtering the solution, sanitizing or sterilizing the containers and equipment, filling measured quantities of product into the sterile containers, stoppering (either completely or partially for products to be freeze-dried), freeze-drying, terminal sterilization (if possible), and final sealing of the final primary container.

Packaging normally consists of the labeling and cartoning of filled and sealed primary containers. Control of quality begins with the incoming supplies, being sure that specifications are met. Careful control of labels is vitally important, as errors in labeling can be dangerous for the consumer. Each step of the process involves checks and tests to ensure the required specifications at the respective step are being met. Labeling and final packaging operations are becoming more automated.

The quality control unit is responsible for reviewing the batch history and performing the release testing required to clear the product for shipment to users. A common FDA citation for potential violation of cGMP is the lack of oversight by the quality control unit in batch testing and review and approval of results.

## Components

The components of parenteral products include the active ingredient, formulation additives, vehicle(s) and primary container and closure. Establishing specifications to ensure the quality of each of these components of an injection is essential. Secondary packaging is relevant more to marketing considerations, although some drug products might rely on secondary packaging for stability considerations, such as added protection from light exposure for light-sensitive drugs and antimicrobial preservatives.

The most stringent chemical-purity requirements will normally be encountered with aqueous solutions, particularly if the product is sterilized at an elevated temperature where reaction rates will be accelerated greatly. Dry preparations pose relatively few reaction problems but may require definitive physical specifications for ingredients that must have certain solution or dispersion characteristics when a vehicle is added.

Containers and closures are in prolonged, intimate contact with the product and may release substances into, or remove ingredients from, the product. Rubber closures are specially problematic (sorption, leachables, air and moisture transmission properties), if not properly evaluated for compatibility with the final product. Assessment and selection of containers and closures are essential for final product formulation, to ensure the product retains its purity, potency and quality during the intimate contact with the container throughout its shelf life.

Administration devices (e.g. syringes, tubing, transfer sets) that come in contact with the product should be assessed and selected with the same care as are containers and closures, even though the contact period is usually brief.

### *1. Water for injection (WFI) preparation*

The source water can be expected to be contaminated with natural suspended mineral and organic substances, dissolved mineral salts, colloidal material, viable bacteria, bacterial endotoxins, industrial or agricultural chemicals, and other particulate matter. The degree of contamination varies with the source and will be markedly different, whether obtained from a well or from surface sources, such as a stream or lake. Hence, the source water must be pretreated by one or a combination of the following treatments: chemical softening, filtration, deionization, carbon adsorption, or reverse osmosis purification.

Water for injection can be prepared by distillation or by membrane technologies (i.e. reverse osmosis or ultrafiltration). The EP (EUROPEAN PHARMACOPEIA) only permits distillation as the process for producing WFI. The USP and JP (JAPANESE PHARMACOPEIA) allow all these technologies to be applied.

i. **Distillation**: Distillation is a process of converting water from a liquid to its gaseous form (steam). Since steam is pure gaseous water, all other contaminants in the feed water are removed. A conventional still consists of a boiler (evaporator), containing feed water (distilland); a source of heat to vaporize the water in the evaporator; a headspace above the level of distilland, with condensing surfaces for refluxing the vapor, thereby returning nonvolatile impurities to the distilland; a means for eliminating volatile impurities (demister/separation device) before the hot water vapor is condensed; and a condenser for removing the heat of vaporization, thereby converting the water vapor to a liquid distillate.
ii. **Reverse osmosis (RO)**: As the name suggests, the natural process of selective permeation of molecules through a semipermeable membrane separating two aqueous solutions of different concentrations is reversed. Pressure, usually between 200 and 400 psig, is applied to overcome osmotic pressure and force pure water to permeate

through the membrane. Membranes, usually composed of cellulose esters or polyamides, are selected to provide an efficient rejection of contaminant molecules in raw water. The molecules most difficult to remove are small inorganic molecules, such as sodium chloride. Passage through two membranes in series is, sometimes, used to increase the efficiency of removal of these small molecules and decrease the risk of structural failure of a membrane to remove other contaminants, such as bacteria and pyrogens.

Several WFI installations utilize both RO and distillation systems for generation of the highest quality water. Since feed water to distillation units can be heavily contaminated and, thus, affect the operation of the still, water is first run through RO units to eliminate contaminants.

### Pyrogens (endotoxins)

Water and packaging materials are the greatest sources of pyrogens (pyrogenic contamination). Pyrogens are the metabolic products of micro-organisms. Bacteria, molds and viruses produce pyrogens. Chemically, pyrogens are lipid substances associated with carrier molecules which are usually a polysaccharide but may be a peptide (lipopolysaccharides). Pyrogens are water soluble and nonvolatile.

Gram-negative bacteria (e.g. *Pseudomonas* sp, *Salmonella* sp, *Escherichia coli*) produces most potent pyrogenic substance "Endotoxin". Gram-positive bacteria and fungi also produce pyrogens but of lower potency and of different chemical nature. Endotoxins are lipopolysaccharides that exist in high molecular weight aggregate forms. The lipid portion of the molecule is responsible for the biological activity.

*Pyrogenic reactions*: Pyrogens, when present in parenteral drug products and injected into patients, 1 hour after injection pyrogens produces a marked rise in body temperature, chill, body aches, cutaneous vasoconstriction and rise in arterial blood pressure. Although pyrogenic reactions are rarely fatal, they can cause serious discomfort and, in the seriously ill-patient, shock-like symptoms that can be fatal.

When bacterial (exogenous) pyrogens are introduced into the body, lipopolysaccharides targets circulating mononuclear cells (monocytes and macrophages) that, in turn, produce proinflammatory cytokines, such as interleukin 2, interleukin 6, and tissue necrosis factor. Besides lipopolysaccharides, gram-negative bacteria also release many peptides (e.g. exotoxin A, peptidoglycan and muramyl peptides) that can mimic the activity of lipopolysaccharides and induce cytokine release.

*Control of pyrogens*: It is impractical, if not impossible, to remove pyrogens, once present, without adversely affecting the drug product. Therefore, the emphasis should be on preventing the introduction or development of pyrogens in all aspects of the compounding and processing of the product. There are various methods for achieving apyrogenicity:

- Pyrogens can be destroyed by heating at high temperatures. A typical procedure for depyrogenation of glassware and equipment is maintaining a dry heat temperature of 250°C for 45 minutes. Exposure of 650°C for 1 minute or 180°C for 4 hours, likewise, will destroy pyrogens. The usual autoclaving cycle will not do so.
- Heating with strong alkali or oxidizing solutions destroys pyrogens. It has been claimed that thorough washing with detergent will render glassware pyrogen-free, if subsequently rinsed thoroughly with pyrogen-free water. Rubber stoppers cannot withstand pyrogen-destructive temperatures, so reliance must be on an effective sequence of washing, thorough rinsing with WFI, prompt sterilization, and protective storage to ensure adequate pyrogen control. Similarly, plastic containers and devices must be protected from pyrogenic contamination during manufacture and storage, since known ways of destroying pyrogens affect the plastic adversely.
- Anion-exchange resins and positively-charged membrane filters also remove pyrogens from water. Also, although reverse osmosis membranes will eliminate them, the most reliable method for their elimination from water is distillation.
- Another method that has been used for the removal of pyrogens from solutions is adsorption on adsorptive agents. However, since the adsorption phenomenon may also cause selective removal of chemical substances from the solution, this method has limited application.
- Other in-process methods for destruction or elimination of pyrogen include selective extraction procedures and careful heating with dilute alkali, dilute acid, or mild oxidizing agents.

*Sources of pyrogens*: Through understanding the means by which pyrogens may contaminate parenteral products, their control becomes more achievable. Therefore, it is important to know that water is probably the greatest potential source of pyrogenic contamination, since water is essential for the growth of micro-organisms and frequently contaminated with gram-negative organisms. When micro-organisms metabolize, pyrogens will be produced. Therefore, raw water can be expected to be pyrogenic and only when it is appropriately treated to render it free from pyrogens, such as WFI, should it be used for compounding the product or rinsing product contact surfaces, such as tubing, mixing vessels, and rubber closures. Although proper distillation will provide pyrogen-free water, storage conditions must be such that micro-organisms are not introduced and subsequent growth is prevented.

Other potential sources of contamination are containers and equipment. Pyrogenic materials adhere strongly to glass and other surfaces, specially rubber closures. Residues of solutions used in equipment often become bacterial cultures, with subsequent pyrogenic contamination. Since drying does not destroy pyrogens, they may remain in equipment for long periods. Adequate washing reduces contamination, and subsequent dry heat treatment can render contaminated equipment suitable for use.

Solutes may be a source of pyrogens. For example, the manufacturing of bulk chemicals may involve the use of pyrogenic water for process steps, such as crystallization, precipitation, or washing. Bulk drug substances derived from cell culture fermentation will almost certainly be heavily pyrogenic. Therefore, all lots of solutes used to prepare parenteral products should be tested to ensure that they will not contribute unacceptable quantities of endotoxin to the finished product.

### *2. Storage and distribution*

The rate of production of WFI is not sufficient to meet processing demands; therefore, it is collected in a holding tank for subsequent use. In large operations, the holding tanks may have a capacity of several thousand gallons and be a part of a continuously operating system. In such instances, the USP requires that the WFI be held at a temperature too high for microbial growth, normally a constant 80°C.

The USP also permits the WFI to be stored at room temperature but for a maximum of 24 hours. Under such conditions, the WFI is collected as a batch for a particular use with any unused water discarded within 24 hours. Such a system requires frequent sanitization to minimize the risk of viable micro-organisms being present. The stainless steel storage tanks in such systems are usually connected to a welded stainless steel distribution loop, supplying the various use sites with a continuously circulating water supply. The tank is provided with a hydrophobic membrane vent filter, capable of excluding bacteria and nonviable particulate matter. Such a vent filter is necessary to permit changes in pressure during filling and emptying. The construction material for the tank and connecting lines is usually electro polished 316 L stainless steel with welded pipe. The tanks also may be lined with glass or a coating of pure tin. Such systems are very carefully designed and constructed and often constitute the most costly installation within the plant. When the water cannot be used at 80°C, heat exchangers must be installed to reduce the temperature at the point of use. Bacterial retentive filters should not be installed in such systems, due to the risk of bacterial build up on the filters and the consequent release of pyrogenic substances.

### *3. Containers and closures (Fig. 4.1)*

Injectable formulations are packaged into containers made of glass or plastic. Container systems include ampules, vials, syringes, cartridges, bottles and bags. Ampules are all glass, whereas bags are all plastic. The other containers can be composed of glass or plastic and must include rubber materials, such as rubber stoppers for vials and bottles and rubber plungers and rubber seals for syringes and cartridges. Irrigation solutions are packaged in glass bottles with aluminum screw caps.

#### i. Glass containers

Glass is employed as the container material of choice for most small volume injections (SVIs). It is composed, principally, of silicon dioxide, with varying amounts of other oxides, such as sodium, potassium, calcium, magnesium, aluminum, boron and iron. The basic structural network of glass is formed by the silicon oxide tetrahedron. Boric oxide will enter into this

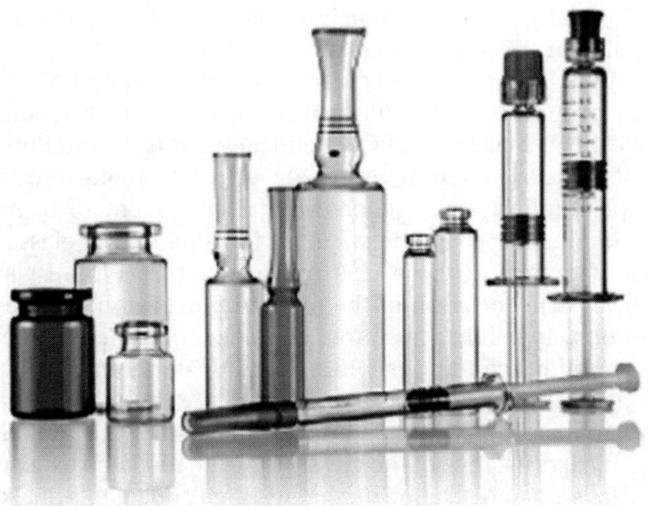

FIGURE 4.1: Various types of packaging for parenterals

structure, but most of the other oxides do not. The latter is only loosely bound, is present in the network interstices, and is relatively free to migrate. These migratory oxides may be leached into a solution in contact with the glass, particularly during the increased reactivity of thermal sterilization. The oxides dissolved may hydrolyze to raise the pH of the solution and catalyze or enter into reactions. Additionally, some glass compounds will be attacked by solutions and, in time, dislodge glass flakes into the solution. Such occurrences can be minimized by the proper selection of the glass composition.

**Types of glass: The USP provides a classification of glass**:

- Type I, a borosilicate glass
- Type II, a soda-lime treated glass
- Type III, a soda-lime glass
- Type IV (Nonparenteral), a soda-lime glass not suitable for containers for parenterals.

Type I glass is composed, principally, of silicon dioxide (~81%) and boric oxide (~13%), with low levels of the non-network forming oxides, such as sodium and aluminum oxides. It is a chemically resistant glass (low leachability), also having a low thermal coefficient of expansion (CoE). The lower the thermal

CoE, the more dimensionally stable the glass against thermal expansion stress that can result in cracking.

Types II and III glass compounds are composed of relatively high proportions of sodium oxide (~14%) and calcium oxide (~8%). This makes the glass chemically less resistant. Both types melt at a lower temperature, are easier to mold into various shapes, and have a higher thermal coefficient of expansion. Although there is no one standard formulation for glass among manufacturers of these USP type categories. Type II glass has a lower concentration of the migratory oxides than Type III. In addition, Type II has been treated under controlled temperature and humidity conditions, with sulfur dioxide or other dealkalizers to neutralize the interior surface of the container. Although it remains intact, this surface increases substantially the chemical resistance of the glass. However, repeated exposures to sterilization and alkaline detergents break down this dealkalized surface and expose the underlying soda-lime compound.

The glass types are determined from the results of two USP tests—The powdered glass test and the water attack test. The latter is used only for Type II glass and is performed on the whole container, due to the dealkalized surface; the former is performed on powdered glass, which exposes internal surfaces of the glass compound. The results are based on the amount of alkali titrated by 0.02 N sulfuric acid, after an autoclaving cycle with the glass sample in contact with a high-purity distilled water. Thus, the Powdered Glass Test challenges the leaching potential of the interior structure of the glass, whereas the Water Attack Test challenges only the intact surface of the container.

Glass can be the source/cause of leachables/extractables, particulates (glass delamination or glass lamellae formation), adsorption of formulation components, specially proteins and cracks/scratches.

*Leachables/extractables*—If the product is sensitive to the presence of ions, such as boron, sodium, potassium, calcium, iron, and magnesium, great care must be taken in selecting the appropriate glass container, as these ions may leach from the glass container and interact with the product, reducing chemical stability, inducing formation of particulate, or altering pH of solution. The presence of formulation components that can act as metal chelating agents, such as EDTA and citrate, is of special concern. Formulation studies involving accelerated aging (increased temperatures) should monitor changes in solution pH, metal content and particulate formation, in addition to drug product stability (purity and potency). Leachables from the glass barrel, such as tungsten (used for the formation of the barrel) and silicone (used for lubrication of the syringe), were shown to have significant impact on the protein stability.

Type I glass will be suitable for all products, although sulfur dioxide treatment is sometimes used for even greater resistance to glass leachables. Because cost must be considered, one of the other, less-expensive types may be acceptable. Type II glass may be suitable, for example, for a solution that is buffered, has a pH below 7, or is not reactive with the glass. Type III glass is usually suitable for anhydrous liquids or dry substances. However, some manufacturer-to-manufacturer variation in glass composition should be anticipated within each glass type. Therefore, for highly chemically sensitive parenteral formulations, it may be necessary to specify both USP type and specific manufacturer.

ii. Plastic containers

Thermoplastic polymers have been established as packaging materials for sterile preparations, such as large-volume parenterals, ophthalmic solutions and increasingly, small-volume parenterals. For such use to be acceptable, a thorough understanding of the characteristics, potential problems and advantages for use must be developed. Three principle problem areas exist in using these materials:

1. Permeation of vapors and other molecules in either direction through the wall of the plastic container.
2. Leaching of constituents from the plastic into the product.
3. Sorption (absorption and/or adsorption) of drug molecules or ions on the plastic material.

Permeation, the most extensive problem, may be troublesome by permitting volatile constituents, water, or specific drug molecules to migrate through the wall of the container to the outside and, thereby, be lost. This problem has been resolved, for example, by the use of an overwrap in the packaging of IV solutions in PVC bags to prevent loss of water during storage. Reverse permeation in which oxygen or other molecules may penetrate to the inside of the container and cause oxidative or other degradation of susceptible constituents may also occur. Leaching may be a problem, when certain constituents in the plastic formulation, such as plasticizers or antioxidants, migrate into the product.

Thus, plastic polymer formulations should have as few additives as possible—an objective characteristically achievable for most plastics used for parenteral packaging. Sorption is a problem on a selective basis, that is, sorption of a few drug molecules occurs on specific polymers. For example, sorption of insulin and other proteins, vitamin A acetate, and warfarin sodium has been shown to occur on PVC bags and tubing, when these drugs were present as additives in IV admixtures.

One of the principle advantages of using plastic packaging materials is that they are not breakable, as is glass; also there is a substantial weight reduction. The flexible bags of polyvinyl chloride or select polyolefins, currently in use for large-volume intravenous fluids, have the added advantage that no air interchange is required; the flexible wall simply collapses as the solution flows out of the bag. Most plastic materials have the disadvantage of not being as clear as glass and therefore, inspection of the contents is impeded.

In addition, many of these materials soften or melt under the conditions of thermal sterilization. However, careful selection of the plastic used and control of the autoclave cycle have made thermal sterilization of some products possible, large-volume injectables, in particular. Ethylene oxide or radiation sterilization may be employed for the empty container with subsequent aseptic filling. However, careful evaluation of the residues from ethylene oxide or its degradation products and their potential toxic effect must be undertaken. Investigation is required concerning potential interactions and other problems that may be encountered when a parenteral product is packaged in plastic.

#### iii. Rubber closures

To permit introduction of a needle from a hypodermic syringe into a multiple-dose vial and provide for resealing as soon as the needle is withdrawn, each vial is sealed with a rubber closure held in place by an aluminum cap. This principle is also followed for single-dose containers of the cartridge type, except that there is only a single introduction of the needle to make possible the withdrawal or expulsion of the contents.

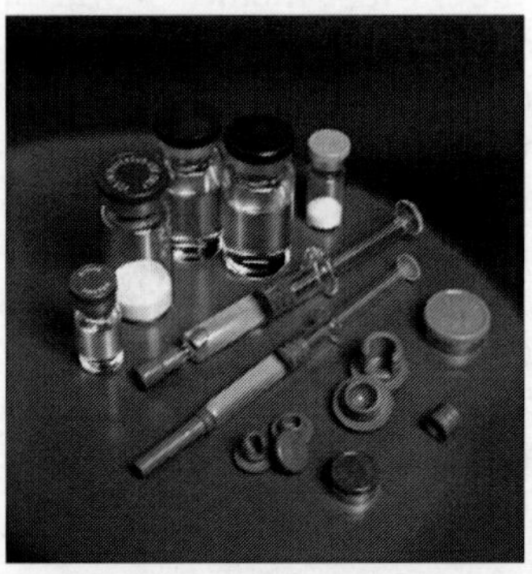

FIGURE 4.2: Rubber closures for vials and syringes

**Table 4.2:** Examples of ingredients found in rubber closures

| *Ingredient* | *Examples* |
|---|---|
| Elastomer | Natural rubber (latex)<br>Butyl rubber<br>Neoprene |
| Vulcanizing (curing agent) | Sulfur<br>Peroxides |
| Accelerator | Zinc dibutyldithiocarbamate |
| Activator | Zinc oxide<br>Stearic acid |
| Antioxidant | Dilauryl thiodipropionate |
| Plasticizer/lubricant | Paraffin oil<br>Silicone oil |
| Fillers | Carbon black<br>Clay<br>Barium sulfate |
| Pigments | Inorganic oxides<br>Carbon black |

Rubber closures are composed of multiple ingredients plasticized and mixed together at an elevated temperature on milling machines. The elastomer primarily used in rubber closures, plungers, and other rubber items used in parenteral packaging and delivery systems is synthetic butyl or halobutyl rubber.

Natural rubber is also used, but, if it is natural rubber latex, then the product label must include a warning statement, due to the potential for allergic reactions from latex exposure. The plasticized mixture is placed in molds and vulcanized (cured) under high temperature and pressure. During vulcanization the polymer strands are cross-linked by the vulcanizing agent, assisted by the accelerator and activator, so that motion is restricted and the molded closure acquires the elastic, resilient character required for its use. Ingredients not involved in the cross-linking reactions remain dispersed within the compound and, along with the degree of curing, affect the properties of the finished closure. Table 4.2 provides examples of rubber closure ingredients.

The physical properties considered in the selection of a particular formulation include elasticity, hardness, tendency to fragment, and permeability to vapor transfer. The elasticity is critical in establishing a seal with the lip and neck of a vial or other opening and in resealing after withdrawal of a hypodermic needle from a vial closure. The hardness should provide firmness, but not excessive resistance to the insertion of a needle through the closure, and minimal fragmentation of pieces of rubber should occur as the hollow shaft of the needle is pushed through the closure. Although vapor transfer occurs to some degree with all rubber formulations, appropriate selection of ingredients makes it possible to control the degree of permeability.

The physical shape of some typical closures may be seen in Figure 4.2. Most of them have a lip and a protruding flange that extends into the neck of the vial or bottle. Many disk closures are being used now, particularly in the high-speed packaging of antibiotics. Slotted closures are used on freeze-dried products to permit the escape of water vapor, since they are inserted only partway into the neck of the vial until completion of the drying phase of the cycle. Also, the top design of the freeze-dry closure is important to minimize sticking of the closure to underneath the dryer shelf after stoppering the vial. Stoppers normally have a small protruding circle at the center of the top of the stopper. Gaps provided within the protruding circle minimize the tendency of the stopper to stick to the freeze-dryer shelf. The plunger type of rubber is used to seal one end of a syringe or cartridge. At the time of use, the plunger expels the product by a needle inserted through the closure at the distal end of the package. Intravenous solution closures often have permanent holes for adapters of administration sets; irrigating solution closures are usually designed for pouring.

Rubber closures must be 'slippery' to move easily through a rubber closure hopper and other stainless steel passages, until they are fitted onto the filled vials. Traditionally, rubber materials are 'siliconized' (silicone oil or emulsion applied onto the rubber) to produce such lubrication. However, advances in rubber closure technologies have introduced closures that do not require siliconization, due to a special polymer coating applied to the outer surface of the closure.

#### iv. Needles

Historically, stainless steel needles have been used to penetrate the skin and introduce a parenteral product inside the body. The advent of needleless injection systems has obviated the need for needles for some injections (e.g. vaccines) and is gaining in popularity over the conventional syringe and needle system. However, needleless injections are more expensive, can still produce pain on injection, are, potentially, a greater source of contamination (and cross-contamination from incessant use), and may not be as efficient in dose delivery.

Needles are hollow devices composed of stainless steel or plastic. Needles are available in a wide variety of lengths, sizes and shapes. Needle lengths range from¼ inch – 6 inches. Needle size is referred to as its gauge (G), or the outside diameter (OD) of the needle shaft. Gauge ranges are 11 – 32 G, with the largest gauge for injection usually being no greater than 16 G. 16 G needles have an OD of 0.065 inches (1.65 mm), whereas 32 G have an OD of 0.009 inches (0.20 mm). Needle-shape includes regular, short bevel, intradermal, and winged. Needle-shape is defined by one end of a needle enlarged to form a hub with a delivery device, such as a syringe, or other administration device. The other end of the needle is beveled, meaning it forms a sharp tip to maximize ease of insertion.

The route of administration, type of therapy and whether the patient is a child or adult dictate the length and size of needle used. Intravenous injections use 1–2 inch 15–25 G needles. Intramuscular injections use 1–2 inch 19–22 G needles. Subcutaneous injections use $^{1}/_{4}$–$^{5}/_{8}$ inch 24–25 G needles. Needle gauge for children rarely is larger than 22 G, usually 25–27G. Winged needles are used for intermittent heparin therapy. Needles are purchased either alone (e.g. Luer-Lock) to be attached to syringes, cartridges and other delivery systems, or for syringes, can be part of the syringe set (stake needle).

## Production facilities

The production facility and its associated equipment must be designed, constructed and operated properly for the manufacture of a sterile product to be achieved at the quality level required for safety and effectiveness. Materials of construction for sterile product production facilities must be 'smooth, cleanable and impervious to moisture and other damage'. Further, the processes used must meet cGMP standards.

### *1. Functional areas*

To achieve the goal of a manufactured sterile product of exceptionally high quality, many functional production areas are involved: warehousing or procurement; compounding (formulation); materials (containers, closures, equipment) preparation; filtration and sterile receiving; aseptic filling; stoppering; packaging; labeling and quarantine.

The extrarequirements for the aseptic area are designed to provide an environment where a sterile fluid may be exposed to the environment for a brief period during subdivision from a bulk container to individual-dose containers, without becoming contaminated. The design and control of an aseptic area is directed toward reducing the presence of contaminants, so they are no longer a hazard to aseptic filling. Although the aseptic area must be adjacent to support areas, so an efficient flow of components may be achieved, barriers must be provided to minimize ingress of contaminants to the critical aseptic area. Such barriers may consist of a variety of forms, including sealed walls, manual or automatic doors, airlock pass-through, ports of various types, or plastic curtains. Adjacent support areas (rooms) consist of glass preparation, equipment wash, capping, manufacturing (compounding), and various storage areas. Figure 4.3 shows an example of a Class 100/Grade A small scale filling room with operators properly gowned and practicing good aseptic techniques.

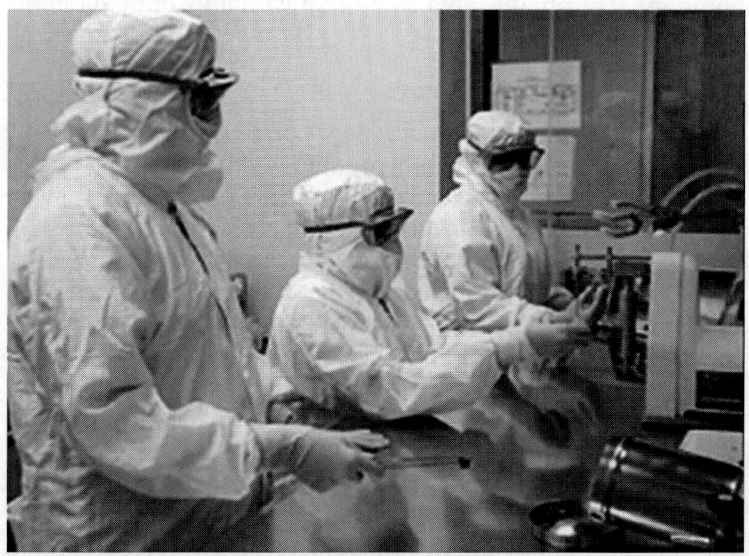

FIGURE 4.3: Properly gowned and trained aseptic processing operators in a class 100/Grade a clean room

## 2. *Flow plan*

In general, the components for a parenteral product flow from the warehouse, after release, to either the compounding area, as for ingredients of the formula, or the materials support area, as for containers and equipment. After proper processing in these areas, the components flow into the security of the aseptic area for filling of the product in appropriate containers. From there, the product passes into the quarantine and packaging area, where it is held until all necessary tests have been performed. If the product is to be sterilized in its final container, its passage is interrupted after leaving the aseptic area for subjection to the sterilization process. After the results from all tests are known, the batch records have been reviewed, and the product has been found to comply with its release specifications, it passes to the finishing area for final release for shipment. There, sometimes, are variations from this flow plan to meet the specific needs of an individual product or to conform to existing facilities. Automated operations have much larger capacity and convey the components from one area to another with little or no handling by operators.

*3. Clean room classified areas*

Due to the extremely high standards of cleanliness and purity that must be met by parenteral products, it has become standard practice to prescribe specifications for the environment (clean rooms) in which these products are manufactured (Table 4.3). Table 4.3 compares US and European classifications and clean room designations assigned by the International Society of Pharmaceutical Engineers. Table 4.3 numbers are based on the maximum allowed number of airborne particles/ft$^3$ or particles/m$^3$ of 0.5 μm or larger size and, for Europe, 5.0 μm or larger size. The classifications used in pharmaceutical practice normally range from Class 100,000 (Grade D) for materials support areas to Class 100 (Grade A) for aseptic areas. To achieve Class 100 conditions, HEPA filters are required for the incoming air, with the effluent air sweeping the downstream environment at a uniform velocity, 100 ft/min along parallel lines (laminar air flow). HEPA filters are defined as 99.99% or more efficient in removing, from the air, 0.3 μm particles. Because so many parenteral products are manufactured at one site for global distribution, air quality standards in aseptic processing areas must meet both US and European requirements.

**Table 4.3**: Clean room classified areas for parenterals

| *European grade* | *US classification* | *International society of Pharm engg. description* | *Max no.of particles per cubic meter* | *Max no.of particles per cubic meter* |
|---|---|---|---|---|
| A | 100 | Critical | 3,500 | 0 |
| B | 100 | Clean | 3,500 | 0 |
| C | 10,000 | Controlled | 3,50,000 | 2,000 |
| D | 100,000 | Pharmaceutical | 35,00000 | 20,000 |

*Air cleaning*—Since air is one of the greatest potential sources of contaminants in clean rooms, special attention must be given to air drawn into clean rooms by the heating, ventilating and air conditioning (HVAC) systems. This may be done by a series of treatments that vary somewhat from one installation to another.

In one such series, air from the outside, first, is passed through a prefilter, usually of glass wool, cloth, or shredded plastic, to remove large particles. Then, it may be treated by passage through an electrostatic precipitator. Such a unit induces an electrical charge on particles in the air and removes them by attraction to oppositely charged plates. The air then passes through the most efficient cleaning device, a HEPA filter.

For personal comfort, air conditioning and humidity control should be incorporated into the system. The clean, aseptic air is introduced into the Class 100 area and maintained under positive pressure, which prevents outside air from rushing into the aseptic area through cracks, temporarily open doors, or other openings.

*Laminar-flow enclosures*—The required environmental control of aseptic areas has been made possible by the use of laminar airflow, originating through a HEPA filter, occupying one entire side of the confined space. Therefore, it bathes the total space with very clean air, sweeping away contaminants. The orientation for the direction of airflow can be horizontal (Fig. 4.4A) or vertical (Fig. 4.4B) and may involve a limited area, such as a workbench, or an entire room.

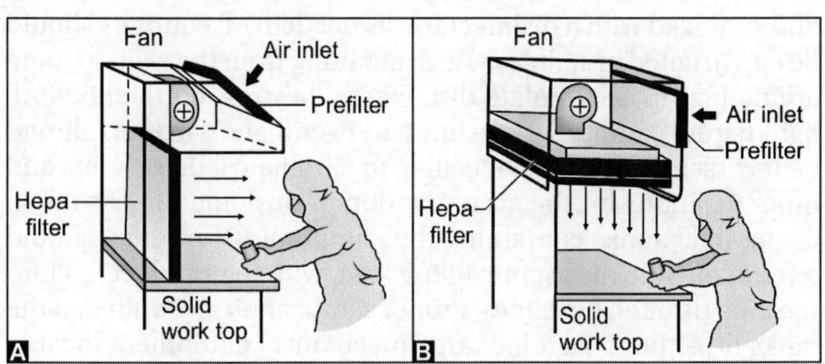


FIGURES 4.4A and B: (A) Horizontal and (B) vertical laminar air flow

Laminar-flow environments provide well-controlled work areas, only if proper precautions are observed. Any reverse air currents or movements exceeding the velocity of the HEPA-filtered airflow may introduce contamination, as may coughing, reaching, or other manipulations of the operator. Therefore, laminar-flow work areas should be protected by being located within controlled environments.

Personnel should be attired for aseptic processing, as subsequently described. All movements and processes should be planned carefully to avoid the introduction of contamination upstream of the critical work area. Checks of the air stream should be performed initially and at regular intervals (usually every 6 months), to be sure no leaks have developed through or around the HEPA filters. Clean room design, traditionally, has Class 100 rooms adjacent to Class 100,000 rooms.

*Compounding area*—Formulations are compounded in this area. Although, it is not essential that this area be aseptic, control of micro-organisms and particulates should be more stringent than in the materials support area. For example, means may be provided to control dust generated from weighing and compounding operations. Cabinets and counters should, preferably, be constructed of stainless steel. They should fit snugly to walls and other furnitures, so there are no catch areas where dirt can accumulate. The ceiling, walls, and floor should be similar to those for the materials support area.

*Aseptic area*—The aseptic area requires construction features designed for maximum microbial and particulate control. The ceiling, walls and floor must be sealed, so they may be washed and sanitized with a disinfectant, as needed. All counters should be constructed of stainless steel and hung from the wall, so there are no legs to accumulate dirt, where they rest on the floor. All light fixtures, utility service lines and ventilation fixtures should be recessed in the walls or ceiling to eliminate ledges, joints and other locations for the accumulation of dust and dirt. As much as possible, tanks containing the compounded product should remain outside the aseptic filling area, with the product fed into the area through hoselines. Proper sanitization is required, if the tanks must be moved in. Large mechanical equipment located in the aseptic area should be housed as completely as possible within a stainless steel cabinet, to seal the operating parts and their dirt-producing tendencies from the aseptic environment. Further, all such equipment parts should be located below the filling line. Mechanical parts that will contact the parenteral product should be demountable, so they can be cleaned and sterilized.

Personnel entering the aseptic area should enter only through an airlock. They should be attired in sterile coveralls with sterile hats, masks, goggles, foot covers and double gloves. Movement within the room should be minimal, and in-and-out movement rigidly restricted during a filling procedure. The requirements for room preparation and the personnel may be relaxed, if the product is to be sterilized terminally in a sealed container. Some are convinced, however, it is better to have one standard procedure meeting the most rigid requirements.

*4. Maintenance of clean rooms*

Maintaining the clean and sanitized conditions of clean rooms, particularly the aseptic areas, requires diligence and dedication of expertly trained custodians. Tools used should be nonlinting, designed for clean room use, held captive to the area, and preferably, sterilizable.

Liquid disinfectants (sanitizing agents) should be selected carefully, due to data showing their reliable activity against inherent environmental micro-organisms. They should be recognized as supplements to good housekeeping, never as substitutes. They should be rotated with sufficient frequency to avoid the development of resistant strains of micro-organisms.

It should be noted that ultraviolet (UV) light rays of 237.5 nm wavelength, as radiated by germicidal lamps, are an effective surface disinfectant. However, it must also be noted that they are only effective, if they contact the target micro-organisms at a sufficient intensity for a sufficient time. The limitations of their use must be recognized, including no effect in shadow areas, reduction of intensity by the square of the distance from the source, reduction by particulates in the ray path and the toxic effect on epithelium of human eyes. It is stated that an irradiation intensity of 20 $\mu w/cm^2$ is required for effective antibacterial activity.

*5. Personnel*

Personnel selected to work on the preparation of a parenteral product must be neat, orderly and reliable. They should be in good health and free from dermatological conditions that might increase the microbial load. If personnel show symptoms of a head cold, allergies, or similar illness, they should not be permitted in the aseptic area, until recovery is complete. Aseptic-area operators should be given thorough, formal training in the principles of aseptic processing and the techniques to be employed. Subsequently, the acquired knowledge and skills should be evaluated, to assure that training has been effective, before personnel are allowed to participate in the preparation of sterile products. Retraining should be performed on a regular schedule to enhance the maintenance of the required level of expertise. An effort should be made to imbue operators with an awareness of the vital role they play in determining the reliability and safety of the final product. The uniform worn is designed to confine the contaminants discharged from the body of the operator, thereby preventing their entry into the production environment. For use in the aseptic area, uniforms should be sterile. Fresh, sterile uniforms should be used after every break period or whenever the individual returns to the aseptic area. Sterile rubber or latex free gloves are also required for aseptic operations, preceded by thorough scrubbing of the hands with a disinfectant soap. Two pairs of gloves are put on, one pair at the beginning of the gowning procedure, the other pair after all other apparel has been donned. Air showers are sometimes directed on personnel entering the processing area to blow loose lint from the uniforms. Gowning rooms should be designed to enhance pregowning and gowning procedures by trained operators, so it is possible to ensure the continued sterility of the exterior surfaces of the sterile gowning components. Degowning should be performed in a separate exit room.

## Production procedures

The processes required for preparing sterile products constitute a series of events initiated with the procurement of approved raw materials (drugs, excipients, vehicles, etc.) and primary packaging components (containers, closures, etc.) and ending with the sterile product sealed in its dispensing package. Each step in the process must be controlled very carefully, so the product has its required quality. To ensure the latter, each process should be validated to ensure it is accomplishing what it is intended to do. The validation of processes requires extensive and intensive effort to be successful and is an integral part of cGMP requirements.

*1. Cleaning containers and equipment*

Containers and equipment coming in contact with parenteral preparations must be cleaned meticulously. It should be obvious that even new, unused containers and equipment are contaminated with such debris as dust, fibers, chemical films and other materials arising from such sources as the atmosphere, cartons, the manufacturing process and human hands. Residues from previous use must be removed from used equipment, before it is suitable for reuse. Equipment should be reserved exclusively for use only with parenteral preparations and, where conditions dictate, only for one product to reduce the risk of contamination. For many operations, particularly with biologic and biotechnology products, equipment is dedicated for only one product.

Containers

Treatments to be employed varies with the condition of the containers to be cleaned. In general, loose debris can be removed by vigorous rinsing with water. Detergents are rarely used for new containers, due to the risk of leaving detergent residues. However, a thermal-shock sequence in the cycle is usually employed to aid, by expansion and contraction, loosening of debris that may be adhering to the container wall. Sometimes, only an air rinse is used for new containers, if only loose debris is present. In all instances, the final rinse, whether air or WFI, must be ultraclean, so no particulate residues are left by the rinsing agent.

A variety of machines are available for cleaning new containers for parenteral products. These vary in complexity from a small, hand loaded, rotary rinsers to large, automatic washers capable of processing several thousand containers per hour. The selection of the particular type is determined largely by the physical type of containers, the type of contamination, and the number to be processed in a given period of time.

In one manual loading type, the jet tubes are arranged on arms like the spokes of a wheel, which rotate around a center post through which the treatments are introduced. An operator places the unclean containers on the jet tubes, as they pass the loading point, and removes the clean containers as they complete one rotation. The vials are fed into the rotary rinser in the foreground, transferred automatically to the covered sterilizing tunnel in the center, conveyed through the wall in the background, and discharged into the filling clean room.

The wet, clean containers must be handled in such a way that contamination is not reintroduced. A wet surface will collect contaminants much more readily than a dry surface will. For this reason, wet, rinsed containers must be protected (e.g. by a laminar flow of clean air until covered, within a stainless steel box, or within a sterilizing tunnel). In addition, microorganisms are more likely to grow in the presence of moisture. Therefore, wet, clean containers should be dry-heat sterilized, as soon as possible after washing. Doubling the heating period is also adequate to destroy pyrogens. For example, increasing the dwell time at 250°C from 1–2 hours, however, the actual time temperature conditions required must be validated. The clean, wet containers are protected by filtered, laminar-flow air from the rinser, through the tunnel, and until they are delivered to the filling line.

### Closures

The rough, elastic and convoluted surface of rubber closures renders them difficult to clean. In addition, any residue of lubricant from molding or surface 'bloom' of inorganic constituents must be removed. The normal procedure calls for gentle agitation in a hot solution of a mild water softener or detergent. The closures are removed from the solution and rinsed several times, or continuously for a prolonged period, with filtered WFI. The rinsing is done in a manner that flushes away loosened debris. The wet closures are carefully protected from environmental contamination, sterilized, usually by steam sterilization (autoclaving), and stored in closed containers, until ready for use. Actually, it is the cleaning and final, thorough rinsing with WFI that must remove pyrogens, since autoclaving does not destroy pyrogens. If the closures were immersed during autoclaving, the solution is drained off, before storage, to reduce hydration of the rubber compound.

The equipment used for washing large numbers of closures is usually an agitator or horizontal basket-type automatic washing machine. Due to the risk of particulate generation from the abrading action of these machines, some procedures simply call for heating the closures in kettles in detergent solution, followed by prolonged flush rinsing. The final rinse should always be with low-particulate WFI.

### Equipment

All equipment should be disassembled as much as possible to provide access to internal structures. Surfaces should be scrubbed thoroughly with a stiff brush, using an effective detergent and paying particular attention to joints, crevices, screw threads and other structures where debris is apt to collect. Exposure to a stream of clean steam aids in dislodging residues from the walls of stationary tanks, spigots, pipes, and similar structures. Thorough rinsing with distilled water should follow the cleaning steps.

Such an approach involves designing the system, normally of stainless steel, with smooth, rounded internal surfaces and without crevices. That is, for example, with welded, rather than threaded connections. Cleaning is accomplished with the scrubbing action of high-pressure spray balls or nozzles delivering hot detergent solution from tanks captive to the system, followed by thorough rinsing with WFI. The system is often extended to allow sterilizing-in-place (SIP), to accomplish sanitizing or sterilizing as well.

Rubber tubing, rubber gaskets and other rubber parts may be washed in a manner as described for rubber closures. Thorough rinsing of tubing must be done by passing WFI through the tubing lumen. However, due to the relatively porous nature of rubber compounds and the difficulty in removing all traces of chemicals from previous use, it is considered by some inadvisable to reuse rubber or polymeric tubing. Rubber tubing must be left wet when preparing for sterilization by autoclaving.

### *2. Product preparation*

The basic principles employed in the compounding of the product are essentially the same as those used, historically, by pharmacists. However, large-scale production requires appropriate adjustments in the processes and their control.

Parenteral dispersions, including colloids, emulsions and suspensions, provide particular problems. In addition to the problems of achieving and maintaining proper reduction in particle size under aseptic conditions, the dispersion must be kept in a uniform state of suspension throughout the preparative, transfer, and subdividing operations. Biopharmaceuticals are usually extremely sensitive to many environmental and processing conditions exposed to during production such as temperature, mixing time and speed, order of addition of formulation components, pH adjustment and control, and contact time with various surfaces, such as filters and tubing. Development studies must include evaluation of manufacturing conditions to minimize adverse effects of the process on the activity of the protein.

### *3. Filtration*

After a product has been compounded, it must be filtered, if it is a solution. The primary objective of filtration is to clarify a solution. A further step, removing particulate matter down to 0.2µm in size, would eliminate micro-organisms and would accomplish cold sterilization. A solution with a high degree of clarity conveys the impression of high quality and purity, desirable characteristics for a parenteral solution.

Membrane filters are used exclusively for parenteral solutions, due to their particle-retention effectiveness, nonshedding property, nonreactivity and disposable characteristics. However, it should be noted that nonreactivity does not apply in all cases. For example, polypeptide products may show considerable adsorption through some membrane filters, but those composed of polysulfone and polyvinylidine difluoride (PVDF) have been developed to be essentially nonadsorptive for these products. The most common membranes are composed of cellulose esters, nylon, polysulfone, polycarbonate, PVDF, or polytetrafluoroethylene (Teflon). Although membrane filters are disposable and, thus, discarded after use, the holders must be cleaned thoroughly between uses. Today, clean, sterile, pretested, disposable assemblies for small, as well as large, volumes of solutions are available commercially.

### *4. Filling*

During the filling of containers with a product, the most stringent requirements must be exercised to prevent contamination, particularly if the product has been sterilized by filtration and will not be sterilized in the final container. Under the latter conditions, the process is called an 'aseptic fill'. During the filling operation, the product must be transferred from a bulk container or tank and subdivided into dose containers. This operation exposes the sterile product to the environment, equipment and manipulative technique of the operators, until it can be sealed in the dose container. Therefore, this operation is carried out with a minimum exposure time, even though maximum protection is provided by filling under a blanket of HEPA-filtered laminar-flow air within the aseptic area.

Most frequently, the compounded product is in the form of a liquid. However, products are also compounded as dispersed systems (e.g. suspensions and emulsions) and as powders. A liquid is more readily subdivided uniformly and introduced into a container having a narrow mouth than that of a solid. Mobile liquids are considerably easier to transfer and subdivide than viscous, sticky liquids, which require heavy-duty machinery for rapid production filling. Although many devices are available for filling containers with liquids, certain characteristics are fundamental to them all. A means is provided for repetitively forcing a measured volume of the liquid through the orifice of a delivery tube introduced into the container.

**Liquids**: There are three main methods for filling liquids into containers with high accuracy—Volumetric filling, time-pressure dosing, and net weight filling.

Volumetric filling machines, employing pistons or peristaltic pumps, are most commonly used. When high-speed filling rates are desired but accuracy and precision must be maintained, multiple filling units are often joined in an electronically co-ordinated machine. When the product is sensitive to metals, a peristaltic-pump filler may be used, because the product comes in contact only with silicone rubber tubing. However, this sacrifices filling accuracy.

Time-pressure (or time-gravity) filling machines are gaining popularity in filling sterile liquids (Fig. 4.5). A product tank is connected to the filling system equipped with a pressure sensor. Product flow occurs when tubing is mechanically unpinched and stops when tubing is mechanically pinched. The main advantage of time-pressure filling operations is that these filling apparatuses do not contain mechanical moving parts in the product stream. The product is driven by pressure (usually nitrogen) with no pumping mechanism involved. Thus, specially for proteins that are quite sensitive to shear forces, time-pressure filling is preferable. Most high-speed fillers for large-volume solutions use the bottle as the measuring device, transferring the liquid either by vacuum or by positive pressure from the bulk reservoir to the individual unit containers. Therefore, a high accuracy of fill is not achievable.

The USP requires that each container be filled with a sufficient volume in excess of the labeled volume to ensure withdrawal of the labeled volume and provides a table of suggested fill volumes. The filling of a small number of containers may be accomplished with a hypodermic syringe and needle, the liquid drawn into the syringe and forced through the needle into the container.

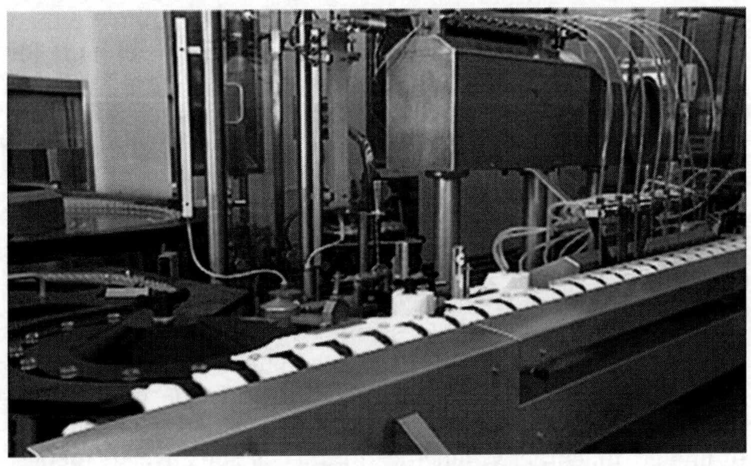

FIGURE 4.5: Vial filling machine

**Solids:** Sterile solids such as antibiotics, are more difficult to subdivide evenly into containers than are liquids. The rate of flow of solid material is slow and often irregular. Even though a container with a larger-diameter opening is used to facilitate filling, it is difficult to introduce the solid particles, and the risk of spillage is ever-present. Some sterile solids are subdivided into containers by individual weighing. A scoop is usually provided to aid in approximating the quantity required, but the quantity filled into the container is finally weighed on a balance. This is a slow process.

When the solid is obtainable in a granular form, so it will flow more freely, other methods of filling may be employed. In general, these involve the measurement and delivery of a volume of the granular material that has been calibrated in terms of the weight desired. In the machine shown in Figures 4.6A and B, an adjustable cavity in the rim of a wheel is filled by vacuum and the contents held by vacuum, until the cavity is inverted over the container. The solid material is then discharged into the container by a puff of sterile air.

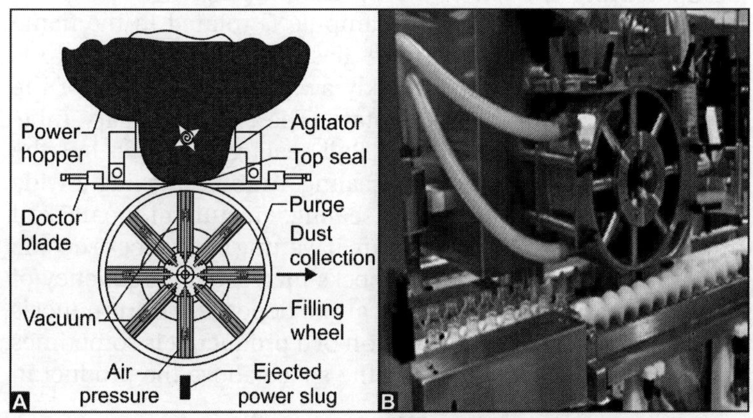


FIGURES 4.6A and B: Sterile powder filling machine
(A) Principle of operation (B) Close up view of filler

## *5. Sealing of ampules, vials and bottles*

### Ampules

Filled containers should be sealed as soon as possible, to prevent the contents from being contaminated by the environment. Ampules are sealed by melting a portion of the glass neck. Two types of seals are employed normally: Tip-seals (bead-seals) or Pull seals (Fig. 4.7).

Tip-seals are made by melting enough glass at the tip of the neck of an ampule to form a bead and close the opening. These can be made rapidly in a high-temperature gas-oxygen flame. To produce a uniform bead, the ampule neck must be heated evenly on all sides, such as by burners on opposite sides of stationary ampules or by rotating the ampule in a single flame. Care must be taken to properly adjust the flame temperature and the interval of heating to completely close the opening with a bead of glass. Excessive heating results in the expansion of the gases within the ampule against the soft bead seal, which causes a bubble to form. If the bubble bursts, the ampule is no longer sealed; if it does not, the wall of the bubble will be thin and fragile. Insufficient heating will leave an open capillary through the center of the bead. An incompletely sealed ampule is called a 'leaker'.

Pull-seals are made by heating the neck of the ampule below the tip, leaving enough of the tip for grasping with forceps or other mechanical devices. The ampule is rotated in the flame from a single burner. When the glass has softened, the tip is grasped firmly and pulled quickly away from the body of the ampule, which continues to rotate. The small capillary tube, thus, formed is twisted closed. Pull sealing is slower, but the seals are more secure than tip-sealing. Ampules having a wide opening must be sealed by pull sealing. Fracture of the neck of ampules during sealing may occur, if wetting of the necks occurs at the time of filling. Also, wet necks increase the frequency of bubble formation and unsightly carbon deposits, if the product is organic. To prevent decomposition of a product, it is sometimes necessary to displace the air in the space above the product in

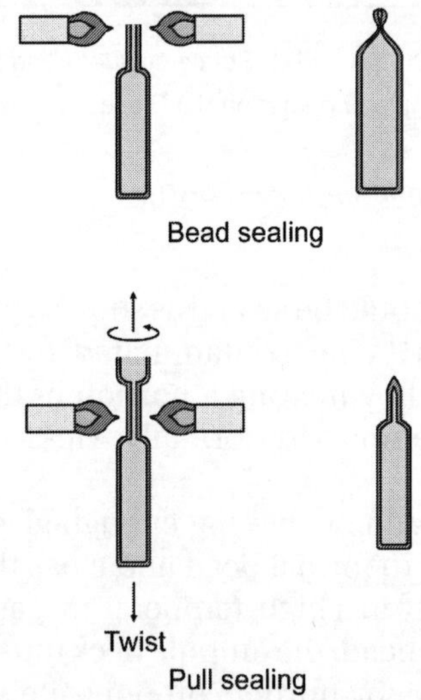


FIGURE 4.7: Sealing of ampoules

the ampule with an inert gas, by introducing a stream of the gas such as nitrogen or carbon dioxide, during or after filling with the product. Immediately thereafter, the ampule is sealed, before the gas can diffuse to the outside.

### Vials and bottles

Glass or plastic vials and bottles are sealed by closing the opening with a rubber closure (stopper). This must be accomplished as rapidly as possible after filling to prevent contamination of the contents. The large opening makes the introduction of contamination much easier than with ampules.

The closure must fit the mouth of the container snugly enough, so its elasticity seals rigid to slight irregularities in the lip and neck of the container. However, it must not fit so snugly that it is difficult to introduce into the neck of the container. Preferably, closures are inserted mechanically, using an automated process, specially with high-speed processing. To reduce friction, the closure may slide more easily through a chute and into the container opening, the closure surfaces are halogenated or treated with silicone. When the closure is positioned at the insertion site, it is pushed mechanically into the container opening. When small lots are encountered, manual stoppering with forceps may be used, but such a process poses greater risk of introducing contamination than automated processes.

Rubber closures are held in place by means of aluminum caps. The caps cover the closure, crimped under the lip of the vial or bottle to hold them in place. The closure cannot be removed without destroying the aluminum cap; it is tamperproof. Therefore, an intact aluminum cap is proof that the closure has not been removed intentionally or unintentionally. Such confirmation is necessary to ensure the integrity of the contents, as to sterility and other aspects of quality.

The aluminum caps are designed so the outer layer of double-layered caps, or the center of single-layered caps, can be removed to expose the center of the rubber closure, without disturbing the band that holds the closure in the container. Rubber closures for use with intravenous administration sets often have a permanent hole through the closure. In such cases, a thin rubber disk, overlaid with a solid aluminum disk, is placed between an inner and outer aluminum cap, thereby providing a seal of the hole through the closure. Single-layered aluminum caps may be applied using a hand crimper. Double- or triple-layered caps require greater force for crimping, therefore, heavy-duty mechanical crimpers are required.

*6. Sterilization*

Whenever possible, the parenteral product should be sterilized, after being sealed in its final container (terminal sterilization) and within as short a time as possible after filling and sealing are completed. Since this usually involves a thermal process, although there is a trend in applying radiation sterilization to finished products, due consideration must be given to the effect of the elevated temperature, upon the stability of the product. Many products, both pharmaceutical and biological, are affected adversely by elevated temperatures required for thermal sterilization. Heat-labile products must, therefore, be sterilized by a nonthermal method, usually by filtration through bacteria retaining filters. Subsequently, all operations must be carried out in an aseptic manner, so contamination is not introduced into the filtrate.

## FREEZE-DRYING (LYOPHILIZATION)

Lyophilization is the process in which water is removed from liquid products by sublimation (also known as sublimation drying). In sublimation on heating, a solid gets converted to vapors without intermediate formation of liquid state and on condensation the vapors gets converted back to the solid state. The products obtained after this sublimation drying known as sublimate.

As the dried product has greater affinity for water (lyophilic—liquid loving), therefore this process is also known as lyophilization.

Many pharmaceutical products lose their viability in the liquid and readily detoriate if dried in air at normal atmospheric pressure. These pharmaceutical materials may be thermolabile or unstable in aqueous solution for prolong storage period or they react readily with oxygen, so that in order to be stabilized they must be dehydrated to a solid state.

## Applications

Method is applicable for the preservation of:

1. Biological preparations such as blood serum, plasma and vaccines.
2. Tissue sections
3. Viable micro-organisms
4. Multivitamin combinations
5. Antibiotics and hormonal preparations.

*Advantages*

1. Product is stored in dry form, few stability problems.
2. Product is dried without elevating temperature.
3. Good for oxygen and air sensitive drugs.
4. Rapid reconstitution time.
5. Constituents of the dried material remain homogeneously dispersed.
6. Product is procesed in liquid form.
7. Sterility of product can be achieved and maintained.

*Disadvantages*

1. Method is not suitable for volatile compounds which may be removed by high vacuum.
2. Single most expensive unit operation.

*Desired characteristics of freeze-dried products*

1. It should be in the form of intact cake
2. It should have sufficient strength
3. It should be sufficiently dry
4. It should be porous
5. It should be sterile
6. It should be free from particulate matter
7. It should be free from pyrogens
8. It should be chemically stable.

*Process*

Product to be freeze-dried is prepared and handled as an aqueous solution or suspension. Freeze-drying is carried out at temperature and pressure below its eutectic point (the temperature and pressure at which frozen solid vaporizes without conversion to a liquid is known as eutectic point). Freeze-drying is carried out at this point to prevent the frozen solid from melting into liquid which would result in frothing. In freeze-drying process liquid is first frozen to ice before application of vacuum to avoid frothing then sublimation of frozen ice is carried out under reduced pressure. The frozen dried product can be readily redissolved or resuspended by the addition of water prior to use (known as reconstitution).

Freeze-drying is carried out in a mechanical refrigeration device by freezing the product in a container kept on the shelves of a chamber by circulating refrigerants like freon, ammonia or ethylene glycol from the compressor through the pipes fitted along the sides of the shelves.

When the product is completely frozen and properly cooled, the chamber is sealed and evacuated by means of vacuum pump. Heat is then supplied to the product by heating coils or by circulating water vapor. Water vapor is removed from the drying chamber by condensers. Removed water vapors condensed in the form of a thin layer of ice in the condenser. As the ice leaves the product, the drying residue maintains its original volume and become porous, owing to the loss of the ice molecules. This process is continued till the product is dry and spongy solid material is left behind (Fig. 4.8).

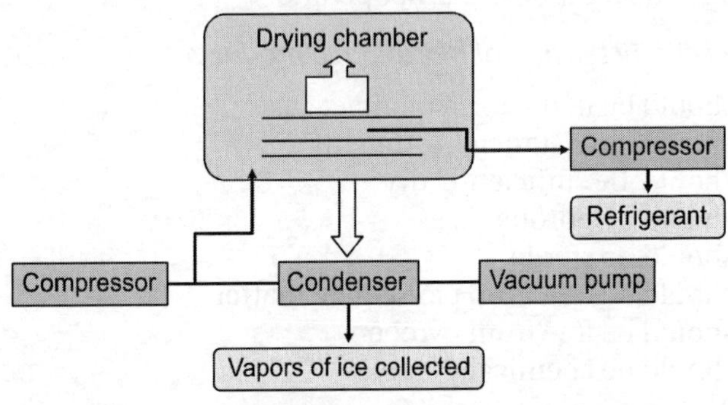


FIGURE 4.8: Freeze dryer

The product is usually processed until there is less than 1% moisture in the dried material. After completion of the drying cycle, reabsorption of moisture must be prevented. The product must, therefore, be removed from the chamber and sealed as rapidly as possible under controlled low humidity conditions.

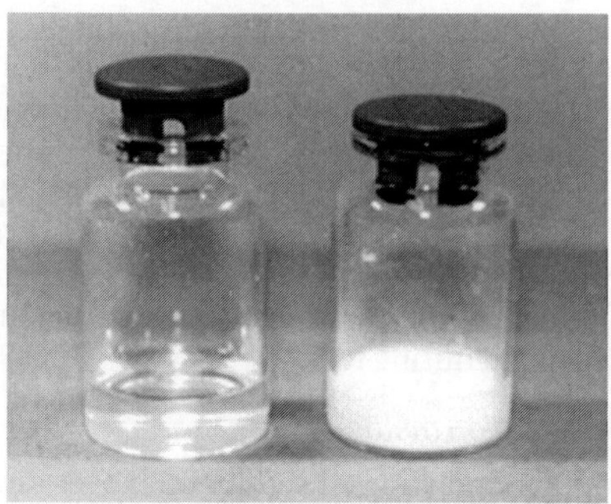

FIGURE 4.9: Vials used for lyophilization showing slotted stopper in open and closed position

Freeze driers also equipped for stoppering vials within the drying chamber, special slotted rubber closures are partially inserted into the neck of the vials prior to freezing the product. The slot permit the escape of water vapor from the vials during the drying cycle (Fig. 4.9). At the end of the drying cycle a hydraulically operated plates or an expandable rubber diaphagram press the closure firmly into the neck of the vials and seals them under vacuum. A butyl rubber compound is used for these rubber closures because of its low water vapor permeability.

## QUALITY CONTROL TESTS FOR PARENTERAL PRODUCTS

The basic quality control tests which are performed on parenteral products include:

### 1. Sterility tests

Sterility test is performed to check the presence of aerobic and anaerobic viable forms of bacteria, fungi and yeast in parenteral products. The methods which are used to perform sterility tests are—direct transfer method and membrane filtration method.

#### *a. Direct transfer method*

It is a traditional sterility test method which involves a direct inoculation of required volume of a sample in two tests tube containing a culture medium that is FTM (fluid thioglycollate medium) and SCDM (soyabean-casein digest medium).

**Procedure**: Suitable amount of material under test is transfered into sterile nutrient media and incubated for suitable period of time at optimum temperature. It is believed that living microbes present, if any, are expected to grow under favorable conditions like nutrient media, pH, temperature (Table 4.4) and incubation time, etc. After incubation, media is examined for the presence or absence of any microbes. Entire procedure is carried out under aseptic conditions so as to preclude entry of any micro-organism during test.

*b. Membrane filtration method*

It is more popular and widely used method over direct transfer method. Successful employment requires more skill and knowledge than direct transfer method.

**Procedure:** This method basically involves filtration of sample through membrane filters of porosity 0.22μ and diameter 47mm with hydrophobic characteristics. The filtration is assisted under vacuum. After filtration completion, the membrane is cut into two halves and one halve is placed in two test tubes containing FTM, SCDM medium.

***Interpretation**: If not any growth of microbes seen, product is considered to be sterile. If growth of microbes occurs, test is repeated 2nd and 3rd time to account for any accidental contamination. If test fails after 2nd and 3rd time, product is declared nonsterile and discarded.

**Table 4.4**: Time and temperature of incubation requirement for USP sterility test

| *Medium* | *Test* | *Time (days)* | *Temperature (°C)* | *Sterilization method* |
|---|---|---|---|---|
| FTM | Direct transfer | 14 | 30–35 | Aseptic process |
| | Membrane filtration | 7 | 30–35 | Terminal sterilization |
| | Membrane filtration | 14 | 30–35 | Aseptic process |
| SCDM | Direct transfer | 14 | 20–25 | Aseptic process |
| | Membrane filtration | 7 | 20–25 | Terminal sterilization |
| | Membrane filtration | 14 | 20–25 | Aseptic process |

## 2. Clarity test

Clarity test is performed to detect presence of any particulate matter. Particulate matter can be defined as any "extraneous, mobile, undissolved substances other than gas bubbles" unintendedly present in injections. Particulate matter is primary concern in the parenteral products given by IV route. Particulate matter can be checked by various methods:

*i. By clarity test apparatus (Fig. 4.10)*

This method involves direct lightning on container against black and white background to check presence of any particulate matter.

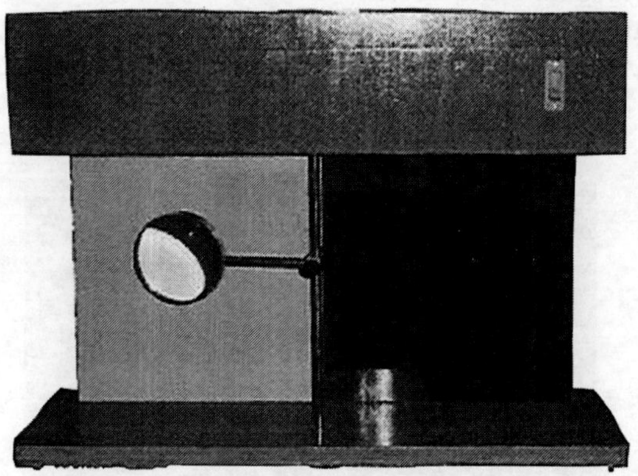

FIGURE 4.10: Clarity test apparatus

*ii. By filter paper method*

This method involve passing solution through filter paper and examine the filter paper microscopically.

*iii. By image analysis devices*

Automatic image analysis devices are also available in which image of the particle focused on the screen.

*iv. Other methods*

Light absorption, light scattering, change in electrical resistance is also used to detect particulate matter.

### 3. Leaker test (Fig. 4.11)

The leaker test is intended to detect incompletely sealed ampules, so that they may be discarded. Tip sealed ampules are more prone to leak than pull sealed. In addition, to that sometimes cracks may present around seal or at the base of ampule as a result of improper handling.

**Procedure**: Test is performed by dipping the ampules in a deeply colored dye solution for which 1% solution of methylene blue is used. The whole process is carried out in a vacuum chamber under negative pressure. When the vacuum is released the color solution will enter the ampules with defective sealing. After careful washing of ampules from outside, the dye can be seen in the leaker ampules.

This test is not performed on vials and bottles because of flexibility of rubber, moreover, the dye will badly stain the rubber stopper.

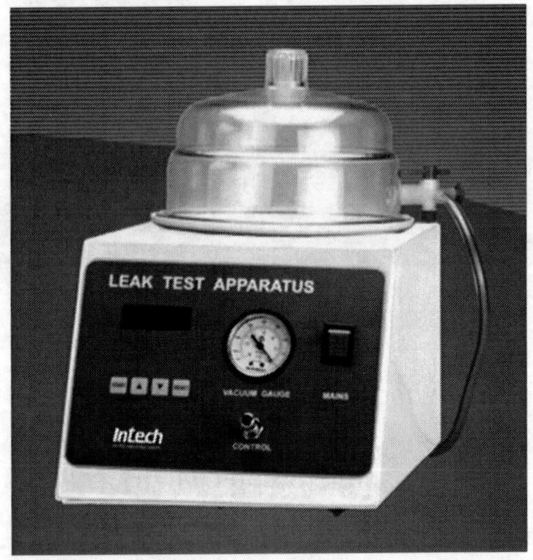


FIGURE 4.11: Leaker test apparatus

### 4. Pyrogen test

The presence of pyrogenic substances in parenteral preparations is determined by qualitative biologic tests: Rabbit and LAL test.

*a. Rabbit test*

This test is performed to check the presence of pyrogenic substance. Pyrogen test is performed on all aqueous parenteral products. In this test, rabbits are used as test animals because they show same physiological response to pyrogenic substances like that of man but the rabbits are very sensitive to external stimuli, therefore they must be handled very carefully.

**Principle**: If pyrogenic substance present in the product, it causes increase in body temperature of test animal.

**Procedure**: Test sample is injected into ear vein of three rabbits. 3 hours after injection, body temperature of test animals are measured by rectal thermocouple inserted into rabbits and temperature is measured by employing electronic thermometer.

***Interpretation**: If no single rabbit shows rise in temperature, product is declared as nonpyrogenic but if anyone rabbit shows the rise in temperature of 0.6°C or more above the normal temperature which has been taken before giving the injection then the test is repeated on 5 additional rabbits with same preparation administered to initial first 3 rabbits. Test requirements are met if not more than 3 of 8 rabbits show an individual rise in temperature of 0.6°C and sum of maximum rise in temperature of 8 rabbits is not more than 3.7°C.

*b. Limulus amebocyte lysate test (LAL)*

This test is performed to check the presence of any bacterial endotoxin.

**Principle**: Amebocyte of horseshoe crab contains enzyme or protein system that coagulates in the presence of small amount of lipopolysaccharide.

**Procedure**: The basic procedure is the combination of 0.1 ml of test sample with cell lysate from amebocyte (blood cell) of the horseshoe crab. After incubation for 1 hour at 37°C the mixture is analyzed for the presence of gel clot.

***Interpretation**: If any endotoxin present, causes coagulation of test solution with protein fraction of the amebocyte and result in formation of gel. If no any endotoxin present, no coagulation occurs, no gel is form.

Advantages of LAL test

- It is in vitro and does not require animal handling, thus is more convenient.

- It is 10 times more sensitive than that of the in vivo rabbit test.
- It is economical.
- It consumes less time, i.e. 1 vs. 3 hours required by rabbits test.
- It requires less laboratory facilities and minimum equipments.
- It requires less test volume.
- It is more accurate.

## PACKAGING

The USP includes certain requirements for the packaging and storage of injections:

1. The volume of injection in single-dose containers is defined as that which is specified for parenteral administration at one time and is limited to a volume of 1 L.
2. Parenterals intended for intraspinal, intracisternal, or peridural administration are packaged only in single-dose containers.
3. Unless an individual monograph specifies otherwise, no multiple-dose container shall contain a volume of injection more than sufficient to permit the withdrawal and administration of 30 ml.
4. Injections packaged for use as irrigation solutions or for hemofiltration or dialysis or for parenteral nutrition are exempt from the foregoing requirements relating to packaging. Containers for injections packaged for use as hemofiltration or irrigation solutions may be designed to empty rapidly and may contain a volume in excess of 1 L.
5. Injections intended for veterinary use are exempt from the packaging and storage requirements concerning the limitation to single-dose containers and to volume of multiple-dose containers.

# Chapter 5

# Novel Drug Delivery Systems

## ORAL CONTROLLED RELEASE DRUG DELIVERY SYSTEMS

### Introduction

During the last two decades, there has been remarkable increase in interest in controlled release drug delivery system. This has been due to various factors, viz. the prohibitive cost of developing new drug entities, expiration of existing international patents, discovery of new polymeric materials suitable for prolonging the drug release, and the improvement in therapeutic efficiency and safety achieved by these delivery systems.

**Modified release dosage forms**: The term 'modified release dosage forms' is used to denote the dosage forms for which the drug release characteristics of time course and/or location are chosen to accomplish therapeutic objectives not offered by the conventional dosage forms. Two types of modified release dosage forms are recognized.

1. Extended release dosage forms: It is defined as the one that allows at least a twofold reduction in the dosing frequency as compared to that of conventional dosage form.
2. Delayed release dosage forms: It is defined as one that releases the drug at a time other than "immediately" after administration.

*Rationale of controlled drug delivery*

The basic rationale for controlled drug delivery is to alter the pharmacokinetics and pharmacodynamics of pharmacologically active moieties by using novel drug delivery system or by modifying the molecular structure and/or physiological parameters inherent in a selected route of administration.

### *Terminology*

The general consensus is that controlled release denotes systems, which can provide some control, whether this is of a temporal or spatial nature, or both, of drug release in the body. In other words, the systems attempt to control drug concentration in the target tissue or cells. Thus, prolonged release or sustained release systems, which only prolong therapeutic blood or tissue levels of the drug for an extended period of time, cannot be considered as controlled release systems by this definition. They are distinguished from rate-controlled drug delivery systems, which are able to specify the release rate and duration in vivo precisely, on the basis of simple in vitro tests. Drug targeting, on the other hand, can be considered as a form of controlled release in that exercises spatial control of drug release within the body.

In general, controlled delivery attempts to:

- Sustain drug action at a predetermined rate by maintaining a relatively constant, effective drug level in the body with concomitant minimization of undesirable side effects associated with a saw tooth kinetic pattern.
- Localize drug action by spatial placement of a controlled release system (usually rate-controlled) adjacent to or in the diseased tissue or organ.
- Target drug action by using carriers or chemical derivatization to deliver drug to a particular "target" cell type.

In practice, very few of the applied systems embrace all of these actions. In most cases, the release systems create constant concentration of drug within the body over an extended period of time. The assumption is that there is steady state drug levels in plasma and in target tissue or cells are correlated. Ideally, it is desirable to place the drug at the target, be it a tissue, a population of cells or receptors, leaving the rest of body drug free. Obviously this would be quite difficult, specially if the target is sheltered from systemic circulation by various barriers. For example, drug targeting to the brain via systemic administration is severely limited by selectivity of the blood brain barrier. Figure 5.1 shows comparative blood level profiles obtained from administration of conventional, controlled and sustained release dosage forms. The conventional tablet or capsule provides only a single and transient burst of drug. A pharmacological effect is seen as long as the amount of drug is within the therapeutic range. Problems occur when the peak concentration is above or below this range, specially for drugs with narrow therapeutic windows. Indeed, prolonged release dosage forms reduce fluctuations in plasma drug levels by slowing down the absorption rate due to slower drug release rate.

The term "sustained release" is known to have existed in the medical and pharmaceutical literature for many decades. It has been constantly used to describe a pharmaceutical dosage form formulated to retard the release of therapeutic agent such that its appearance in the systemic circulation is delayed and/or prolonged and its plasma profile is sustained in duration.

The term "controlled release", on the other hand, has a meaning that goes beyond the scope of sustained drug action. It also implies a predictability and reproducibility in the drug release kinetics, which means that the release of drug from controlled release drug delivery system proceeds at a rate profile that is not predictable kinetically, but also reproducible from one unit to another.

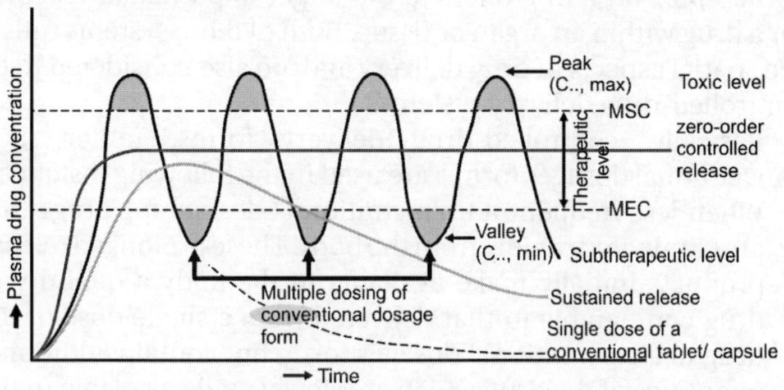


FIGURE 5.1: Comparative blood level profiles obtained from administration of conventional, controlled and sustained release dosage forms

### *Theoretical overview*

The basic goal of therapy is to achieve a steady-state blood or tissue level that is therapeutically effective and nontoxic for extended period of time. Modified-release delivery systems may be divided conveniently into four categories:

1. Delayed release
2. Sustained release
3. Site-specific targeting
4. Receptor targeting.

***Delayed release systems*** are those that use repetitive, intermittent dosing of a drug from one or more immediate-release units incorporated into a single dose form. For example, delayed release system include repeat action tablets, capsules and enteric coated tablet where timely release is achieved by barrier coating.

***Sustained release system*** includes any drug delivery system that achieves slow release of drug over an extended period of time. If the system provides some control, whether this is of temporal or spatial nature, or both, of drug release in the body, or in other words, the system is successful at maintaining constant drug levels in the target tissue or cells, it is considered a controlled-release system.

***Site-specific targeting*** refers to targeting of drug directly to a certain biological locations. In the case of site-specific release, the target is adjacent to or in the diseased organ or tissue.

***Receptor targeting*** refers to the target in particular receptor for a drug within an organ or tissue. Both of these systems satisfy the spatial aspects of drug delivery and are also considered to be controlled-drug delivery systems.

Basically, controlled-drug delivery forms, rather than conventional dosages forms, are used in the following instances:

1. When less frequent administration is desired for drugs that are eliminated rapidly from the body. These prolonged release products initially make available to the body a quantity of drug comparable to that delivered from a single dose of the drug in a conventional dosages form, but contain additional quantities of the drug which are slowly made available to the body so as to prolong the clinical effect beyond that attainable with a single dose. The prolonged-release dosage forms should be most useful for drugs that are used chronically but that have relatively short half lives and must be administered several times a day.
2. When high peak blood levels due to rapid drug absorption from conventional dosages forms are associated with adverse side effects. Thus, the use of certain drugs with relatively long

half lives in slow release dosages forms may also be rational and advantageous if there is question regarding the safety of giving the entire daily dose in a single administration of conventional dosages forms.

Ideally with sustained and controlled drug delivery forms, the drug absorption into the body should be determined by dosages form factors rather than by physiological factors. Basically, the drugs delivered into the systemic circulation are a function of the rate of drug release from the dosages form and the rate of drug passage through biological membranes. The slower of the two processes will be rate determining. In conventional dosages forms the physiologic factors are often rate controlling. But in controlled drug delivery forms the dosages formulation is rate controlling.

It is important to understand physiologic factors while designing controlled drug delivery systems. For example, the most used route of drug administration is oral, yet the gastrointestinal tract presents a very challenging variety of physiologic factors that affect dosages form performance, e.g. gastric acidity and more neutral intestinal fluids, thick membranes with small surface area and poor blood supply (gastric) and thinner membranes with large surface area and good blood supply (duodenal), highly liquid environments and semisolid environments, etc. these variations are made even more challenging by changing transit times and the probability of first pass metabolism. To render these physiologic factors less important to the rate of drug absorption than the dosages form factors is sometimes not possible, e.g. for drugs that are not absorbed throughout the gastrointestinal tract or for some drugs that undergo extensive first pass metabolism. The majority of oral controlled release systems rely on dissolution, diffusion or a combination of both mechanisms, to generate slow release of drug to the gastrointestinal milieu. Theoretically and desirably a controlled release delivery device, should release the drug by a zero-order process which would result in a blood-level time profile similar to that after intravenous constant rate infusion.

### *Potential advantages and disadvantages of sustained and controlled release dosage forms*

#### Advantages

1. **Patient compliance**: Lack of compliance is generally observed with long-term treatment of chronic disease, as

success of drug therapy depends upon the ability of patient to comply with the regimen. Patient compliance is affected by a combination of several factors, like awareness of disease process, patient faith in therapy, his understanding of the need to adhere to a strict treatment schedule and also the complexity of therapeutic regimens, the cost of therapy and magnitude of local and or systemic side effect of the dosage form. The problem of lack of patient compliance can be resolved to some extent by administering controlled release drug delivery system.

2. **Reduced 'see-saw' fluctuation**: Administration of a drug in a conventional dosage form [except via intravenous infusion at a constant rate] often results in 'see-saw' pattern of drug concentration in the systemic circulation and tissue compartments. The magnitudes of these fluctuations depend on drug kinetics such as the rate of absorption, distribution, elimination and dosing intervals. The 'see-saw' or 'peak and valley' pattern is more striking in case of drugs with biological half lives of less than four hours, since prescribed dosing intervals are rarely less than four hours. A well-designed controlled release drug delivery system can significantly reduce the frequency of drug dosing and also maintain a steadier drug concentration in blood circulation and target tissue cells.
3. **Reduced total dose**: Controlled release drug delivery systems have repeatedly been shown to use less amount of total drug to treat a diseased condition. By reducing the total amount of drug, decrease in systemic or local side effects are observed. This would also lead to greater economy.
4. **Improved efficiency in treatment**: Optimal therapy of a disease requires an efficient delivery of active drugs to the tissues, organs that need treatment. Very often doses far in excess to those required in the cells have to be administered in order to achieve the necessary therapeutically effective concentration. This unfortunately may lead to undesirable, toxicological and immunological effects in nontarget tissue. A controlled release dosage forms leads to better management of the acute or chronic disease condition.
5. **Economy**:
   a. In comparison with conventional dosage forms the average cost of treatment over an extended period may be less.

   b. Economy also may result from a decrease in nursing time and hospitalization.
6. **Improved therapy**:
   a. *Sustained blood level*: The dosage form provides uniform drug availability/blood levels unlike peak and valley pattern obtained by intermittent administration.
   b. *Attenuation of adverse effects*: The incidence and intensity of undesirable effects caused by excessively high peak drug concentration resulting from the administration of conventional dosage forms is reduced.
   c. It is seldom that a dose is missed because of non-compliance by the patient.

Disadvantages

1. **Dose dumping**: Dose dumping is a phenomenon where by relatively large quantities of drug in a controlled release formulation is rapidly released, introducing potential toxic quantities of the drug into the systemic circulation. Dose dumping can lead to fatalities in case of potent drug, which has a narrow therapeutic index, e.g. phenobarbital.
2. **Less flexibility in accurate dose adjustment**: In conventional dosage forms, dose adjustments are much simpler, e.g. tablet can be divided into two fractions. In case of controlled release dosage forms, this appears to be much more complicated. Controlled release property may get lost, if dosage form is fractured.
3. **Poor in vitro–in vivo correlation**: In controlled release dosage form, the rate of drug release is deliberately reduced to achieve drug release possibly over a large region of gastrointestinal tract. Here the so called 'Absorption window' becomes important and may give rise to unsatisfactory drug absorption in vivo despite excellent in vitro release characteristics.
4. **Patient variation**: The time period required for absorption of drug released from the dosage form may vary among individuals. Co-administration of other drugs, presence or absence of food and residence time in gastrointestinal tract is different among patients. This also gives rise to variation in clinical response among the patient.

## Factors considered in designing of sustained/controlled release dosage forms

The therapeutic efficacy of drug under clinical conditions is not simply a function of its intrinsic pharmacological activity but also depends upon the path of the drug molecule from the site of administration to the target site. Different conditions encountered by the drug molecule while traversing the path of distribution may alter either the effectiveness of the drug or affect the amount of the drug reaching the receptor site.

*Biopharmaceutical factors*

1. **Dose size**: For orally administered systems, there is an upper limit to the bulk size of the dose to be administered. In general, a single dose of 0.5–1.0 gm is considered maximal for a conventional dosage form. This also holds for sustained-release dosage forms. Those compounds that require large dosing size can sometimes be given in multiple amounts or formulated into liquid system. Another consideration is the margin of safety involved in administration of large amounts of a drug with narrow therapeutic range.
2. **Dissociation constant "pKa"**: A drug to be absorbed, it first must dissolve in the aqueous phase surrounding the site of administration and then partition in the absorbing membrane. Two of the most important physicochemical properties of a drug that influence its absorptive behavior are its aqueous solubility and if it is a weak acid or base it is pKa. These properties pay an influential role in the performance of controlled release systems.
3. **Partition coefficient**: When a drug is administered to the GI tract, it must cross a variety of biological membranes to produce a therapeutic effect in another area of the body. It is common to consider that these membranes are lipidic, therefore, the partition coefficient of oil-soluble drugs becomes important in determining the effectiveness of membrane barrier penetration. Partition coefficient is generally defined as the ratio of the fraction of drug in an oil phase to that of an adjacent aqueous phase. Accordingly, compounds with a relatively high partition coefficient are predominantly lipid-soluble and, consequently, have very low aqueous solubility.

4. **Drug stability**: The stability of the drugs at the site of its release and exposure bio milieu is one more drug property that can influence the design of oral controlled drug delivery. Drugs that are unstable in gastric pH can be developed as slow release dosage form and drug release can be delayed till the dosage form reaches the intestine. Drugs that undergo gut-wall metabolism and show instability in small intestine are not suitable for controlled drug delivery systems.
5. **Protein binding**: It is well-known that many drugs bind to plasma proteins with concomitant influence on the duration of drug action. Since blood proteins are for the most part recirculated and not eliminated, drug protein binding can serve as the depot for drug producing a prolonged release profile, specially if high degree of drug binding occurs. There are, however, other drug-protein interaction that has bearing on drug performance.

*Pharmacokinetic factors*

1. **Absorption**: The rate, extent and uniformity of absorption of a drug are important factors when considering its formulation into a controlled-release system. Since, the rate limiting step in drug delivery from a controlled-release system is its release from a dosage form, rather than absorption, a rapid rate of absorption of drug relative to its release is essential if the system is to be successful.
2. **Distribution**: The distribution of a drug into vascular and extravascular spaces in the body is an important factor in its overall elimination kinetics. Two parameters that are used to describe the distribution characteristics of a drug are its apparent volume of distribution and the ratio of drug concentration in the tissue to that in plasma at the steady state is called T/P ratio. The magnitude of the apparent volume of distribution can be used as a guide for additional studies and as a predictor for a drug dosing regimen and hence the need to employ a controlled-system.
3. **Metabolism**: Drugs that are significantly metabolized before absorption either in the lumen or tissue of the intestine can show decreased bioavailability from slower-releasing dosage forms. Formulation of these enzymatically susceptible compounds as prodrug is another viable solution.

4. **Elimination half-life**: Smaller the $t_{1/2}$, larger the amount of drug to be incorporated in the controlled release dosages forms. For drugs with $t_{1/2}$ less than 2 hours, a very large dose may be required to maintain the high release rate. Drugs with half- life in the range of 2–4 hours make good candidates for such a system, e.g. propranolot. Drugs with long half-life need not be presented in such a formulation, e.g. amlodipine.

## Criteria to be met by drug proposed to be formulated in sustained/controlled release dosage forms

*1. Desirable half-life*

The half-life of a drug is an index of its residence time in the body. If the drug has a short half-life (less than 2 hours) the dosage form may contain a prohibitively large quantity of the drug. On the other hand, drugs with elimination half-life of 8 hours or more are sufficiently sustained in the body, when administered in conventional dosage form, and controlled release drug delivery system is generally not necessary in such cases. Ideally, the drug should have half-life of 3–4 hours.

*2. High therapeutic index*

Drugs with low therapeutic index are unsuitable for incorporation in controlled release formulations. If the system fails in the body, dose dumping may occur, leading to fatalities, e.g. digitoxin.

*3. Small dose*

If the dose of a drug in the conventional dosage form is high, its suitability as a candidate for controlled-release is seriously undetermined. This is chiefly because the size of a unit dose controlled-release formulation would become too big, to administer without difficulty.

*4. Desirable absorption and solubility characteristics*

Absorption of poorly water-soluble drug is often dissolution rate limited. Incorporating such compounds into controlled-release formulations is, therefore, unrealistic and may reduce overall absorption efficiency.

*5. Desirable absorption window*

Certain drugs when administered orally are absorbed only from a specific part of gastrointestinal tract. This part is referred to as the absorption window. Drugs exhibiting an absorption window like fluorouracil, thiazide diuretics, if formulated as controlled-release dosage form, are unsuitable.

## Design and formulation of oral controlled release drug delivery system

Advances in oral controlled-release technology are attributed to the development of novel biocompatible polymers and machineries that allow preparation of novel design dosage forms in a reproducible manner. The main oral drug-delivery approaches that have survived through the ages are as follows:

1. Diffusion controlled systems
   i. Reservoir type
   ii. Matrix type
2. Dissolution controlled systems
   i. Reservoir type
   ii. Matrix type
3. Methods using ion-exchange
4. Methods using osmotic pressure
5. pH independent formulations
6. Altered density formulations
7. Mucoadhesive systems
8. Intestinal release systems
9. Colonic release systems.

### *1. Diffusion controlled systems*

Diffusion systems are characterized by the release rate of drug being dependent on its diffusion through an inert membrane barrier. Usually, this barrier is an insoluble polymer. In general, two types or subclasses of diffusional systems are recognized reservoir devices and matrix devices.

#### i. Reservoir devices

Reservoir devices, as the name implies, are characterized by a core of drug, the reservoir surrounded by a polymeric membrane. The nature of the membrane determines the rate of release of drug from the system (Fig. 5.2). It is also possible to use polymer coatings to achieve sustained release. For this purpose the polymer itself should not dissolve, but rather should allow the drug to diffusion through the polymer membrane to the outside, in the case of oral drug delivery, into the gastrointestinal tract.

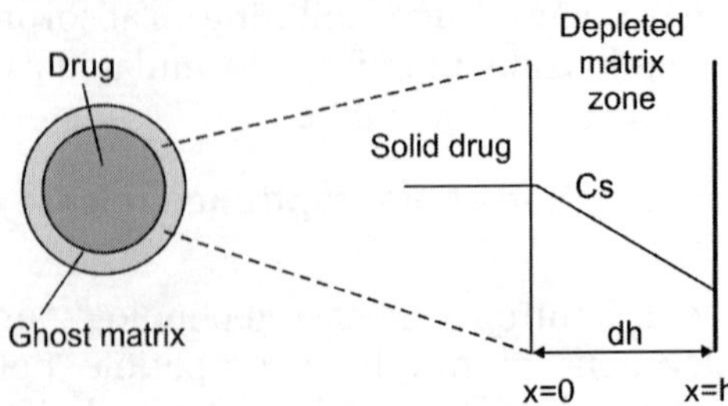


FIGURE 5.2: Schematic representation of a reservoir diffusional device

## ii. Matrix devices (Fig. 5.3)

A matrix device, as the name implies, consist of drug dispersed homogeneously throughout a polymer matrix. In the model, drug in the outside layer exposed to the bathing solution is dissolved first and then diffuses out of the matrix (Fig. 5.3). This process continues with the interface between the bathing solution and the solid drug moving towards the interior, obviously, for this system to be diffusion controlled, the rate of dissolution of drug particles within the matrix must be much faster than the diffusion rate of dissolved drug leaving the matrix.

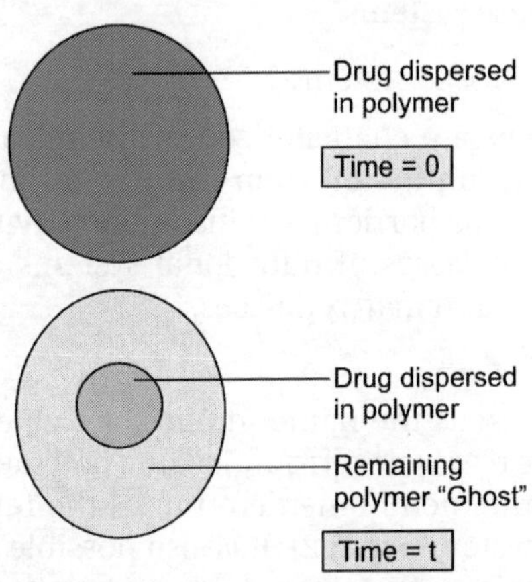


FIGURE 5.3: Matrix diffusional system before drug release (time = 0) and after partial drug release (time = t)

*Matrix systems*

One of the least complicated approaches to the manufacture of sustained release dosage forms involves the direct compression of blends of drug, retardant materials and additives to form a tablet in which drug is embedded in matrix core of the retardant. Alternately, retardant drug blends may be granulated prior to compression.

*Types of matrix*

a. Hydrophobic matrices

These matrices are mixed composite of one or more drugs with a gelling agent (hydrophilic polymer). These systems are called swellable controlled release systems. The polymers used in the preparation of hydrophilic matrices are divided into two broad groups:

i. *Cellulose derivatives*: Methylcellulose 400 and 4000cPs, Hydroxyethylcellulose; Hydroxypropyl methylcellulose (HPMC) 25, 100, 4000 and 15000cPs; and Sodium carboxy methylcellulose.
ii. *Noncellulose natural or semisynthetic polymers*: Agar-Agar, alginates, polysaccharides of mannose and galactose, chitosan and modified starches.

b. Lipid matrices

These matrices prepared by the lipid waxes and related materials. Drug release from such matrices occurs through both pore diffusion and erosion. Release characteristics are, therefore, more sensitive to digestive fluid composition than to totally insoluble polymer matrix. Carnauba wax in combination with stearyl alcohol or stearic acid has been utilized as retardant base for many sustained release formulation.

*2. Dissolution controlled systems*

It seems inherently obvious that a drug with a slow dissolution rate will demonstrate sustaining properties, since the release of drug will be limited by the rate of dissolution. This being true, sustained-release preparation of drugs could be made by decreasing their rate of dissolution. The approaches to achieve this include preparing appropriate salts or derivatives, coating the drug with a slowly dissolving material, or incorporating it into a tablet with a slowly dissolving carrier (Figs 5.4A and B).

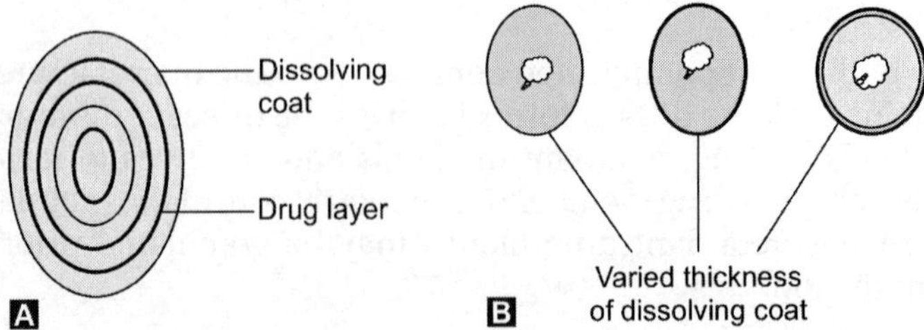


FIGURES 5.4A and B: Two types of dissolution-controlled delivery system (A) Single bead type device with alternating drug and rate controlling layer, (B) Beads containing drug with differing thickness of dissolving coats

### 3. *Osmotic controlled systems*

Osmotic pressure is employed as the driving force to generate a constant release of drug. Consider semipermeable membrane that is permeable to water, but not to drug. When this device is exposed to water or any body fluid, water will flow into the tablet owing to the osmotic pressure difference. These systems generally appear in two different forms. The first contains the drug as a solid core together with electrolyte, which is dissolved by the incoming water. The electrolyte provides the high osmotic pressure difference. The second system contains the drug in solution in an impermeable membrane within the device (Fig. 5.5).

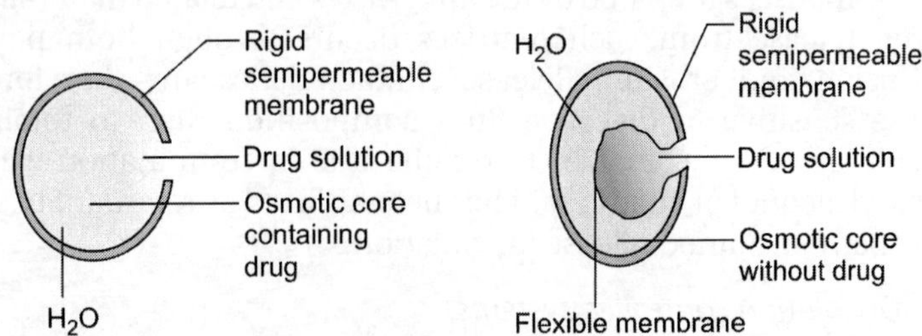


FIGURE 5.5: Diagrammatic representation of two types of osmotically controlled system

### 4. *Ion-exchange systems*

Ion-exchange systems generally use resins composed of water-insoluble cross-linked polymers. These polymers contain salt-forming functional groups in repeating positions on the polymer chain. The drug is bound to the resin and released by exchanging with appropriately charged ions in contact with the ion-exchange groups.

$$\text{Resin}^{+} \text{ - drug}^{-} + X^{-} \text{ resin}^{+} = X^{-} + \text{drug}^{-}$$

Conversely,

$$\text{Resin}^{-} \text{ - drug}^{+} + Y^{+} \text{ resin}^{-} = Y^{+} + \text{drug}^{+}$$

The free drug diffuses out of the resin. The drug-resin complex is prepared either by repeated exposure of the resin to the drug in a chromatography column, or by prolonged contact in solution.

*5. Swelling and expansion systems (hydrogels)*

Conventional hydrogels swell slowly upon contact with water due to their small pore size, which usually ranges in the nanometers and low-micrometer scale. However, if the hydrogel has a pore size of more than 100 μm, swelling is much faster and may lead to a large increase in size. Swelling ratios of over 100 can be achieved. These swollen systems become too large to pass through the pylorus and thus may be retained in the stomach even after housekeeper wave, provided they have a sufficiently high mechanical strength to withstand the peristaltic movement in the antrum of the stomach.

*6. Muco (Bio) adhesive drug delivery systems*

Mucosal drug delivery technologies are expanding exponentially with applications in every imaginable route of administration. Because of the indisputable therapeutic benefit this delivery system brings benefits include site-specific targeting, less frequent dosing and maintaining effective plasma concentration without increased consumption.

Bioadhesion may be defined as the state in which two materials, at least one of which is of a biological nature, are held together for extended period of time by interfacial forces. For drug delivery purposes, the term bioadhesion implies attachment of a drug carrier system to a specific biological location. The biological surface can be epithelial tissues, or the mucous coat on the surface of a tissue. If adhesive attachment is to a mucous coat, the phenomenon is referred as mucoadhesion (Fig. 5.6).

The mucosal layer lines a number of the body including the gastrointestinal tract, urogenital tract, ear, nose and eye. These represent potential sites for the attachment of any bioadhesive system and hence, the mucoadhesive drug delivery system includes the following:

a. Buccal delivery system
b. Oral delivery system
c. Vaginal delivery system
d. Rectal delivery system
e. Nasal delivery system
f. Ocular delivery system.

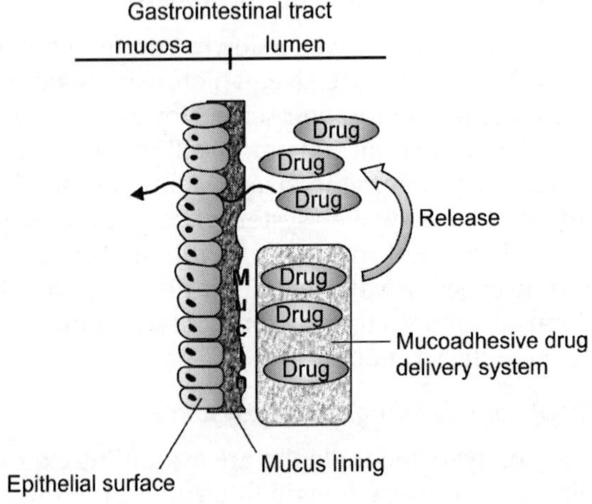


FIGURE 5.6: Diagrammatic representation of bioadhesive or mucoadhesive systems

### *7. Gastroretentive drug delivery systems*

Oral sustained drug delivery system is complicated by limited gastric residence times (GRTs). Rapid GI transit can prevent complete drug release in the absorption zone and reduce the efficacy of the administered dose since the majority of drugs are absorbed in stomach or the upper part of small intestine. To overcome these limitations, various approaches which have been proposed to increase gastric residence of drug delivery systems in the upper part of the gastrointestinal tract, includes floating drug dosage systems (FDDS), swelling or expanding systems, mucoadhesive systems, modified-shape systems, high-density system and other delayed gastric emptying devices. Among these systems, FDDS has been most commonly used.

Dosage forms that can be retained in the stomach are called gastroretentive drug delivery systems (GRDDS). GRDDS can improve the controlled delivery of drugs that have an absorption window by continuously releasing the drug for a prolonged period of time before it reaches its absorption site (Figs 5.7A and B), thus ensuring its optimal bioavailability. GRDDS provides a rational approach to enhanced bioavailability and improve pharmacokinetic and pharmacodynamic profile is to retain the drug reservoir above its absorption area, i.e. in the stomach and to release the drug in a controlled manner, so as to achieve a zero order kinetic (i.e. oral infusion) for a prolong period of time. Another group of drugs that can benefit from retained and controlled release in the stomach are those which are meant for the treatment of pathologies located in the stomach, the duodenum or the small intestine. Gastroretentive systems can remain in the gastric region for several hours and hence significantly prolong the gastric residence time of drugs. Prolonged gastric retention improves bioavailability, reduces drug waste and improves solubility for drugs that are less soluble in a high pH environment. It has applications also for local drug delivery to the stomach and proximal small intestines. Gastro-retention helps to provide better availability of new products with new therapeutic possibilities and substantial benefits for patients.

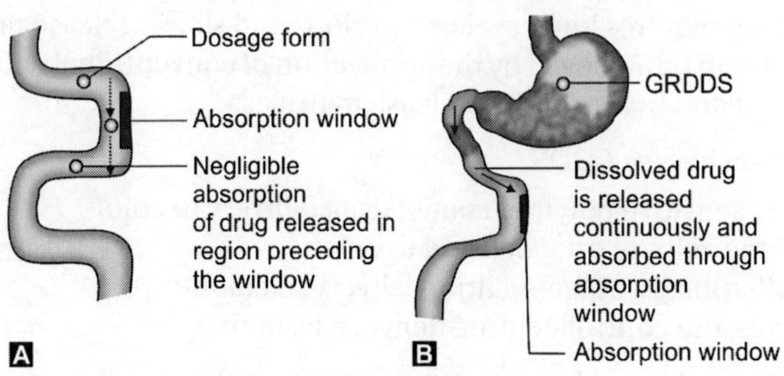


FIGURES 5.7A and B: Drug absorption in the case of (A) Conventional dosage forms (B) Gastroretentive drug delivery systems

Several approaches have been developed to prolong the residence time of drug delivery system in the gastrointestinal tract:

- **High density approach**: In this approach, the density of the pellets must exceed that of normal stomach content and should, therefore, be at least 1–4 gm/cm.
- **Low density approach**: Globular shells which have an apparent density lower than that of gastric fluid can be used as a carrier of drug for sustained release purpose.

*8. Colon specific drug delivery systems*

The colon is advisable site where both local or systemic drug delivery can be achieved. The topical treatment of inflammatory bowel disease (IBD) includes ulcerative colitis or Crohn's disease, irritable bowel syndrome, etc. Colon specific drug delivery is having capability to protect the drug from the acidic environment and the release of drug is only possible at the colonic environment. The use of hydrophilic gums which degrade in the colon helps in release of drug from the formulation. The colon is believed to be an absorption site for proteins and peptide drugs and protects them from the enzymatic degradation in duodenum and jejunum. Among all the routes being used, oral route is preferable route for colon specific drug delivery. The colon has a long retention time and appears highly responsive to agents that enhance the absorption of poorly absorbed drugs.

To achieve the successful colon drug delivery a drug need to be protected from the environment of upper GIT. Colon drug delivery requires longer release periods and slower release rates, which can be achieved by the application of conventional enteric coating and by use of slow release matrices.

Approaches for CDDS

1. pH sensitive polymer coated drug delivery to colon
2. Time-release drug delivery to colon
3. Microbially triggered drug delivery to colon
4. Pressure controlled drug delivery systems.

1. **pH- and time-dependent systems**: A multiparticulate dosage form was prepared to deliver active molecules to colonic region, which combines pH dependent and controlled drug

release properties. Enteric coating has traditionally been used to prevent drug release in the upper GI tract.

2. **Microbially controlled systems**: Natural hydrophilic polymer includes chondroitin sulfate, guar gum, pectin and dextran are commonly useful in this system, all of which undergo microbial degradation at colonic environment where the site is rich of microbial load.
3. **Pressure controlled drug delivery systems**: Such systems develop pressure controlled drug delivery, where the release of drug takes place as a result of peristalsis. It is the pressure difference which makes the release of the drug only at the site of colon, as low pressure existing in the small intestine prevents the drug release. Here, the drug is placed in the form of liquid into the ethylcellulose capsules, whose thickness is the major factor for the disintegration.

## PARENTERAL CONTROLLED DRUG DELIVERY SYSTEMS

### Introduction

The parenteral administration route is the most effective and common form of delivery for active drug substances with poor bioavailability and the drugs with a narrow therapeutic index. Drug delivery technology that can reduce the total number of injection throughout the drug therapy period will be truly advantageous not only in terms of compliance, but also to improve the quality of the therapy and also may reduce the dosage frequency. Such reduction in frequency of drug dosing is achieved by the use of specific formulation technologies that guarantee the release of the active drug substance in a slow and predictable manner.

A number of technological advances have been made in the area of parenteral drug delivery, leading to the development of sophisticated systems that allow drug targeting and the sustained or controlled release of parenteral medicines. Parenteral formulations, particularly intravascular ones, offer a unique opportunity for direct access to the bloodstream and rapid onset of drug action as well as target to specific organ and tissue sites.

**Ideal properties of parenteral controlled drug delivery system:**

a. Safe from accidental release
b. Simple to administer and remove

c. Inert
d. Biocompatible
e. Mechanically strong
f. Comfortable for the patient
g. Capable of achieving high drug loading
h. Readily processable
i. Easy to fabricate and sterilize
j. Free of leachable impurities.

*Advantages*

a. Convenience
b. Compliance potential for controlled release
c. Avoiding the peak (risk of toxicity) at troughs (risk of ineffectiveness of conventional therapy)
   i. Reducing the dosing frequency
   ii. Increasing patient compliance
d. Improved drug delivery
e. Flexibility.

*Disadvantages*

a. Invasive
b. Danger of device failure
c. Limited to potent drug
d. Commercial disadvantage.

## Polymers used in parenteral controlled drug delivery system

Generally, biodegradable polymers are used for the preparation of parenteral controlled drug delivery system as it gets degraded in the body and hence does not require removal from the body. Biodegradable polymers investigated for controlled drug delivery are polylactide/polyglycolide polymers, polyanhydrides, polycaprolactone, polyorthoesters, pseudopolyamino acid, polyphosphazenes and natural polymers.

*Desirable characteristics of an ideal parenteral drug carrier*:

a. Versatility in that carrier can deliver a variety of agents.
b. High capacity to carry a sufficient quantity of drug per unit carrier to release therapeutic concentration to the target site without excessively loading host with the carrier.
c. Restricting drug distribution to the desired target tissue.

d. Uniform distribution within the capillary vasculature of the target tissue.
e. Affording drug ready access to the parenchyma of target tissue.
f. Restricting drug activity at the target site over a prolonged period.
g. Minimizing systemic drug release during intravascular transit.
h. Protecting drug from inactivation by plasma enzymes.
i. Being biocompatible and minimally antigenic.
j. Undergoing biologic degradation with prompt elimination and minimal toxicity of the breakdown products.

### Classification of parenteral controlled drug delivery system

1. Injectables (depot)
   I. Solution
   II. Colloidal dispersion
      a. Liposome
      b. Noisome
      c. Polymeric/mixed micelle
      d. Nanoparticle
         i. Nanosuspension
         ii. Nanoemulsion
         iii. Solid lipid nanoparticle
   III. Microparticle
      a. Microsphere
      b. Microcapsule
      c. Microemulsion
   IV. Resealed erythrocytes
2. Implants
3. Infusion devices
   a. Osmotic pumps
   b. Vapor pressure powered pumps
   c. Battery powdered pumps.

### Parenteral depot system (PDS)

**Depot**: Long-acting parenteral drug formulation, designed ideally to provide slow constant, sustained, prolonged action.

*Reason for development of PDS*

1. No surgical removal of depleted system is required as it is metabolized in nontoxicological byproduct.
2. The drug release from this system can be controlled by following:
   – Diffusion of drug through the polymer.
   – Erosion of the polymer surface with concomitant release of physically entrapped drug.
   – Cleavage of covalent bond between the polymer bulks or at the surface followed by diffusional drug loss.
   – Diffusion controlled release at the physically entrapped drug with bioadsorption of the polymer until drug depletion.

*Approaches used in depot formulation:*

1. Use of low aqueous soluble salt.
2. Use of largest particle with crystallinity.
3. The suspension of the drug particle in vegetable oil and specially of gels with substances such as aluminum monasteries produces prolonged absorption rates.

*Mechanism of controlled drug release based depot formulations*:

On the basis of different mechanism, depot formulation categories are divided into four types:

1. Dissolution controlled depot formulation
2. Adsorption type depot formulation
3. Encapsulation type depot formulation
4. Esterification type depot formulation.

*1. Dissolution controlled depot formulations*

In this depot formulation, the rate limiting step of drug absorption is the dissolution of drug particles in the formulation or in the tissue fluid surrounding the drug formulation. So drug absorption can control by slow dissolution of drug particle. The rate of drug dissolution (Q/t)d under sink conditions is defined by

$$(Q/t)d = S_a D_s C_s / hd$$

Where $S_a$ is the surface area of the drug particles in contact with the medium; $D_s$ is the diffusion coefficient of drug molecules in the medium; $C_s$ is the saturation solubility of drug in the medium and hd is the thickness of the hydrodynamic diffusion layer surrounding each of the drug particle.

Basically, two approaches can be utilized to control the dissolution of drug particle to prolong the absorption and hence the therapeutic activity of the drug.

i. *Formation of salt or complexes with low aqueous solubility*: For example, preparations of penicillin G procaine ($C_s$ = 4 mg/ml) and penicillin G benzathine ($C_s$ = 0.2 mg/ml) from the highly water-soluble alkali salts of penicillin G and preparations of naloxone pamoate and naltrexone-zinc-tannate from the water-soluble hydrochloride salts of naloxone and naltrexone respectively.
ii. *Suspension of Macrocrystals*: Macrocrystals (large crystals) are known to dissolve more slowly than microrystals (small crystals). This is called the macrocrystal principle and can be applied to control the rate of drug dissolution. For example, the aqueous suspension of testosterone isobutyrate for intramuscular administration.

### 2. *Adsorption type depot preparation*

This depot preparation is formed by the binding of drug molecules to adsorbents. In this case only the unbound, free species of the drug is available for absorption. As soon as the unbound drug molecules are absorbed a fraction of the bound drug molecules is released to maintain equilibrium. This depot preparation is exemplified by vaccine preparations in which the antigens are bound to highly dispersed aluminum hydroxide gel to sustain their release and hence prolong the duration of stimulation of antibody formation.

### 3. *Encapsulation type depot preparations*

This depot preparation is prepared by encapsulating drug solids within a permeation barrier or dispersing drug particles in a diffusion matrix. The release of drug molecule is controlled by the rate of permeation across the permeation barrier and the rate of biodegradation of the barrier macromolecules. Both permeation barrier and diffusion matrix are fabricated from biodegradable or bioabsorbable macromolecules, such as gelatin, dextran, polylactic acid, lactide-glycolide copolymers, phospholipids and long-chain fatty acids and glycerides. For examples naltrexone pamoate-releasing biodegradable microcapsule, liposomes and norethindrone-releasing biodegradable lactide-glycolide copolymer beads.

*4. Esterification type depot preparations*

This depot preparation is produced by esterifying a drug to form a bioconvertible prodrug-type ester and then formulating it in an injectable formulation. This chemical approach depends upon number of enzyme (esterase) present at the injection site. This formulation forms a drug reservoir at the site of injection. The rate of drug absorption is controlled by the interfacial partitioning of drug esters from the reservoir to the tissue fluid and the rate of bioconversion of drug esters to regenerate active drug molecules. It is exemplified by the fluphenazine enanthate, nandrolone decanoate in oleaginous solution.

*Classification of depot systems*

1. Injectables
   I. **Solutions**: Both aqueous as well as oil solutions may be used for parenteral controlled drug release. With aqueous solutions (given IM), the drug release may be controlled in three ways:
      - By increasing the viscosity of vehicle by use of MC, CMC, or PVP and thus, decreasing molecular diffusion and localizing the injected drug.
      - By forming a complex with macromolecules like MC, CMC, or PVP from which the drug dissociates at a controlled rate (only free drug will get absorbed).
      - By forming complexes that control drug release not by dissociation but by reducing the solubility of parent drug, e.g. protamine zinc insulin and cyanocobalamin zinc tannate.

   Oil solutions control the release by partitioning the drug out of the oil in the surrounding aqueous biofluids. Vegetable oils like arachis oil, cottonseed oil, etc. are used for such a purpose. The method is applicable only to those drugs which are oil-soluble and have optimum partition coefficient.

   II. **Colloidal dispersions**
      a. **Liposomes**: Liposomes are formed by the self-assembly of phospholipid molecules in an aqueous

environment. The amphiphilic phospholipid molecules form a closed bilayer sphere in an attempt to shield their hydrophobic groups from the aqueous environment while still maintaining contact with the aqueous phase via the hydrophilic head group (Fig. 5.8). When suitably dispersed they consist of a series of concentric bilayers alternating with aqueous compartments. Water or lipid soluble substances can be entrapped within their aqueous or lipid phase respectively. Depending on the phospholipids used and the ionic composition of the medium, liposomes of various sizes and shapes can be obtained. Furthermore, antibodies can be covalently coupled to liposomes to enhance their cell specificity.

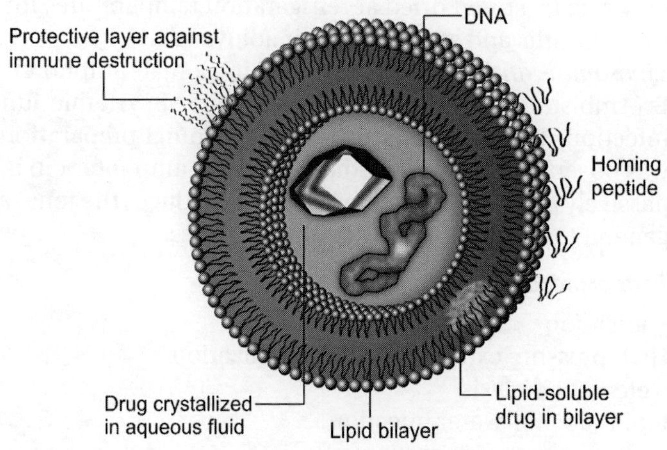


FIGURE 5.8: Liposome structure

*Applications*

a. *Liposomal anticancer agent*: The use of liposomes as anticancer drug delivery systems was originally hampered by the realization that liposomes are rapidly cleared from the circulation and largely taken up by the liver macrophage. It was observed that doxorubicin-loaded stealth liposomes circulate for prolonged periods, accumulate and extravagate within tumors and also improve tumoricidal activity in mice. In one study, it has been reported that in patients, liposomal doxorubicin accumulates within Kaposi's sarcoma lesions and produces a good therapeutic response. Liposomal doxorubicin is now licensed as Caelyx for the treatment of Kaposi's sarcoma. This formulation is currently in clinical trials for ovarian cancer and could be approved shortly for use in ovarian cancer patients who have failed to respond to paclitaxel and cisplatin.

b. *Liposomes as vaccine adjuvants*: Liposomal vaccines can be made by associating microbes, soluble antigens, cytokines, or DNA with liposomes, the latter stimulating an immune response on expression of the antigenic protein. Liposomes encapsulating antigens are subsequently encapsulated within alginate lysine microcapsules to control the antigen release and to improve the antibody response. Liposomal vaccines may also be stored dried at refrigeration temperatures for up to 12 months and still retain their adjuvanticity.

c. *Liposomal anti-infective agents*: Liposomal amphotericin B (Ambisome) is used for the treatment of systemic fungal infection. This is the first licensed liposomal preparation. It was observed in one study that liposomal amphotericin B, by passively targeting the liver and spleen, reduces the renal and general toxicity of the drug at normal doses.

*Methods of preparation*

a. Sonication
b. High pressure extrusion or homoginization
c. Detergent dialysis
d. Lipid-alcohol-water injection
e. Reverse phase evaporation
f. Dehydration-rehydration.

b. **Niosomes**: Niosomes are nonionic surfactant vesicles obtained on hydration of synthetic nonionic surfactants of the alkyl or dialkyl polyglycerol ether class, with or without incorporation of cholesterol or other lipids. These are bilayered structure which can entrap both hydrophilic and lipophilic drugs either in an aqueous layer or in vesicular membrane, made up of lipids (Fig. 5.9). Niosomal dispersion in an aqueous phase can be emulsified in a nonaqueous phase to regulate the delivery rate of drug and administer normal vesicle in external nonaqueous phase.

Various drugs incorporated into niosomes by different methods are shown in Table 5.1.

**Table 5.1**: Drugs incorporated into noisome by various methods

| *Method of preparation* | *Drugs incorporated* |
|---|---|
| Ether injection | Doxorubicin, sodium stibogluconate |
| Hand shaking | Methotrexate |
| Sonication | Vasopressin, estradiol, 8-arginine, 9-desglycinamide |

*Advantages of niosomes (Fig. 5.9)*

- They entrap solute in a manner analogous to liposomes.
- They are osmotically active and stable.
- Handling and storage of surfactants require no special conditions.
- They possess an infrastructure consisting of hydrophobic and hydrophilic moieties together and as a result can accommodate drug molecules with a wide range of solubilities.
- They exhibit flexibility in their structural characteristics (composition, fluidity and size) and can be designed according to desired application.
- They improve oral bioavailability of poorly absorbed drugs and enhance skin penetration of drugs.
- They allow their surface for attachment of hydrophilic group and can incorporate hydrophilic moieties in bilayer to bring about changes in their in vivo behavior.
- The surfactants are biodegradable, biocompatible and nonimmunogenic.

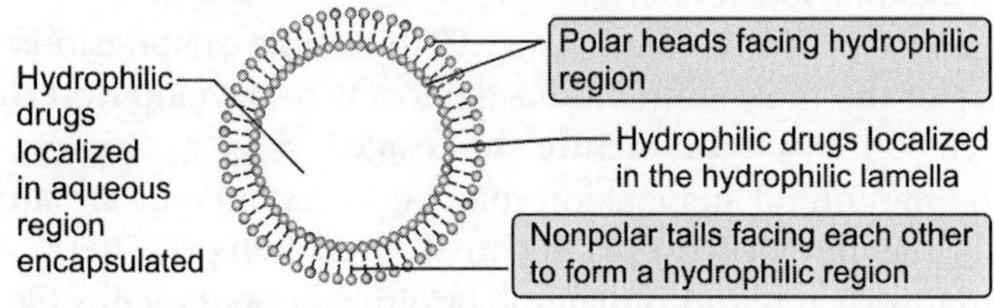


Figure 5.9: Niosome structure

- They improve the therapeutic performance of the drug molecules by delaying the clearance from the circulation, protecting the drug from biological environment, and restricting effects to target cells.

**c. Polymeric/mixed micelles**

Polymeric micelles are nanosized core/shell assemblies of amphiphilic block copolymers that are suitable for the delivery of hydrophobic and amphiphilic agents. Among different micelle-forming block copolymers, those with poly ethylene oxide (PEO) as the shell forming block and poly(l-amino acid)s (PLAA) s and poly(ester)s as the core forming block are most popular in drug development. Hydrophobic core of polymeric micelles provides an excellent host for the incorporation and stabilization of anticancer agents that are mostly hydrophobic. Nanosize of these micelles enables them to escape the phagocytic effects of reticuloendothelial system (RES), enhance their circulation life and penetration into tumor tissues.

**d. Nanoparticles**

*i. Nanosuspension*

A nanosuspension is a submicron colloidal dispersion of drug particles that are produced by suitable methods and stabilized by surfactants. A pharmaceutical nanosuspension can be defined as the nano-sized drug particle which is finely dispersed in an aqueous vehicle for either oral and topical use or parenteral and pulmonary administration. In general, the particle size in nanosuspension is always less than 1µm (usually lies between 200–600 nm).

*Characteristics of nanosuspension*

- They should be sterile, pyrogen free, stable, resuspendable, syringable, injectable, isotonic and nonirritating.
- Because of above requirements injectable suspensions are one of the most difficult dosage forms to develop in term of their stability, manufacture and usage.
- The parenteral suspension may be formulated as already to use injection or require a reconstitution step prior to use.
- They are usually administered by either subcutaneous (SC) or intramuscular nerve suspension delivery systems containing

drug in microparticulate or nanoparticle can be injected by intravenously or intra-arterially.

- These suspensions usually contain between 0.5% and 5.0% solid and should have particle size less than 5 μm for IM or SC administration.
- Certain antibiotic preparation (for example, procaine, Penicillin G) may contain upto 30% solids.

*Preparation of nanosuspension*

Nanosuspension is generally prepared by two methods that are "Bottom up technology" and "Top down technology". "Bottom up technology" follows precipitation method where the drug is dissolved in a solvent, which is then added to a nonsolvent which precipitates crystals. Precipitation technique uses simple and low cost equipments. The basic challenge of this technique is that during the precipitation procedure the growing of the drug crystals needs to be controlled by addition of surfactant to avoid formation of microparticles. The limitation of this technique lies, in the fact, that the drug needs to be soluble in at least one solvent and this solvent needs to be miscible with the nonsolvent. Moreover, precipitation technique is not applicable to drugs, which are simultaneously poorly soluble in aqueous and nonaqueous media. Some nanosuspensions of carbamazepine, cyclosporin, griseofulvin and retinoic acid have already been developed by precipitation method.

The "Top down technology" follows the method of disintegration which is preferred over the conventional precipitation technology. Technologies like media milling (nanocrystals), high pressure homogenization in water (dissocubes), high pressure homogenization in nonaqueous media (nanopure), combination of precipitation and high-pressure homogenization (nanoedge) and others like emulsion solvent diffusion method and microemulsion as templates are various examples of "Top down technology".

- Media milling
- Emulsion method
- Nanojet technology
- Nanoedge technology

– High pressure homogenization
– Microemulsion template
– Dry cogrinding
– Supercritical fluid method.

*Application of nanosuspension as parenteral administration*

Nanosuspension can be delivered either intra-articular or intravenous route. But in case of parenteral administration, solute should be remained in solubilized form or particle or globule size below 5 μm to avoid capillary blockage. Some current approaches have come to resolve the drawbacks of poorly soluble drug for parenteral delivery. These are salt formation, solubilization using cosolvent, miceller solution, complexation with cyclodextrin and vesicular system (liposome and transfersome). In recent time, vesicular systems like liposome have been accepted for parenteral delivery but they have some limitations in terms of physical instability, high manufacturing cost and difficulties in scale-up. However, nanosuspension has still been considered as a useful dosage form which employs better efficacy for parenteral administered drugs. More for example, paclitaxel nanosuspension has been found better responses in treating tumor than taxol.

*ii. Nanoemulsion/Microemulsion*

Nanoemulsion/microemulsion are liquid dispersions of water and oil that are made homogeneous, transparent (or translucent) and thermodynamically stable by the addition of relatively large amounts of a surfactant and a cosurfactant and having diameter of the droplets in the range of 100–1000 A (10–100 nm).

*Components of nanoemulsion*: The main three components of nanoemulsions are as follows:

1. Oil-like myristic acid isopropyl ester, glyceryl tricaprylate (Tricaprylin), glyceryl tricaprylate/caprate
2. Surfactant/cosurfactant
3. Aqueous phase-water for injection

Methods of preparation

1. High-pressure homogenisation
2. Microfluidization.

*Application*

i. They can also be used as intravenous delivery systems for the fat soluble vitamins and lipids in parenteral nutrition.
ii. They are generally not dilutable with aqueous fluids, such as certain bodily fluids and buffer solutions.
iii. They are also sensitive to temperature and are not stable outside of room temperature conditions.
iv. O/W microemulsions/nanoemulsions were characterized by their small particle size and their wide range of temperature stability, typically from about –20°–50°C. They could be administered by intravenous, intra-arterial, intrathecal, intraperitoneal, intraocular, intra-articular, intramuscular or subcutaneous injection.

*iii. Solid lipid nanoparticles (SLNs)*

Melt-emulsified nanoparticles based on lipids (or waxes) are solid at room temperature and generally prepared by hot high pressure homogenization.The concept of lipid nanoparticles for injectable delivery was developed from submicron sized parenteral fat o/w emulsion used for parenteral nutrition, viz intralipid in 1960s. This gave birth to the idea of encapsulating lipophilic drugs into oil droplets. The only drawback associated with these submicron emulsions was the low viscosity of the droplets, causing fast release and susceptibility of the incorporated actives towards degradation by the aqueous continuous phase.

SLNs are colloidal particles composed of a biocompatible/biodegradable lipid matrix that is solid at body temperature and exhibit size range in between 100 and 400 nm.

*Advantages*

- Particulate nature.
- Amenability to encapsulate hydrophilic and hydrophobic drugs.
- Ability to sustain the release of incorporated drug.
- Ability to prevent chemical, photochemical, or oxidative degradation of drug.
- Ability to immobilize drug in the solid matrix.
- Ease of scale-up and manufacture.
- Low cost of solid lipids as compared with phospholipids and biodegradable polymers.

*Application of lipid nanoparticles for parenteral drug delivery*

i. *Treatment of cancer*: SLN have been shown to improve the efficacy and residence time of the cytotoxic drugs, with concomitant reduction in the side effects associated with them. The salient features of SLN which make them a suitable carrier for antitumor drug delivery, are their ability to encapsulate antitumor agents of diverse physiochemical properties, improved stability of the drug, less in vitro toxicity, enhanced drug efficacy and improved pharmacokinetics.

ii. *Transfection*: Cationic SLN have been shown to be efficacious in transfecting $COS^{-1}$ cells in vitro. These, 100 nm SLN were able to bind deoxyribonucleic acid (DNA) to form a stable complex of 300–800 nm size. The transfection efficacy was determined using $COS^{-1}$ cells.

iii. *Liver targeting*: Particulate carriers (including SLN) usually accumulate in the liver by passive targeting on parenteral administration. However, passive targeting leads to entrapment of the drug in the Kupffer cells and not in the hepatocytes, which is the major target for the treatment of hepatic diseases such as cancers. Hence, for liver targeting, SLN containing galactosylated or mannosylated lipids are employed.

iv. *Targeting the central nervous system*: Various drugs ranging from antipsychotics, antiparkinson, anti-ischemic to antibiotics have been encapsulated in lipid nanoparticles with the aim to either modify the biodistribution or for brain targeting. Recently, potential of surface-modified SLN has been demonstrated in the treatment of brain diseases such as cerebral malaria. Fabricated transferrin-conjugated SLN and studied their ability to target quinine hydrochloride to brain by studying biodistribution.

v. *Treatment of cardiovascular diseases*: Tanshinone IIA, a lipophilic natural drug product, has the ability to dilate coronary arteries and increase myocardial contractility. Liu and coworkers studied the ability of SLN to improve the delivery of Tanshinone IIA by in vitro and in vivo studies.

vi. *Treatment of parasitic diseases*: Antiparasitic agents represent a class of drugs which had been neglected as a model for drug delivery systems for a long time. As compared with other therapeutic agents, relatively fewer reports are published on the delivery of antiparasitic agents. Transferrin-conjugated SLN of quinine dihydrochloride, an antimalarial drug, was prepared to target it to the brain for the management of cerebral malaria.

vii. *Treatment of rheumatoid arthritis*: SLN by passive targeting were shown to enhance the therapeutic efficacy with concomitant reduction in the various adverse effects such as nephrotoxicity and gastrointestinal disorders.

*iv. Nanostructured lipid carriers (NLC)*

NLC are oil loaded solid-lipid nanoparticles. NLC offers several advantages over SLN such as:

- Greater degree of drug loading
- Reduced burst release of drug
- Better control of drug release.

*v. Lipid drug conjugate (LDC) nanoparticles*

Covalent bonding or salt formation of a hydrophilic drug with lipid is done to:

- Enhance in vivo stability
- Improve membrane permeability
- Control drug release.

## III. **Microparticles**

### a. Microspheres

Microspheres are free flowing powders consisting of spherical particles of size ideally less than 125 μm that can be suspended in a suitable aqueous vehicle and injected by an 18 or 20 number needle. Each particle is basically a matrix of drug dispersed in a polymer form which release occurs by a first order process. The polymers used are biocompatible and biodegradable, e.g. PLA, PLGA, etc. Drug release is controlled by dissolution/degradation of matrix. Small matrices release drug at a faster rate and thus, by using particles of different sizes, various degrees of controlled-release can be achieved.

The system is ideally suited for controlled-release of peptide/protein drugs such as LHRH which have short half-lives and otherwise need to be injected once or more, daily, as conventional parenteral formulations. In comparison to peptides, proteins are difficult to formulate because of their higher molecular weight, lower solubility and the need to preserve their conformational structure during manufacture. In order to overcome uptake of intravenously administered microsphere by the RES and promote drug targeting to tumors with good perfusion, magnetic microspheres were developed. They are prepared from albumin and magnetite ($Fe_2O_3$) and have a size of 1.0 µm to permit intravascular injection. The system is infused into an artery that perfuses the target site and a magnet is placed over the area to localize it in that region. Magnetic microspheres have specifically been used to target anticancer drug such as doxorubicin to tumors and as diagnostics/contrast agent for magnetic resonances imaging (MRI).

*Disadvantages of microspheres for controlled release parenterals include*:

- Difficulty of removal from the site
- Low drug loading (maximum of 50%)
- Possible drug degradation within the microspheres
- Changes in drug crystallinity or polymorphic form during microsphere processing.

### b. Microcapsules

Drug is centrally located within the polymeric shell of finite thickness and release may be controlled by dissolution, diffusion or both. Quality microcapsules with thick walls generally release their medicaments at a zero order rate. Steroids, peptides and antineoplastic have been successfully administered parenterally by use of controlled release microcapsules. The methods used for preparing microcapsules (for parenterally or per-os delivery) can be classified into two categories:

1. **Type A processes**: These are defined as those in which capsule formation occurs entirely in a liquid filled stirred tank or tubular reactor, e.g.
   - Complex coacervation
   - Polymer incompatibility
   - In situ polymerization

- Solvent evaporation or in liquid drying
- Submerged nozzle extrusion.

2. **Type B processes**: These are processes in which capsule formation occurs because a coating is sprayed or deposited in some manner onto the surface of a liquid or solid core material dispersed in a gas phase or vacuum, e.g.
   - Spray drying
   - Fluidized bed coating
   - Centrifugal extrusion
   - Extrusion or spraying into a desolvation bath
   - Rotational suspension separation (spinning disk).

IV. **Resealed erythrocytes**

Drug is loaded into body's own erythrocytes when used to serve as controlled delivery systems.

*Advantages*

- Fully biodegradable, biocompatible and nonimmunogenic.
- Longer lifespan in circulation
- Drug protected from enzymatic inactivation
- Ability to target the organs of the RES.

Drug loading can be done by immersing the cell in buffered hypotonic solution of drug which causes them to rupture and release hemoglobin and trap the medicament. On restoration of isotonicity and incubation at 37°C, the cells reseal and are ready for use upon reinjection; the drug loaded erythrocytes serve as slow circulating depots. Damaged erythrocytes are removed by the liver and spleen. These organs can, thus be specifically targeted by drug loaded erythrocytes and is used in the therapy such as enzyme replacement, treating liver tumors, eradication of parasites, etc.

2. Implants

Implants are generally cylindrical devices injected into the subcutaneous tissue with a large bore needle (trocar). Comparing to other controlled delivery devices, these formulations have the advantages that they can be designed and prepared easily and with high uniformity. A major disadvantage is the need of a painful injection for their application. Implants are manufactured by standard techniques such as extrusion, melt compression, or injection molding. In these cases, the drug is distributed in a melt of biodegradable polymer and subsequently the device is formed. For most biodegradable polyesters temperature between 80°C and 175°C is necessary for manufacturing implants. This high temperature may affect the polymer stability and encapsulated active ingredients specially for labile macromolecules.

Despite these disadvantages, implants are useful tools for systemic and local drug delivery. For example, sustained systemic delivery of LH-RH agonists, somatostatin analogue and sustained local delivery of anesthetics, antibiotics have been achieved using biodegradable polymer implant systems. PLGA based implant systems for controlled delivery of LH-RH agonists are available on the market under the brand names Zoladex® and Profact® for treatment of prostate cancer. They are manufactured by a melt extrusion method.

*Advantages*

i. Improved control of drug level at the specific site of action.
ii. Preservation of the medication that are rapidly destroyed but the body.
iii. Less fluctuation in plasma drug level during therapy.
iv. Possible reduction in therapy costs because patient care and the potentially lower drug dose required.
v. Improved special compliance.
vi. Administration of drugs with short biological half-life may be facilitated.
vii. Minimal harmful side effect of systemic administration through local therapy.

*Disadvantages*

i. Toxicity or lack of biocompatibility of the material used for the implant.
ii. Harmful by product may be formed from the system, particularly for biodegradable types.
iii. Dose dumping and variable imprecise drug release may occur if not formulated properly.
iv. Pain and discomfort may be caused by the presence of implant.

v. These systems can be more expensive than the conventional dosage form.
vi. Most implantable controlled drug delivery system requires minor surgery to implant and to remove from the administered site, if it is not biodegradable type.
vii. Possibility of the tissue and the body reaction to implant.
viii. Danger of toxic effect in case of leakage or burst release of drug.

### Mechanism of drug released from implantable therapeutic system:

A. Controlled drug released by diffusion:
   – Membrane permeation-controlled drug delivery
   – Matrix diffusion-controlled drug delivery
   – Microreservoir dissolution controlled drug delivery.
B. Controlled drug release by activation:
   – Osmotic pressure activated drug delivery
   – Magnetism activated drug delivery
   – Ultrasound activated drug delivery
   – Vapor pressure activated drug delivery
   – Hydrolysis activated drug delivery.

#### *Polymers used for implants*

Many polymers can be used to prepare rate-limiting membrane for controlled release; few are employed for implantation purpose. The polymer used should be biocompatible and sterilizable implantable polymers can be classified into biodegradable and nonbiodegradable polymers. Nonpolymeric material such as fatty substance like cholesterol and metal like titanium, stainless steel may be used in implantation device. Nonbiodegradable polymers like silicon polymers, cellulose acetate and polyethylene vinyl acetate are used.

**Silicone polymers**: Silicone polymers are widely used in controlled drug delivery. They provide advantages like biocompatibility resistance to heat sterilization, high permeability for lipophilic drugs. Therapeutic products prepared with silicon elastomers includes: Norplant, a subdermal implant to deliver levonorgestrel for contraception, a dual-release vaginal ring.

**Polyethylene vinyl acetate**: Ethylene vinyl acetate copolymer is used in the Alza ocular insert and in IUD reservoir type system (Progestasert).

**Cellulose acetate**: Cellulose derivatives are used in controlled drug delivery devices. Application to implants is restricted to cellulose acetate. Cellulose acetate is formed by the acetylation of hydroxyl groups in glucose.

## Classification of implants

Implants can be classified as:

### *i. Solid implants*

Solid implants typically exhibit biphasic release kinetics, with initial burst of drug. It is usually due to the release of drug deposited on the surface of the implant. Although zero order kinetics may be achieved by, e.g. coating the implant drug impermeable material. Overall drug release may be controlled by varying polymer composition, an increase in the level of lactic acid in a polylactic acid coglycolic acid copolymer retards drug release and increase in polymer molecular weight also retards drug release and prolongs drug effects.

In order to achieve high drug doses in traditionally inaccessible areas such as CNS, bone tissue and beyond the blood retinal barrier implants could effectively be used clinically. Ethylene vinyl acetate copolymer dexamethasone intracranial base implants produce high drug levels in brain with plasma levels remain normal. Additionally polylactic acid coglycolic acid sclera implants containing ganciclovir for the treatment of cytomegalovirus infection could maintain effective therapeutic levels of the drug in vitreous humor and retina/choroid for over a period of 3–5 months. It is concluded that implant systems offer a means of achieving high drug concentration in areas that are usually inaccessible to peripherally or vascularly administered drug. In addition, the high drug levels are maintained in sustained manner in these areas.

### *ii. In situ forming implants*

Biodegradable injectable in situ forming drug delivery systems represent an attractive alternative to microspheres and implants as parenteral depot systems. The controlled release of bioactive macromolecules via semisolid in situ forming systems has a number of advantages, such as:

- Ease of administration
- Less complicated fabrication
- Less stressful manufacturing conditions for sensitive drug molecules.

From a manufacturing point of view, in situ forming depot systems offer the advantage that they are relatively simple to manufacture from polymers adapted for this approach. Compared with microspheres, which have to be washed and isolated after preparation, operating expenses for the production of in situ forming applications are marginal, thus lowering investment and manufacturing costs.

### Infusion devices

These are also implantable devices but are versatile in the sense that they are intrinsically powered to release the medicament at a zero-order rate and the drug reservoir can be replenished from time to time. Depending upon the mechanism by which these implantable pumps are powered to release the contents, they are classified into following types:

i. Osmotic pressure activated drug delivery systems
ii. Vapor pressure activated drug delivery systems
iii. Battery powered drug delivery systems.

#### *1. Osmotic pressure activated drug delivery systems (Osmotic pumps)*

The pump is made up of three concentric layers—The innermost drug reservoir contained in a collapsible impermeable polyester bag followed by a sleeve of dry osmotic energy source (sodium chloride) and the outer most rigid, the rate controlling semi permeable membrane fabricated from substituted cellulosic polymers. An additional component flow modulator, comprising of cap and a tube made up of stainless steel, is inserted into the body of osmotic pump after filling (Fig. 5.10).

After implantation, water from the surrounding tissue fluids is imbibed through the semipermeable membrane at a controlled rate that dissolves the osmogen creating an osmotic pressure differential across the membrane. The osmotic sleeve thus expands sand since the outer shell is rigid, it squeezes the inner flexible drug reservoir and drug solution is expelled in a constant volume per unit time fashion. The drug delivery continues until the reservoir is completely collapsed. Ionized drugs macromolecules, steroids and peptides (insulin) can be delivered by such a device.

Sodium chloride is a typical osmotic agent used in such systems. Membranes are usually constructed from cellulosic polymers. Pumps are available with a variety of delivery rates between 0.1–10 μl/hour for periods of 3 days to 4 weeks. Systems are marketed empty (Alzet osmotic pump), allowing formulation of choice of any concentration. The osmotic pump has been designed for oral, subcutaneous or rectal drug delivery and is specially well-suited for preliminary screening of new drugs in assessing their pharmacokinetic and pharmacodynamic properties. Results from the studies are invaluable in the rational development of an optimized drug delivery system.

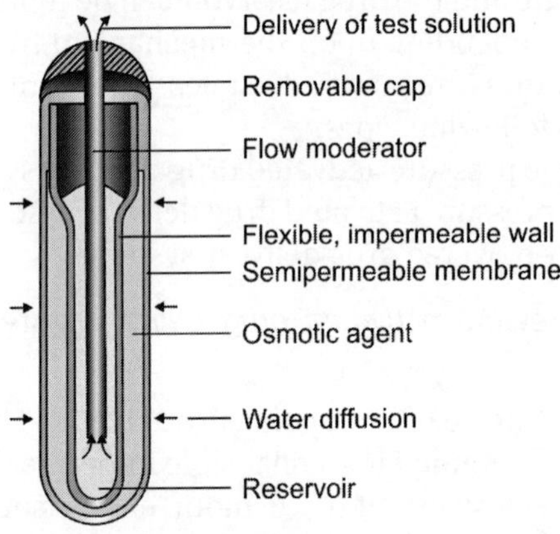


FIGURE 5.10: Osmotic pump

## Advantages

1. Osmotic pump can be used as a useful experimental tool to determine important pharmacokinetic parameters of new drugs, which ultimately find use in the development of an optimized delivery system.

2. Osmotic systems deliver the drug at zero order release kinetic, so they are superior to older sustained release technologies in many instances because of better control over their in vivo performance is possible.
3. Drug release from osmotic system is independent of variation in environment pH and hydrodynamic conditions.
4. It is possible to attain substantially higher release rates than with diffusion base drug delivery systems.
5. Osmotic systems are able to deliver very large volumes.
6. In osmotic system reformulation is not required for different drugs.

### Disadvantages

1. Osmotic system can be much more expensive than conventional systems.
2. Implantation is required for osmotic implants.
3. The drug which are unstable in solution that may be inappropriate because the drug remains in solution form for extended periods before release.

#### *2. Vapor pressure powered pump (infusaid)*

This device is based on the principle that at a given temperature, a liquid in equilibrium with its vapor phase exerts a constant pressure that is independent of enclosing volume. The disk shaped device consists of 2 chambers—An infusate chamber containing the drug solution which is separated by a freely movable flexible bellow and the vapor chamber containing inexhaustible vaporizable fluid such as fluorocarbons.

After implantation, the volatile liquid vaporizes at the body temperature and creates a vapor pressure that compresses the bellows and expels the infusate through a series of flow regulators at a constant rate. Insulin for diabetics and morphine for terminally ill cancer patients have been successfully delivered by such a device.

#### *3. Battery powered pump*

The two types of battery powered implantable programmable pumps used successfully to deliver insulin are—Peristaltic pumps and solenoid driven reciprocating pumps, both with electronic controls. The system can be programmed to deliver drug at desired rate. Their design is such that the drug moves towards the exit and there is no backflow of the infusate.

## TARGETED DRUG DELIVERY SYSTEMS

### Introduction

Targeted drug delivery system is a special form of drug delivery system where the pharmacologically active agent or medicament is selectively targeted or delivered only to its site of action or absorption and not to the nontarget organs or tissues or cells. Targeted drug delivery implies for selective and effective localization of pharmacologically active moiety at preidentified (preselected) target in therapeutic concentration, while restricting its access to nontarget normal cellular linings, thus minimizing toxic effects and maximizing therapeutic index. Targeting of drugs to special cells and tissues of the body without their becoming a part of systemic circulation is a very novel idea. If a drug can be administered in a form such that it reaches the receptor sites in sufficient concentration without disturbing in extraneous tissue cells.

Such products are prepared by considering specific properties of target cells, nature of markers or transport carriers or vehicles, which convey drug to specific receptors, ligands and physically modulated components.

*Advantages of drug targeting*

i. Drug administration protocols may be simplified.
ii. Drug quantity may be greatly reduced as well as the cost of therapy.
iii. Drug concentration in the required sites can be sharply increased without negative effects on nontarget compartments.

*Disadvantages of drug targeting*

i. Rapid clearance of targeted systems.
ii. Immune reactions against intravenous administered carrier systems.
iii. Insufficient localization of targeted systems into tumor cells.
iv. Diffusion and redistribution of released drugs.

*Ideal characteristics of targeted drug delivery system*

i. Targeted drug delivery system should be biochemically inert (nontoxic), nonimmunogenic.
ii. Both physically and chemically stable in vivo and in vitro.
iii. Restrict drug distribution to target cells or tissues or organs and should have uniform capillary distribution.
iv. Controllable and predictable rate of drug release.
v. Drug release should not affect the drug action.
vi. Therapeutic amount of drug release.
vii. Minimal drug leakage during transit.
viii. Carriers used must be biodegradable or readily eliminated from the body without any problem.
ix. The preparation of the delivery system should be easy or reasonably simple, reproductive and cost effective.

## Types of drug targeting

An ideal targeted drug delivery approach would not only increase therapeutic efficacy of drugs but also decrease the toxicity associated with drug to allow lower doses of the drug to be used in therapy. Two approaches are used—Passive targeting and active targeting.

i. **Passive targeting**: Passive targeting refers to the accumulation of drug or drug-carrier system at a particular site due to physicochemical or pharmacological factors. Drug or drug carrier nanosystems can be passively targeted making use of the pathophysiological and anatomical opportunities, e.g. include targeting of antimalarial drugs for treatment of leishmiansis, brucellosis, candiadsis.
ii. **Active targeting**: Active targeting employs specific modification of drug/drug carrier nanosystems with active agents having selective affinity for recognizing and interacting with a specific cell, tissue or organ in the body. Direct coupling of drugs to targeting ligand, restricts the coupling capacity to a few drug molecules. In contrast, coupling of drug carrier nanosystems to ligands allows import of thousands of drug molecules by means of one receptor targeted ligand. For example, active targeting is the use of monoclonal antibody of the treatment of cancer.

This active targeting approach can be further classified into three different levels of targeting:

- First order targeting, it refers to restricted distribution of the drug carrier systems to the capillary bed of a predetermined target site, organ or tissue. Examples include compartmental targeting in lymphatics, peritoneal cavity, plural cavity, cerebral ventricles, eyes, joints, etc.
- Second order targeting, selective delivery of drugs to specific cell types such as tumor cells and not to the normal cells is referred as second order targeting, For example selective drug delivery to Kupffer cells in the liver.
- Third order targeting, defined as drug delivery specifically to the intracellular site of targeted cells, e.g. receptor based ligand mediated entry of a drug complex into a cell by endocytosis.

## Drug carriers

Drug carrier is the important entity required for successful transportation of the loaded drug.

*Properties of ideal drug carriers*

i. It must be able to cross anatomical barriers and in case of tumor chemotherapy, tumor vasculature.
ii. It must be recognized specifically and selectively by the target cells and must maintain the specificity of the surface ligands.
iii. The linkage of the drug and the directing unit (ligand) should be stable in plasma, interstitial and other biofluids.
iv. Carrier should be nontoxic, nonimmunogenic and biodegradable particulate or macromolecule.
v. After recognition and internalization, the carrier system should release the drug moiety inside the target organs, tissues or cells.
vi. The biomodules used as carrier should not be ubiquitous (existing or being everywhere at the same time).

*Type of drug carriers*

- Liposomes
- Monoclonal antibodies and fragments

- Modified (plasma) proteins
- Soluble polymers
- Lipoproteins
- Microspheres and nanoparticles
- Polymeric micelles
- Cellular carriers.

*Targeting moieties*

- Antibodies
- Lectins and other proteins
- Lipoprotein
- Hormones
- Charged molecules
- Polysaccharides
- Low-molecular-weight ligands.

## Drug immobilization techniques

### *1. Liposomes*

Liposomes are small vesicles composed of unilamellar or multilamellar phospholipid bilayers surrounding one or several aqueous compartments. Charge, lipid composition and size (ranging from 20–10, 000 nm) of liposomes can be varied and these variations strongly affect their behavior in vivo. Many liposome formulations are rapidly taken up by macrophages. They are exploited either for macrophage-specific delivery of drugs or for passive drug targeting, allowing slow release of the drug overtime from these cells into the general circulation. Cationic liposomes and lipoplexes have been extensively investigated for their application in nonviral vector mediated gene therapy. The use of molecules such as polyethylene glycol (PEG) to prevent liposome recognition by phagocytic cells led to the development of so called 'stealth' liposomes with longer circulation times and increased distribution to peripheral tissues in the body. Although liposomes do not easily extravasate from the systemic circulation into the tissues, enhanced vascular permeability during an inflammatory response or proangiogenic conditions in tumors can favor local accumulation. Another approach is the design of target sensitive liposomes or fusogenic liposomes that become destabilized after binding and/or internalization to/ into the target cells.

*2. Monoclonal antibodies and fragments*

The development of monoclonal antibodies by Kohler and Milstein in 1975 passed the way to antibody therapy for disease. In the last 25 years, the number of preclinical and clinical studies with monoclonal antibodies and derivatives has greatly increased. The majority of strategies based on antigen recognition by antibodies have been developed for cancer therapy. These strategies are mostly aimed at tumor associated antigens being present on normal cells but over-expressed by tumor cells. More recently, antibodies against other molecules have been developed for clinical application. For examples, anti-TNFα antibodies for treatment of chronic inflammatory diseases and anti-VEGF (vascular endothelial growth factor) antibodies which inhibit new blood vessel formation or angiogenesis. The advent of recombinant DNA technology led to the development of antibodies and fragments that are tailored for optimal behavior in vivo. Humanized and chimeric antibodies can be constructed to circumvent the human antimouse antibody response elicited by mouse antibody treatment of patients, which severely hampers the application of these powerful molecules.

*3. Modified (plasma) proteins*

Modified plasma proteins are attractive carriers for drug targeting as they are soluble molecules with a relatively small molecular weight. They can easily be modified by covalent attachment of peptides, sugars and other ligands, as well as drugs of interest. Particularly in the case of liver cell targeting, quite extensive modifications of protein backbones, such as albumins, have been carried out.

*4. Soluble polymers*

Soluble synthetic polymers have been widely employed as versatile drug carrier systems. Polymer chemistry allows the development of tailor made conjugates in which target moieties as well as drugs are introduced into the carrier molecule. In the case of enhanced permeability retention in, e.g. tumor vasculature, the introduction of drugs into the polymer may suffice, as nonspecific adherence to cells is an undesirable property, excessive charge or hydrophobicity should be avoided in the design of polymeric carriers. For cancer therapy, the well-established N (-2-hydroxypropyl)methacrylamide (HMPA) polymers have been extensively studied.

*5. Lipoproteins*

Endogenous lipid particles such as LDL and HDL containing a lipid and apoprotein moiety can be seen as natural targeted liposomes. The lipid core can be used to incorporate lipophilic drugs or lipophilic prodrugs, covalent binding of the drug to the carrier is not necessary here. The apolipoprotein moiety of these particles can be glycosylated or modified with other (receptor) targeting ligands. Furthermore, modifications at the level of glycolipid incorporation can be employed to introduce targeting moieties. As with the liposomes, the size and charge of the particles determine their behavior in vivo. Large particles will not easily pass the endothelial barrier of organs containing blood vessels with a continuous endothelial cell lining. The majority of the research on the use of LDL and HDL particles has been devoted to the targeting of drugs to the liver.

*6. Microspheres and nanoparticles*

Microspheres and nanoparticles often consist of biocompatible polymers and belong either to the soluble or the particle type carriers. Besides the aforementioned HPMA polymeric backbone, carriers have also been prepared using dextrans, ficoll, sepharose or poly-L-lysine as the main carrier body. More recently, alginate nanoparticles have been described for the targeting of antisense oligonucleotides. As with other polymeric carrier systems, the backbone can be modified with, e.g. sugar molecules or antibody fragments to introduce cellular specificity. Nanoparticles are smaller (0.2–0.5 μm) than microspheres (30–200 μm) and may have a smaller drug loading capacity than the soluble polymers. Formulation of drugs into the nanoparticles can occur at the surface of the particles and at the inner core, depending on the physicochemical characteristics of the drug.

The site of drug incorporation significantly affects its release rate from the particle. After systemic administration they quickly distribute to and subsequently become internalized by the cells of the phagocytic system. Even coating of these carriers with PEG does not completely divert them from distribution to the phagocytes in liver and spleen. Consequently, intracellular infections in Kupffer cells and other macrophages are considered a useful target for these systems. Besides parenteral application of microspheres and nanoparticles for cell selective delivery of drugs, they have more recently been studied for their application in oral delivery of peptides and peptidomimetics.

*7. Polymeric micelles*

Polymeric micelles are characterized by a core-shell structure. They have a diblock structure with a hydrophilic shell and a hydrophobic core. The hydrophobic core generally consists of a biodegradable polymer that serves as a reservoir for an insoluble drug. If a water-soluble polymeric core is used, it is rendered hydrophobic by chemical conjugation with a hydrophobic drug. The viscosity of the micellar core may influence the physical stability of the micelles as well as drug release. The biodistribution of the micelle is mainly dictated by the nature of the shell which is also responsible for micelle stabilization and interactions with plasma proteins and cell membranes. The micelles can contain functional groups at their surface for conjugation with a targeting moiety. Polymeric micelles are mostly small (10–100 nm) in size and drugs can be incorporated by chemical conjugation or physical entrapment. For efficient delivery activity, they should maintain their integrity for a sufficient amount of time after injection into the body. Most of the experience with polymeric micelles has been obtained in the field of passive targeting of anticancer drugs to tumors.

*8. Cellular carriers*

Cellular carriers may have the advantage of their natural biocompatibility. However, they will encounter endothelial barriers and can rather easily invoke an immunological response. Most of the approaches on cellular carriers have been applied to the field of cancer therapy.

## NANOPARTICLES

### Introduction

Nanoparticles (NPs) are submicron sized polymeric colloidal particles with a therapeutic agent of interest encapsulated within their polymeric matrix or adsorbed or conjugated onto the surface. The particles size ranges from 10–1000 nm in diameter.

Recent years have witnessed unprecedented growth of research and applications in the area of nanoscience and nanotechnology. There is increasing optimism that nanotechnology, as applied to medicine, will bring significant advances in the diagnosis and treatment of disease. Anticipated applications in medicine include drug delivery, both in vitro and in vivo diagnostics, nutraceuticals and production of improved biocompatible materials. Engineered nanoparticles are an important tool to realize a number of these applications. It has to be recognized that not all particles used for medical purposes comply with the recently proposed and now generally accepted definition of a size ≤ 100 nm.

#### *Advantages*

Pharmaceutical nanoparticles are being increasingly used as drug delivery systems and have a number of advantages over more conventional delivery systems:

- Applications in controlled and targeted delivery (e.g. for gene therapy).
- Excellent administration performance via oral, injection, or dermal routes.
- Enhanced bioavailability and a high level of pharmacological action.
- It may be stabilized to give long shelf lives.

#### *Applications*

There are many potentially valuable prospects for nanotechnology in the drug delivery area and great strides are already being made for some applications. The key areas in which nanotechnology efforts are being focused are:

- Systems that improve the solubility and bioavailability of poorly water-soluble drugs.

- Delivery vehicles that can enhance the circulatory persistence of drugs and/or target drugs to specific cells.
- Controlled release delivery systems.
- Vaccine adjuvants and delivery systems.
- Nanostructured materials that can be used in a diverse range of drug delivery applications such as orthopedics and wound management.

## Polymeric nanoparticles (PNPs)

As name only suggests polymeric nanoparticles are nanoparticles which are prepared from polymers. The drug is dissolved, entrapped, encapsulated, or attached to a nanoparticles and depending upon the method of preparation, nanoparticles, nanospheres, or nanocapsules can be obtained. Nanocapsules are vesicular systems in which the drug is confined to a cavity surrounded by a polymer membrane, while nanospheres are matrix systems in which the drug is physically and uniformly dispersed.

In recent years, biodegradable polymeric nanoparticles have attracted considerable attention as potential drug delivery devices in view of their applications in drug targeting to particular organs/tissues, as carriers of DNA in gene therapy, and in their ability to deliver proteins, peptides and genes through a per oral route of administration.

### *Polymers used in nanoparticles*

Classification: Polymers are classified as:

A. Natural polymers:
   - Gums (e.g. acacia, guar gum, etc.)
   - Chitosan
   - Gelatin
   - Sodium alginate
   - Albumin
B. Synthetic polymers:
   a. Nonbiodegradable:
      - Cellulosics
      - Poly (2-hydroxyethyl methacrylate)
      - Poly (N-vinyl pyrrolidone)

- Poly (methyl methacrylate)
- Poly (vinyl alcohol)
- Poly (acrylic acid)
- Polyacrylamide
- Poly (ethylene-covinyl acetate)
- Poly (ethylene glycol)
- Poly (methacrylic acid).

b. Biodegradable
   - Polylactides (PLA)
   - Polyglycolides (PGA)
   - Poly(lactide-coglycolides) (PLGA)
   - Polyanhydrides
   - Polyorthoesters
   - Polycyanoacrylates
   - Polycaprolactone.

## Mechanisms of drug release

The polymeric drug carriers deliver the drug at the tissue site by anyone of the three general physicochemical mechanisms.

i. By the swelling of the polymer nanoparticles by hydration followed by release through diffusion.
ii. By an enzymatic reaction resulting in rupture or cleavage or degradation of the polymer at site of delivery, there by releasing the drug from the entrapped inner core.
iii. Dissociation of the drug from the polymer and its de-adsorption/release from the swelled nanoparticles.

## Techniques of preparation

The properties of polymeric nanoparticles have to be optimized depending on the particular application. In order to achieve the properties of interest, the mode of preparation plays a vital role. Thus, it is highly advantageous to have preparation techniques at hand to obtain polymeric nanoparticles with the desired properties for a particular application.

A. *Methods for preparation of nanoparticles from dispersion of preformed polymer*

Dispersion of drug in preformed polymers is a common technique used to prepare biodegradable nanoparticles from poly (lactic acid) (PLA), poly (D, L-glycolide) (PLG), poly (D, L-lactide-coglycolide) (PLGA) and poly (cyanoacrylate) (PCA). These can be accomplished by different methods described below.

i. Solvent evaporation
ii. Nanoprecipitation
iii. Emulsification/solvent diffusion
iv. Salting out
v. Dialysis
vi. Supercritical fluid technology (SCF).

B. Methods for preparation of nanoparticles from polymerization of monomers
   i. Emulsion
   ii. Miniemulsion
   iii. Microemulsion
   iv. Interfacial polymerization
   v. Controlled/living radical polymerization (C/LRP).

### *A. Methods for preparation of nanoparticles from dispersion of preformed polymer*

#### i. Solvent evaporation

Solvent evaporation was the first method developed to prepare NPs. In this method, polymer solutions are prepared in volatile solvents and emulsions are formulated. The emulsion is converted into a nanoparticle suspension on evaporation of the solvent for the polymer, which is allowed to diffuse through the continuous phase of the emulsion (Fig. 5.11). In the conventional methods, two main strategies are being used for the formation

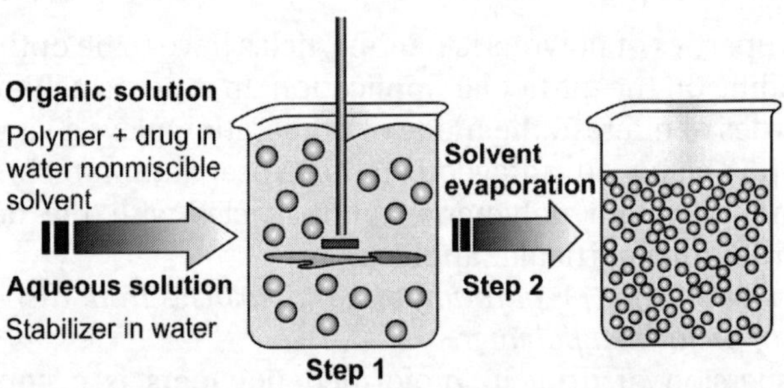


FIGURE 5.11: Solvent evaporation technique

of emulsions, the preparation of single-emulsions, e.g. oil-in-water (o/w) or double-emulsions, e.g. (water-in-oil)-in-water (w/o)/w. These methods utilize high-speed homogenization or ultrasonication, followed by evaporation of the solvent, either by continuous magnetic stirring at room temperature or under reduced pressure. Afterwards, the solidified nanoparticles can be collected by ultracentrifugation and washed with distilled water to remove additives such as surfactants. Finally, the product is lyophilized.

### ii. Nanoprecipitation

Nanoprecipitation is also called solvent displacement method. It involves the precipitation of a preformed polymer from an organic solution and the diffusion of the organic solvent in the aqueous medium in the presence or absence of a surfactant. The polymer generally PLA, is dissolved in a water-miscible solvent of intermediate polarity, leading to the precipitation of nanospheres. This phase is injected into a stirred aqueous solution containing a stabilizer as a surfactant. Polymer deposition on the interface between the water and the organic solvent, caused by fast diffusion of the solvent, leads to the instantaneous formation of a colloidal suspension. To facilitate the formation of colloidal polymer particles during the first step of the procedure, phase separation is performed with a totally miscible solvent that is also a nonsolvent of the polymer (Fig. 5.12). The solvent displacement technique allows the preparation of nanocapsules when a small volume of nontoxic oil is incorporated in the organic phase. Considering the oil-based central cavities of the nanocapsules, high loading efficiencies are generally reported for lipophilic drugs when nanocapsules are prepared. The usefulness of this simple technique is limited to water-miscible solvents, in which the diffusion rate is enough to produce spontaneous emulsification. Then, even though some water-miscible solvents produce certain instability when mixed in water, spontaneous emulsification is not observed if the coalescence rate of the formed droplets is sufficiently high. Although, acetone/dichloromethane (ICH, class 2) are used to dissolve and increase the entrapment of drugs, the dichloromethane increases the mean particle size and is considered toxic. This method is basically applicable to lipophilic drugs because of the miscibility of the solvent with the aqueous phase, and it is not an efficient means to encapsulate water-soluble drugs. This method has been applied to various polymeric materials such as PLGA, PLA, PCL and poly (methyl vinyl ether-co-maleic anhydride) (PVM/MA). This technique was well adapted for the incorporation of cyclosporin A, because entrapment efficiencies as high as 98% were obtained. Highly loaded nanoparticulate systems based on amphiphilic h-cyclodextrins to facilitate the parenteral administration of the poorly soluble antifungal drugs Bifonazole and clotrimazole were prepared according to the solvent displacement method.

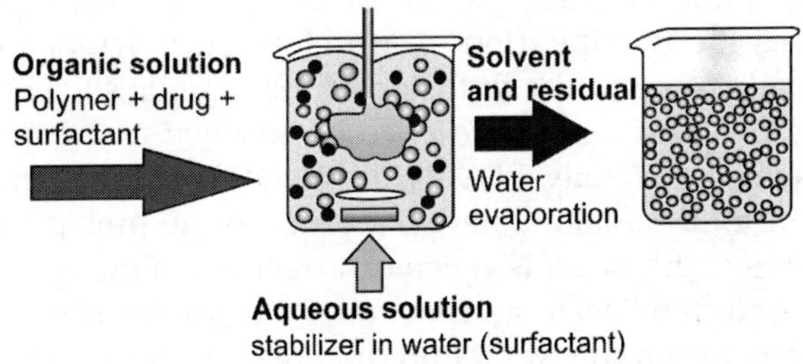


FIGURE 5.12: Nanoprecipitation technique

### iii. Emulsification/solvent diffusion (ESD)

This is a modified version of solvent evaporation method. The encapsulating polymer is dissolved in a partially water- soluble solvent such as propylene carbonate and saturated with water to ensure the initial thermodynamic equilibrium of both liquids. In fact, to produce the precipitation of the polymer and the consequent formation of nanoparticles, it is necessary to promote the diffusion of the solvent of the dispersed phase by dilution with an excess of water when the organic solvent is partly miscible with water or with another organic solvent in the opposite case. Subsequently, the polymer-water saturated solvent phase is emulsified in an aqueous solution containing stabilizer, leading to solvent diffusion to the external phase and the formation of nanospheres or nanocapsules, according to the oil-to-polymer ratio (Fig. 5.13). Finally, the solvent is eliminated by evaporation or filtration, according to its boiling point. This technique presents several advantages, such as high encapsulation efficiencies (generally >70%), no need for homogenization, high batch-to-batch reproducibility, ease of scale-up, simplicity and narrow size distribution. Disadvantages are the high volumes of water to be eliminated from the suspension and the leakage of water-soluble drug into the saturated-aqueous external phase during emulsification, reducing encapsulation efficiency. As with some of the other techniques, this one is efficient in encapsulating lipophilic drugs. Several drug-loaded nanoparticles were produced by the ESD technique, including mesotetra(hydroxyphenyl)porphyrin-loaded PLGA (p-THPP) nanoparticles 30,31, doxorubicin-loaded PLGA nanoparticles, plasmid DNA-loaded PLA nanoparticles 33, coumarin-loaded PLA nanoparticles, indocyanine, cyclosporine (Cy-A)-loaded gelatin and cyclosporin (Cy-A)-loaded sodium glycolate nanoparticles.

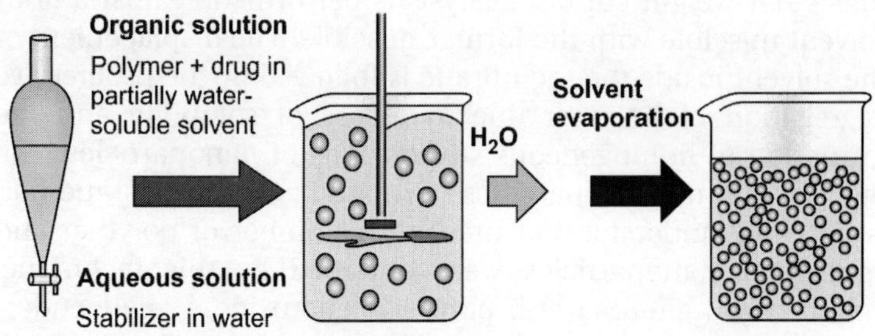


FIGURE 5.13: Emulsification/solvent diffusion technique

## iv. Salting-out procedure

In this method, the use of potentially toxic solvents is avoided. Here only acetone is used and it can be easily removed in the final step by cross-flow filtration. The preparation method consists of adding, under mechanical stirring, an electrolyte saturated solution containing a hydrocolloid, generally poly (vinyl alcohol) as a stabilizing and viscosity increasing agent to an acetone solution of polymer. After the preparation of an oil-in-water emulsion, sufficient water or an aqueous solution of PEG is added to allow complete diffusion of acetone into the aqueous phase, thus inducing the formation of nanospheres (Fig. 5.14).

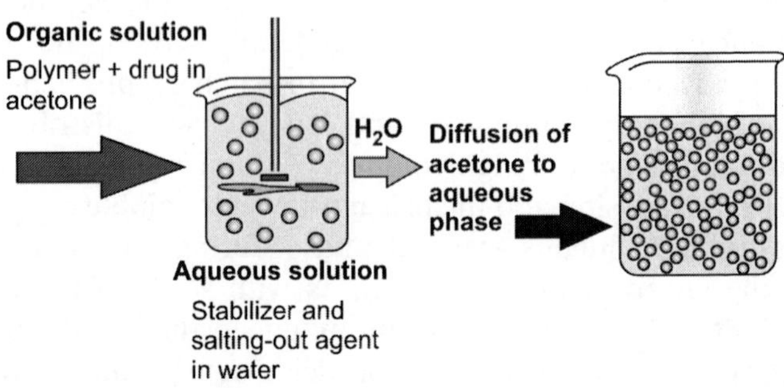


FIGURE 5.14: Salting-out technique

### v. Dialysis

Dialysis offers a simple and effective method for the preparation of small, narrow-distributed nanoparticles. Polymer is dissolved in an organic solvent and placed inside a dialysis tube with proper molecular weight cut off. Dialysis is performed against a non-solvent miscible with the former miscible. The displacement of the solvent inside the membrane is followed by the progressive aggregation of polymer due to a loss of solubility and the formation of homogeneous suspensions of nanoparticles. The mechanism of nanoparticles formation by dialysis method is not fully understood at present. A number of polymer and copolymer nanoparticles were obtained by this technique. Poly(benzyl-l-glutamate)-b-poly(ethylene oxide), Poly(lactide)-b-poly(ethylene oxide) nanoparticles were prepared using DMF as the solvent. The solvent used in the preparation of the polymer solution affects the morphology and particle size distribution of the nanoparticles.

### vi. Supercritical fluid technology

The need to develop environmentally safer methods for the production of nanoparticles has motivated research on the utility of supercritical fluids as more environmental friendly solvents, with the potential to produce nanoparticles with high purity and without any trace of organic solvent. Supercritical fluid and dense gas technology are expected to offer an interesting and effective technique of particle production, avoiding most of the drawbacks of the traditional methods.

Two principles have been developed for the production of nanoparticles using supercritical fluids:

a. Rapid expansion of supercritical solution (RESS).
b. Rapid expansion of supercritical solution into liquid solvent (RESOLV).

a. **Rapid expansion of supercritical solution**: In traditional RESS, the solute is dissolved in a supercritical fluid to form a solution, followed by the rapid expansion of the solution across an orifice or a capillary nozzle into ambient air. The high degree of super saturation, accompanied by the rapid pressure reduction in the expansion, results in homogenous nucleation and thereby, the formation of well-dispersed particles (Fig. 5.15). Results from mechanistic studies of different model solutes for the RESS process indicate that both nanometer and micrometer-sized particles are present in the expansion jet. A few studies were carried out on the production of nanoparticles using RESS. Poly (perfluoropolyether diamide) droplets are produced from the rapid expansion of $CO_2$ solutions. The RESS experimental apparatus consists of three major units: a high-pressure stainless steel mixing cell, a syringe pump and a pre-expansion unit. A solution of polymer in $CO_2$ is prepared at ambient temperature. The

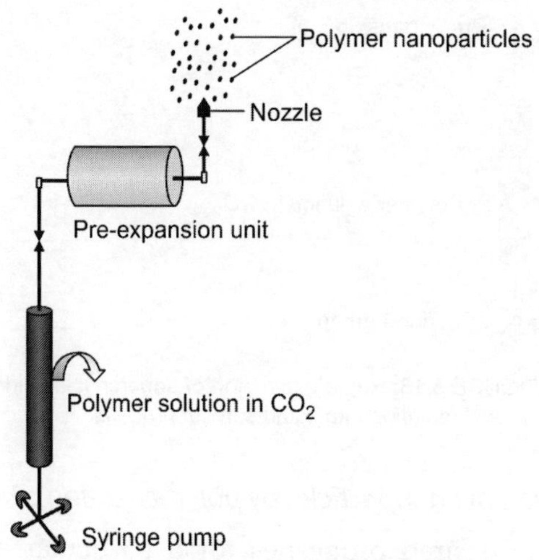


FIGURE.5.15: Rapid expansion of supercritical fluid solution

supercritical solution is now allowed to expand through the nozzle, at ambient pressure. The concentration and degree of saturation of the polymer have a considerable effect on the particle size and morphology of the particles for RESS.

b. **Rapid expansion of supercritical solution into liquid solvent**: A simple, but significant modification to RESS involves expansion of the supercritical solution into a liquid solvent instead of ambient air, termed as RESOL. Even though in RESS technique no organic solvents used for the formation of nanoparticles, the prime products obtained using this technique are microscaled rather than nanoscaled, which is the main drawback of RESS. In order to overcome, this drawback a new supercritical fluid technology known as RESOLV has been developed. In RESOLV the liquid solvent apparently suppresses the particle growth in the expansion jet, thus making it possible to obtain primarily nanosized particles (Fig. 5.16).

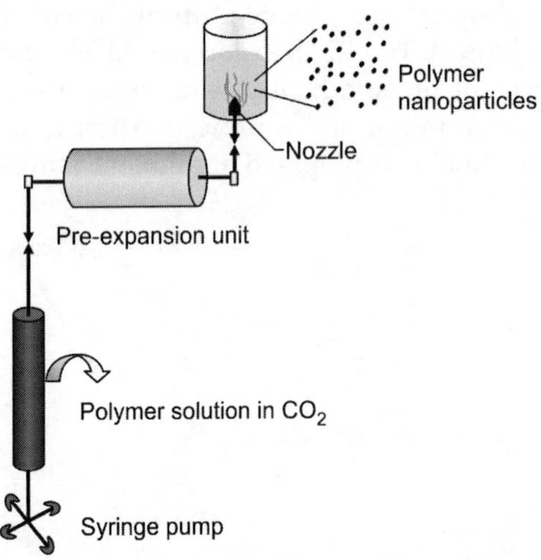


FIGURE 5.16: Rapid expansion of supercritical fluid solution into liquid solvent process

## *B. Preparation of nanoparticles by polymerization of a monomer*

To attain the desired properties for a particular application, suitable polymer nanoparticles must be designed, which can be done during the polymerization of monomers. Processes for the production of nanoparticles through the polymerization of monomers are discussed below:

i. **Emulsification polymerization**

   In case of conventional emulsification polymerization the continuous phase is aqueous (o/w emulsion), whereas in inverse emulsification polymerization the continuous phase is organic (w/o emulsion). In both cases, the monomer is emulsified in nonsolvent phase with surfactant molecules, leading to the formation of monomer-swollen micelles and stabilized monomer droplets. The polymerization reaction takes place in the presence of a chemical or physical initiator. The drug to be associated to the nanospheres may be present during polymerization or can be added to preformed nanospheres, so that the drug can be either incorporated into the matrix or simply adsorbed at the surface of the nanospheres.

ii. **Miniemulsion polymerization**

   A typical formulation used in miniemulsion polymerization consists of water, monomer mixture, costabilizer, surfactant and initiator. The key difference between emulsion polymerization and miniemulsion polymerization is the utilization of a low molecular mass compound as the costabilizer and also the use of a high-shear device (ultrasound, etc.). Miniemulsions are critically stabilized, require a high-shear to reach a steady state and have an interfacial tension much greater than zero.

iii. **Microemulsion polymerization**

   Microemulsion polymerization is a new and effective approach for preparing nanosized polymer particles and has attracted significant attention. Although emulsion and microemulsion polymerization appear similar because both methods can produce colloidal polymer particles of high molar mass, they are entirely different when compared kinetically. Both particle size and the average number of chains per particle are considerably smaller in microemulsion polymerization. In microemulsion polymerization, an initiator, typically water-soluble, is added to the aqueous phase of a thermodynamically stable microemulsion containing swollen micelles. The polymerization starts from this thermodynamically stable, spontaneously formed state and relies on high quantities of surfactant systems, which possess an interfacial tension at the oil/water interface close to zero. Furthermore, the particles are completely covered with surfactant because of the utilization of a high amount of surfactant. Initially, polymer chains are formed only in some droplets, as the initiation cannot be attained simultaneously in all micro-droplets. Later, the osmotic and elastic influence of the chains destabilize the fragile microemulsions and typically lead to an increase in the particle size, the formation of empty micelles and secondary nucleation. Very small latexes, 5–50 nm in size, coexist with a majority of empty micelles in the final product. The types of initiator and concentration, surfactant, monomer and reaction temperature are some of the critical factors affecting the microemulsion polymerization kinetics and the properties of nanoparticles.

iv. **Interfacial polymerization**

It is one of the well-established methods used for the preparation of polymer nanoparticles. It involves step polymerization of two reactive monomers or agents, which are dissolved respectively in two phases (i.e. continuous- and dispersed-phase), and the reaction takes place at the interface of the two liquids. Nanometer-sized hollow polymer particles were synthesized by employing interfacial cross-linking reactions as polyaddition and polycondensation 100–102 or radical polymerization. Oil-containing nanocapsules were obtained by the polymerization of monomers at the oil/water interface of a very fine oil-in-water microemulsion. The organic solvent, which was completely miscible with water, served as a monomer vehicle and the interfacial polymerization of the monomer was believed to occur at the surface of the oil droplets that formed during emulsification. To promote nanocapsule formation, the use of aprotic solvents, such as acetone and acetonitrile was recommended. Protic solvents, such as ethanol, n-butanol and isopropanol were found to induce the formation of nanospheres in addition to nanocapsules. Alternatively, water-containing nanocapsules can be obtained by the interfacial polymerization of monomers in water-in-oil micro-emulsions. In these systems, the polymer formed locally at the water-oil interface and precipitated to produce the nanocapsule shell.

v. **Controlled/living radical polymerization**

The primary limitations of radical polymerization include the lack of control over the molar mass, the molar mass distribution, the end functionalities and the macromolecular architecture. The limitations are caused by the unavoidable fast radical-radical termination reactions. The recent emergence of many so-called controlled or 'living' radical polymerization (C/LRP) processes has opened a new area using an old polymerization technique. The most important factors contributing to this trend of the C/LRP process have increased environmental concern and a sharp growth of pharmaceutical and medical applications for hydrophilic polymers. These factors have given rise to "green chemistry" and created a demand for environmentally and chemically benign solvents such as water and supercritical carbon dioxide. Industrial radical polymerization is widely performed in aqueous dispersed systems and specifically in emulsion polymerization. The primary goal was to control the characteristics of the polymer in terms of molar mass, molar mass distribution, architecture and function. Implementation of C/LRP in the industrially important aqueous dispersed systems, resulting in the formation of polymeric nanoparticles with precise particle size and size distribution control, is crucial for future commercial success of C/LRP. The nature and concentration of the control agent, monomer, initiator and emulsion type (apart from temperature) are vital in determining the size of nanoparticles. Of these, the nature of the control agent is critical in determining the particle size of the final product.

## Types of nanoparticles used for drug delivery

Many different types of nanoparticles currently being studied for applications in nanomedicine, they can be carbon-based skeletal-type structures, such as the fullerenes, or micelle-like, lipid-based liposomes, which are already in use for numerous applications in drug delivery and the cosmetic industry. Colloids, typically liposome nanoparticles, selected for their solubility and suspension properties are used in cosmetics, creams and protective coatings. Other examples of carbon-based nanoparticles are chitosan and alginate-based nanoparticles described in the literature for oral delivery of proteins, and various polymers under study for insulin delivery. Additional nanoparticles can be made from metals and other inorganic materials, such as phosphates. Nanoparticle contrast agents are compounds that enhance MRI and ultrasound results in biomedical applications of in vivo imaging. These particles typically contain metals whose properties are dramatically altered at the nanoscale. Gold "nanoshells" are useful in the fight against cancer, particularly soft-tissue tumors, because of their ability to absorb radiation at certain wavelengths. Once the nanoshells enter tumor cells and radiation treatment is applied, they absorb the energy and heat up enough to kill the cancer cells. Positively-charged silver nanoparticles adsorb onto single-stranded DNA and are used for its detection. Many other tools and devices for in vivo imaging (fluorescence detection systems), and to improve contrast in ultrasound and MRI images, are being developed. There are numerous examples of disease-fighting strategies in the literature, using nanoparticles. Often, particularly in the case of cancer therapies, drug delivery properties are combined with imaging technologies, so that cancer cells can be visually located while undergoing treatment.

### *Types of nanoparticles*

1. Gold nanoparticles

Gold nanoparticles can provide effective carriers for biomolecules such as DNA, RNA, proteins and drugs, protecting these materials from degradation and transporting them across the cell-membrane barrier without effective toxicity.

2. Magnetic nanoparticles (MNPs)

These are a class of engineered particulate materials of < 100 nm diameter that can be manipulated under the influence of an external magnetic field. MNPs commonly composed of magnetic elements such as iron, cobalt and their oxides like magnetite, cobalt ferrite and chromium dioxide. Applications of MNPs include targeted drug delivery, gene delivery cell separation and cell labeling.

3. Ceramic nanoparticles

Nanoparticles of silica, titanium, alumina, etc. are normally called as ceramic nanoparticles. The advantages of ceramic nanoparticles preparation are very simple and they are unaffected by change in pH or temperature.

4. Protein nanoparticles

Protein nanoparticles are biodegradable, nonantigenic, metabolizable and can also be easily amenable for surface modification and covalent attachment of drugs and ligands. The proteins used for the preparation of nanoparticles are albumin, gelatin, gliadin and legumin.

5. Solid lipid nanoparticles (SLNs)

These are a new generation of submicron-sized lipid emulsions where the liquid lipid (oil) has been substituted by a solid lipid. SLNs offer unique properties such as small size, large surface area, high drug loading and the interaction of phases at the interfaces, and are attractive for their potential to improve performance of pharmaceuticals, nutraceuticals and other materials.

6. Nanogels

Nanogels are cross-linked nanoscale particles made of flexible hydrophilic polymers. These are soluble in water. Nanogels possess large surface area and a network to allow incorporation of molecules. These are used to incorporate drugs, DNA/RNA and inorganic molecules such as quantum dots. These are also used for pH dependent release.

7. Nanoshells

A nanoshell comprises of a spherical core made from silica or other similar materials, surrounded by a coating of few nanometers thickness. The coatings comprise a metal such as gold or silver. In cancer applications, antibodies or other biomolecules are attached to the gold surface to target at tumor site.

### 8. Dendrimers

Dendrimers are unimolecular, monodisperse, micellar nanostructures with a well-defined regularly branched symmetrical structure and a high density of functional end groups. Dendrimers contain three regions core, branches and surface. The first and most widely studied dendrimers are poly (amidoamino) (PAMAM) dendrimer. The advantage of dendrimers is that they are similar in size to many proteins and biomolecules like insulin, cytochrome C and hemoglobin. These are effective against bacterial and viral infection. Dendrimers hybridized with chitosan have useful antibacterial properties as well as potentially acting as drug delivery agents.

### 9. Carbon nanohorns

Carbon nanohorns have a structure similar to carbon nanotubes except they are closed at one end, forming a cone-shaped cap, or horn.

### 10. Carbon nanotubes

Carbon nanotubes are hexagonal networks of carbon atoms, 1nm in diameter and 1–100 nm in length. Two types of nanotubes are present, i.e. single-walled nanotubes, and multi-walled nanotubes. The advantages of nanotubes are ultra-light weight, high mechanical strength, and high surface area. Due to their size and shape, carbon nanotubes can enter living cells without causing cell death or obvious damage. Carbon nanotubes have the ability to transport drug molecules, protein and nucleotides. Therapeutic applications of carbon nanotubes including boron neutron capture therapy (BNCT), induce immunoresponse, gene and RNA delivery.

### 11. Nanodiamonds

Also called diamond nanoparticles, used to immobilize proteins and deliver drug molecules. Fluorescent nanodiamonds can enter cells, and may have applications in cell tracking and imagining.

12. Cyclodextrin nanosponges

Cyclodextrin nanosponges are complex networks of cross-linked cyclodextrins and formed into a roughly spherical structure, about the size of a protein, with channels and pores inside.

13. Drug carrying implantable thin films

These are nanoscale thin films that can be precisely controlled to release chemical agents by applying an electrostatic field. The advantages are ease of preparation, versatility and capability of incorporating high loading of biomolecules into films. The film can be implanted in the body and can carry discrete packets of drugs that can be released separately, which could be particularly useful for chemotherapy.

14. Quantum dots

Quantum dots (QDs) are semiconducting materials consisting of a semiconductor core ($C_d$, $S_e$), coated by a shell (e.g. ZnS). These are used as diagnostic tools, detection and analysis of biomolecules, immunoassays, DNA hybridization, and development of nonviral vectors for gene therapy, transport vehicles for DNA, protein, drugs or cells.

## TRANSDERMAL DRUG DELIVERY SYSTEMS

### Introduction

Delivering medicine to the general circulation through the skin is seen as a desirable alternative to taking it by mouth. Patients often forget to take their medicine, and even the most faithfully compliant get tired of swallowing pills, specially if they must take several each day. Additionally, bypassing the gastrointestinal (GI) tract would obviate the GI irritation that frequently occurs and avoid partial first-pass inactivation by the liver. Further, steady absorption of drug over hours or days is usually preferable to the blood level spikes and troughs produced by oral dosage forms.

From 1979, when the Food and Drug Administration approved the first transdermal drug delivery system (Transderm Scop® Patch), to the current transdermal delivery systems, there evolved a successful alternative to systemic drug delivery. Despite their relatively higher costs, transdermal delivery systems have proved advantageous for delivery of selected drugs, such as estrogens, testosterone, clonidine, nitroglycerin, scopolamine, fentanyl and nicotine.

Transdermal therapeutic systems are defined as self-contained, discrete dosages forms which when applied to the intact skin, deliver the drug, through the skin, at a controlled rate to the systemic circulation. Transdermal drug delivery systems (TDDS), where applicable, offer several advantages over other conventional dosage forms.

*Advantages*

Using TDDS, it is possible to achieve the following advantages:

1. Avoidance of the 'first pass effect'.
2. A stable and controlled blood level.
3. Comparable characteristics with intravenous infusion.
4. Termination of further administration, if necessary.
5. Long-term duration (ranging from a few hours to one week).
6. No interference with gastric and intestinal fluids.
7. Administration of drugs with:
   – A very short half-life
   – Narrow therapeutic window
   – Poor oral absorption.
8. Improved patient compliance and reduced inter- and intrapatient variability.
9. Self-administration is possible.
10. Systems are noninvasive.

*Limitations*

Transdermal drug delivery systems have some limitations:

1. The drug must have some desirable physicochemical properties for penetration through stratum corneum.
2. Skin irritation or contact dermatitis due to drug or excipients.
3. The barrier function of skin changes from one site to another on the same person, from person to person and with age.

### Percutaneous absorption and kinetics of transdermal permeation

Percutaneous absorption involves passive diffusion of substances through the skin. The mechanism of permeation can involve passage through the epidermis itself (transepidermal absorption) or diffusion through shunt particularly hair follicles and eccrine glands (transfollicular or shunt pathway absorption).

*A. Transepidermal absorption*

Transepidermal pathway is principally responsible for diffusion across skin. Permeation by the transepidermal route first involves partitioning into stratum corneum than diffusion takes place across this tissue. Most substances diffused across the stratum corneum, via the intercellular lipoidal route.

*B. Transfollicular (shunt pathway) absorption*

The skin's appendages offer only secondary route for permeation. Sebaceous and eccrine glands are the only appendages which are seriously considered as shunts bypassing the stratum corneum. The follicular route remains an important route for percutaneous absorption since the opening of follicular pore, where the hair shaft exits the skin, is relatively large and sebum aids in diffusion of penetrants.

Transdermal permeation of a drug involves the following steps:

1. Sorption by stratum corneum
2. Penetration of drug through viable epidermis
3. Uptake of the drug by capillary network in the dermal papillary layer.

This permeation can be possible only if the drug possesses certain physicochemical properties.The rate of permeation across the skin (dQ/dt) is given by—

$$dQ/dt = P_s\ (C_d - C_r)$$

where

$C_d$—The concentrations of skin penetrants in the donor compartment (surface of stratum corneum)

$C_r$—The concentrations of skin penetrants in receptor compartment (body)

$P_s$—Overall permeability coefficient of the skin tissues to the penetrant.

$$P_s = K_s.D_{ss}/h_s$$

where
$K_s$—Partition coefficient
$D_{ss}$—Apparent diffusivity for steady state diffusion
$h_s$—Overall thickness of skin tissues.

A constant rate of drug permeation can be obtained only when $C_d >> C_r$, i.e. the drug concentration at the surface of stratum corneum ($C_d$) is consistently and substantially greater than the drug concentration in the body—

$$dQ/dt = P_s . C_d$$

When $C_d >> C_s$ then maximum rate of skin permeation $(dQ/dt)_m$

$$(dQ/dt)_m = P_s . C_s$$

The maximum rate of skin permeation depends on:
– The skin permeability coefficient ($P_s$)
– Equilibrium solubility in stratum corneum ($C_s$).

Thus, skin permeation appears to be stratum corneum limited.

## Factors affecting transdermal permeability

The factors influencing transdermal permeability of stratum corneum can be classified into three major categories:

1. Physicochemical properties of the penetrants
2. Physicochemical properties of the drug delivery systems
3. Physiological and pathological conditions of the skin.

### *1. Physicochemical properties of the penetrants*

i. *Partition coefficient*—Drugs possessing both water and lipid solubilities are favorably absorbed through skin. Transdermal permeability coefficient shows in linear dependency on partition coefficient. A lipid/water partition coefficient of 1 or greater is generally required for optimal transdermal permeability.
ii. *pH conditions*—pH conditions of skin surface and in drug delivery systems affect the extent of dissociation of ionogenic drug molecules and their transdermal permeability.

iii. *Penetrant concentration*—Transdermal permeability across mammalian skin is a passive diffusion process thus depends on the concentration of penetrant molecules on the surface layers of the skin.

2. *Physicochemical properties of drug delivery systems*
   i. *Release characteristics*—Generally, the more easily the drug is released from the delivery system, the higher the rate of transdermal permeation. The mechanism of drug release depends on whether the drug molecules are dissolved or suspended in the delivery system and on interfacial partition coefficient of the drug from delivery system to the skin tissue.
   ii. *Composition of drug delivery systems*—The composition of drug delivery system has a great influence on percutaneous absorption of a drug molecule. It may affect not only the rate of drug release but also the permeability of stratum corneum by means of hydration, mixing with skin lipids, or other sorption promoting effects.
   iii. *Enhancement of transdermal permeation*—Transdermal permeation of drugs can be improved by the addition of a sorption or permeation promoter in the drug delivery system.
      a. Organic solvents as permeation promotor—For example, dimethylsulfoxide (DMSO), dimethylacetamide (DMAA), dimethylformide (DMFA), ethylene glycol, polyethylene glycol, Ethanol.
      b. Surface active agent as permeation promoter—The anionic surfactants are most effective permeation promoters, e.g. sodium lauryl sulfate, sodium dioctyl sulfosuccinate.

3. *Physiological and pathological conditions of the skin*
   a. *Reservoir effect of horny layer*—The horny layer specially its deeper layer can act as a depot or reservoir and modify transdermal permeation characteristics of some drug.
   b. *Lipid film*—Lipid film on skin surface, formed by product of the excretion of sebaceous gland and epidermal cell lipid maintains the barrier function of stratum corneum.

c. *Skin hydration*—Hydration of stratum corneum can enhance the permeability of the skin by as much as eight fold.
d. *Skin temperature*—Skin permeation of acetyl salicylic acid and glucosteroids was raised ten fold when the environmental temperature raised from 10°–37°C.

## Basic components of TDDS

The components of transdermal devices include:

1. Polymer matrix/ drug reservoir
2. The drug
3. Permeation enhancers
4. Pressure sensitive adhesive (PSA)
5. Backing membrane
6. Release liner.

### *1. Polymer matrix /drug reservoir*

The polymer controls the release of the drug from the device. The following criteria should be satisfied for a polymer to be used in a transdermal system:

i. Polymer should be stable, nonreactive with the drug, easily manufactured and fabricated into the desired product and inexpensive.
ii. The polymer and its degradation products must be nontoxic or nonantagonistic to the host.
iii. The mechanical properties of the polymer should not deteriorate excessively when large amounts of active agent are incorporated into it.

The polymers used for TDDS can be classified as:

**Natural polymers**: Cellulose derivatives, zein, gelatin, shellac, waxes, proteins, gums, natural rubber, chitosan, etc.

**Synthetic elastomers**: Polybutadiene, hydrin rubber, polysiloxane, polyisobutylene, silicon rubber, nitrile, acrylonitrile, neoprene, butylrubber, etc.

**Synthetic polymers**: Polyvinyl alcohol, polyvinylchloride, polyethylene, polypropylene, polyacrylate, polyamide, polyurea, polyvinylpyrrolidone, polymethyl methacrylate, etc.

*2. Drug*

For successfullly developing a transdermal drug delivery system, the drug should be chosen with great care. Transdermal patches offer much to drugs which undergo extensive first pass metabolism, drugs with narrow therapeutic window, or drugs with short half-life which causes noncompliance due to frequent dosing. The foremost requirement of TDDS is that the drug possesses the right mix of physicochemical and biological properties for transdermal drug delivery. It is generally accepted that the best drug candidates for passive adhesive transdermal patches must be nonionic, of low molecular weight (less than 500 Da), have adequate solubility in oil and water (log P in the range of 1–3), a low melting point (less than 200°C) and are potent (dose in mg/day).

*3. Permeation enhancers*

This term refers to an entire family of chemically different substances that all share a common characteristic—They facilitate the permeation of the penetrants through the skin. They increase the permeation rate by several times, by altering the skin as a barrier to the flux of a desired penetrant. This is very important with respect to the feasibility of a system, because most of the penetrants do not enter the skin in the required dosage from a relatively small area. Sometimes, a combination of ingredients is needed to create the correct enhancement effect. These may conveniently be classified under the following headings:

**Solvents**: These compound increase penetration possibly by swelling the polar pathway and/or by fluidizing lipids. The examples include:

- *Alcohols*—Methanol, Ethanol
- *Alkyl methyl sulfoxide*—Dimethylsulfoxide (DMSO), dimethylacetamide (DMAA), dimethylformamide (DMFA)
- *Pyrrolidones*—2-pyrrolidone, N-methyl-2-pyrrolidone

**Surfactants**: These compounds are proposed to enhance polar pathway transport, specially of hydrophilic drugs. The examples of commonly used surfactants are:

- *Anionic surfactants*—Dioctyl sulfosuccinate, sodium lauryl sulfate, dodecyl methyl sulfoxide, etc.
- *Nonionic surfactants*—Pluronic F127, pluronic F68, etc.
- *Bile salts*—Sodium taurocholate, sodium deoxycholate, sodium tauroglycocholate.

**Binary systems**: These systems apparently open up the heterogeneous multilaminate pathway as well as the continuous pathways. The examples include: Propylene glycol-oleic acid and 1, 4 butane diol-linoleic acid.

Miscellaneous: These include urea, ahydrating and keratolytic agent: N, N-dimethyl-m-toluamide; calcium thioglycolate; anticholinergic agents.

*4. Pressure sensitive adhesives*

Pressure sensitive adhesives (PSAs) help in fastening of all transdermal devices to the skin. They can be positioned on the face of the device or in the back of the device and extending peripherally.

The pressure sensitive adhesives used for TDDS, can be classified under three main categories (Table 5.2):

- Rubber-based adhesives
- Acrylics
- Silicon-based adhesives.

**Table 5.2**: Pressure-sensitive adhesives in TDDS

| *Pressure-sensitive adhesives* | *Advantages* | *Disadvantages* |
|---|---|---|
| Rubber-based adhesives | Good adherence to low and high energy surfaces<br>Relatively inert adhesives<br>High initial adhesion<br>Useful in broad temperature range<br>Flexibility<br>Low cost | Poor ageing<br>Low shear and irradiation resistance<br>MW variability<br>Low tack and adhesion without additives |
| Acrylics | Good UV, solvent and hydrolysis resistance<br>Excellent adhesion build up<br>Good shear strength<br>Easy to apply<br>Good service life | Moderate cost<br>Fair initial adhesion<br>Poor creep |
| Silicon-based adhesives | Chemical and biological inertness<br>Extremely low toxicity, sensitization and irritation<br>Retaining of mechanical and physiochemical properties on the skin | Highest cost<br>The need for expensive release liners<br>No aggressive behavior |

*5. Backing membrane*

Backing membranes are flexible and they provide a good bond to the drug reservoir, prevent drug from leaving the dosages form through the top, and accept printing. It is impermeable substance that protects the product during use on the skin, e.g. metallic plastic laminate, plastic backing with absorbent pad and occlusive base plate (aluminum foil), adhesive foam pad (flexible polyurethane) with occlusive base plate (aluminum foil disk), etc.

*6. Release liners*

Generally, a release liner is a film covered with an antiadherent coating. The role of the release liner is to protect the system as long as it is in the package, and it is removed just before the adhesion of the TDDS to the skin. Release liners play a crucial role in the stability of the product and in its safe and functional use. The release liner must, therefore, be chosen very carefully.

The most common films used as release liners are paper-based, plastic film-based and composite films. The two major classes of coating are silicones and fluoropolymers.

## Approaches used in development of transdermal drug delivery systems

Different approaches have been utilized to obtain transdermal drug delivery systems:

1. Membrane permeation-controlled
2. Adhesive dispersion type systems
3. Matrix diffusion controlled systems
4. Microreservoir type or microsealed dissolution controlled system.

*1. Membrane permeation-controlled systems*

In this type of system, the drug reservoir is totally encapsulated in a shallow compartment moulded from a drug impermeable metallic plastic laminate and rate controlling polymeric membrane which may be microporous or nonporous, e.g. ethylene vinyl acetate (EVA) copolymer, with a defined drug permeability property (a cross-sectional view of this system is shown in Figure 5.17).

The constant release of the drug is the major advantage of membrane permeation controlled transdermal system. The examples of this system are:

1. Nitroglycerin releasing transdermal system (transderm-nitro).
2. Scopolamine releasing transdermal system (transderm-scop).

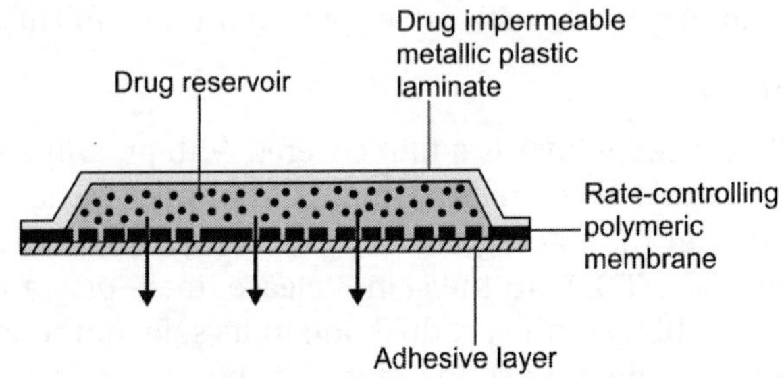


FIGURE 5.17: Membrane moderated transdermal drug delivery system

The intrinsic rate of drug release from this type of system is defined by—

$$dQ/dt = C_R/(1/P_m + 1/P_a)$$

where

$C_R$—The drug concentration in the reservoir compartment

$P_a$—The permeability coefficient of the adhesive layer

$P_m$—The permeability coefficient of rate controlling membrane.

*2. Adhesive dispersion type systems*

This is a simplified form of membrane permeation-controlled system. Drug reservoir is formulated by directly dispersing the drug in an adhesive polymer and then spreading the medicated adhesive, by solvent casting or hot melt, onto a flat sheet of drug impermeable metallic plastic backing to form a thin drug reservoir layer. On top of the drug reservoir layer, thin layer of nonmedicated, rate-controlling adhesive polymer of a specific permeability and constant thickness are applied to produce an adhesive diffusion-controlled delivery system (Fig. 5.18). An example of this type of system is isosorbide dinitrate-releasing transdermal therapeutic system.

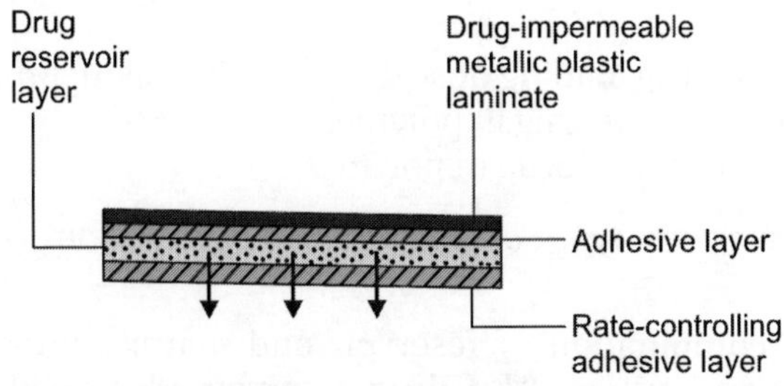


FIGURE 5.18: Adhesive dispersion type transdermal drug delivery system

The rate of drug release from this type of system is defined as—

$$dQ/dt = K_{a/r}.D_a / h_a . C_R$$

where

$K_{a/r}$—Partition coefficient for the interfacial partitioning of the drug from the reservoir layer to adhesive layer.

*3. Matrix diffusion controlled systems*

In this approach, the drug reservoir is prepared by homogeneously dispersing drug particles in a hydrophilic or lipophilic polymer matrix. The resultant medicated polymer is then moulded into a medicated disk with a defined surface area and controlled thickness. This drug reservoir containing polymer disk is then pasted onto an occlusive base plate in a compartment fabricated from a drug impermeable plastic backing. The adhesive polymer is then spread along the circumference to form a strip of adhesive rim around the medicated disk (Fig. 5.19). An example of this type of system is nitroglycerin-releasing transdermal therapeutic system.

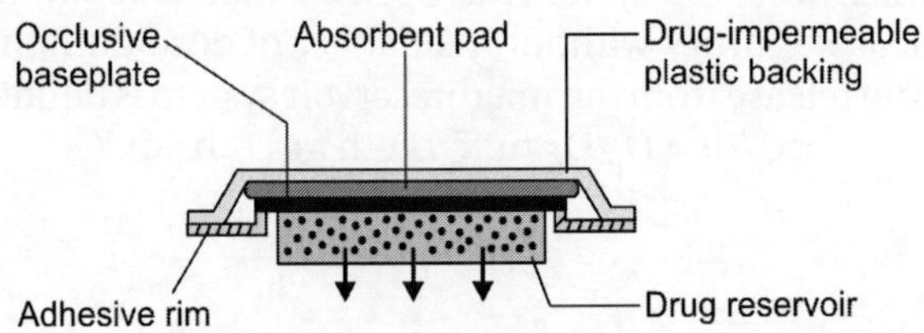


FIGURE 5.19: Matrix diffusion controlled transdermal drug delivery systems

The rate of drug release from this type of system is defined by—

$$dQ/dt = \{AC_p.D_p/2t\}^{1/2}$$

where
A—Initial drug loading dose dispersed in polymer matrix
$C_p$—Solubility of drug in polymer
$D_p$—Diffusivity of drug in polymer.

4. *Microreservoir type or microsealed dissolution controlled system*

This is a combination of reservoir and matrix diffusion type drug delivery system. The drug reservoir is formed by first suspending the drug solids in an aqueous solution of a water-soluble liquid polymer and then dispersing the drug suspension homogeneously in lipophilic polymer, viz silicone elastomers by high energy dispersion technique to form several discrete, unleachable microscopic spheres of drug reservoirs. A transdermal therapeutic system is produced by positioning the medicated disk at the center and surrounding it with an adhesive rim (Fig. 5.20).

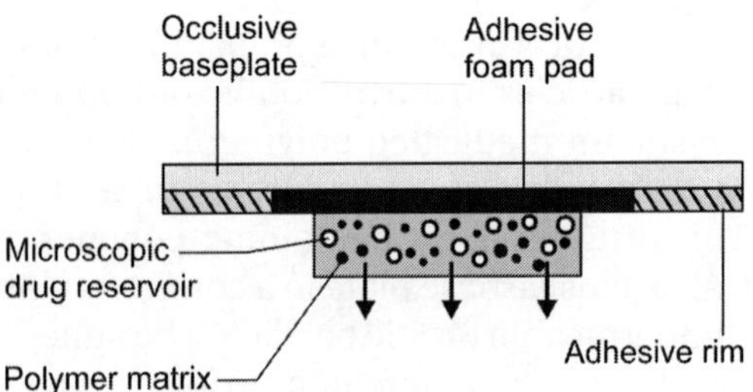


FIGURE 5.20: Microreservoir dissolution controlled transdermal drug delivery system

The microreservoir system has been claimed to follow the zero order release of drugs without the danger of dose dumping. The rate of drug release from the microreservoir system is defined by—

$$dQ/dt = D_p.D_d.m.K_p/D_p.h_d + D_d.h_p.m.K_p$$

$$[n. Sp \quad \frac{D_1.S_1.(1-n)}{h_1} \quad (1/K_1 + 1/K_m)]$$

where
m = a/b, a is the ratio of the drug concentration in the bulk of the elution medium over drug solubility in the same medium and b is the ratio of drug concentration at the outer edge of the

polymer coating over the drug solubility in the same polymer composition.

n = ratio of drug concentration at the inner edge of the interfacial barrier over drug solubility in the polymer matrix.

$D_l$, $D_p$ and $D_d$ are respectively, the drug diffusivities in the liquid layer surrounding the drug particles, polymer coating membrane surrounding the polymer matrix and the hydrodynamic diffusion layer surrounding the polymer coating with respective thickness of $h_l$, $h_p$ and $h_d$.

$K_l$, $K_m$ and $K_p$ are the partition coefficients for the interfacial partitioning of the drug from the liquid compartment to the polymer matrix, from the polymer matrix to the polymer coating membrane and from the polymer coating membrane to the elution solution (or skin) respectively.

$S_l$ and $S_p$ are the solubilities of the drug in the liquid compartment and in the polymer matrix respectively.

## Evaluation of transdermal drug delivery systems

### *A. Physicochemical evaluation*

i. ***Thickness***: The thickness of transdermal film is determined by traveling microscope, dial gauge, screw gauge or micrometer at different points of the film.

ii. ***Uniformity of weight***: Weight variation is studied by individually weighing 10 randomly selected patches and calculating the average weight. The individual weight should not deviate significantly from the average weight.

iii. ***Drug content determination***: An accurately weighed portion of film (about 100 mg) is dissolved in 100 ml of suitable solvent in which drug is soluble and then the solution is shaken continuously for 24 hours in shaker incubator. Then the whole solution is sonicated. After sonication and subsequent filtration, drug in solution is estimated spectrophotometrically by appropriate dilution.

iv. ***Content uniformity test***: 10 patches are selected and content is determined for individual patches. If 9 out of 10 patches have content between 85%–115% of the specified value and one has content not less than

75%–125% of the specified value, then transdermal patches pass the test of content uniformity. But if 3 patches have content in the range of 75%–125%, then additional 20 patches are tested for drug content. If these 20 patches have range from 85%–115%, then the transdermal patches pass the test.

v. ***Moisture content***: The prepared films are weighed individually and kept in a desiccators containing calcium chloride at room temperature for 24 hours. The films are weighed again after a specified interval until they show a constant weight. The percent moisture content is calculated using following formula.

$$\text{Percentage of moisture content} = \frac{\text{Initial weight} - \text{Final weight}}{\text{Final weight}} \times 100$$

vi. ***Moisture uptake***: Weighed film is kept in a desiccator at room temperature for 24 hours. These are then taken out and exposed to 84% relative humidity using saturated solution of potassium chloride in a desiccator until a constant weight is achieved. Percentage of moisture uptake is calculated as given below:

$$\text{Percentage of moisture uptake} = \frac{\text{Final weight} - \text{Initial weight}}{\text{Initial weight}} \times 100$$

vii. ***Water vapor transmission studies (WVT)***: For the determination of WVT weighed 1 gm of calcium chloride and placed it in previously dried empty vials having equal diameter. The polymer films were pasted over the brim with the help of adhesive like silicon adhesive grease and the adhesive was allowed to set for 5 minutes. Then, the vials were accurately weighed and placed in humidity chamber maintained at 68% RH. The vials were again weighed at the end of every 1st day, 2nd day, 3rd day upto 7 consecutive days and an increase in weight was considered as a quantitative measure of moisture transmitted through the patch.

*B. Evaluation of adhesive*

Pressure sensitive adhesive are evaluated for following properties:

i. ***Peel adhesion properties***: Peel adhesion force is required to remove adhesive coating from a test substrate (Fig. 5.21). Peel adhesion properties are affected by the molecular weight of adhesive polymer, the type and amount of additives and polymer composition.

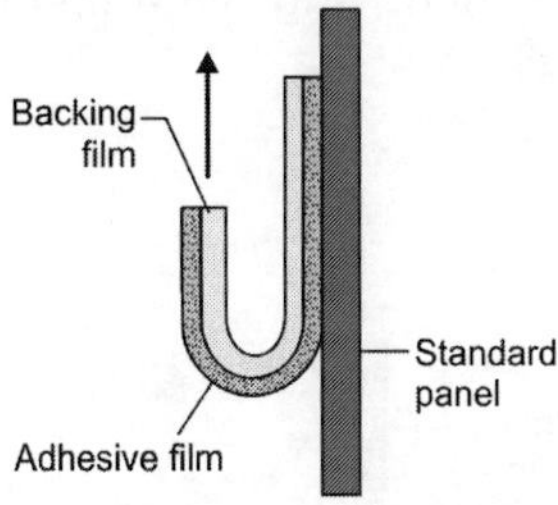


Figure 5.21: Peel adhesion test

It is tested by measuring the force required to pull a single coated tape, applied to a substrate, at a 180° angle. No residue on the substrate indicates adhesive failure which is desirable for transdermal devices.

ii. ***Tack properties***: Tack is the ability of polymer to adhere to a substrate with little contact pressure. It is important in transdermal devices which are applied with finger pressure. Tests for tack include:
   a. Thumb tack test—This is a subjective test in which evaluation is done by pressing the thumb briefly into the adhesive.
   b. Rolling ball tack test—It involves measurement of the distance that a stainless steel ball travels along an upward facing adhesive. The less tacky the adhesive, the farther the ball will travel (Fig. 5.22).

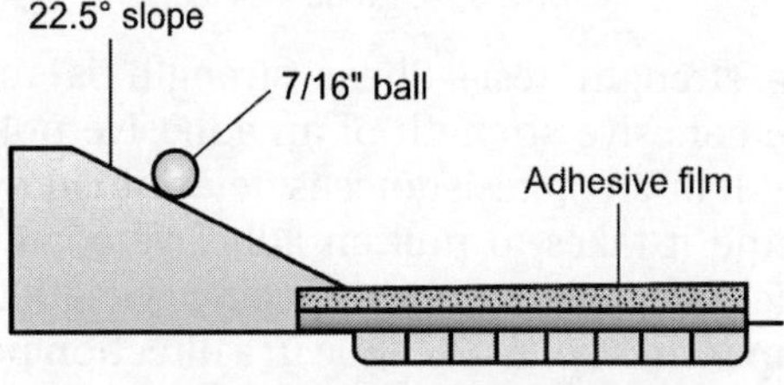


FIGURE 5.22: Rolling ball tack test

c. Quick-stick or peel tack test—The peel force required to break the bond between an adhesive and substrate is measured by pulling the tape away from substrate at 90° at a speed of 12 inch/min (Fig. 5.23). The force is recorded as tack value and is expressed in ounce (or grams) per inch width with higher values indicating increasing tack.

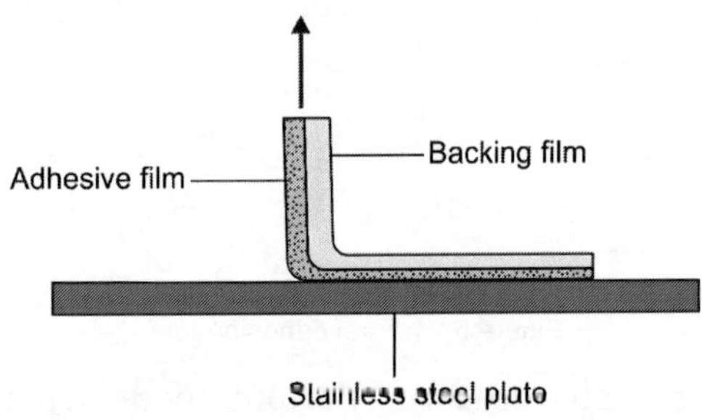


FIGURE 5.23: Quick-stick or peel tack test

d. Probe tack test—The force required to pull a probe away from an adhesive (Fig. 5.24) at a fixed rate is recorded as tack (force is expressed in gm).

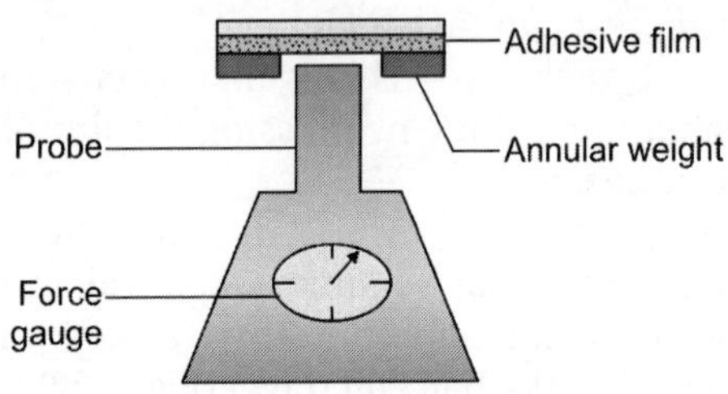


FIGURE 5.24: Probe tack test

iii. Shear strength test—Shear strength is measurement of the cohesive strength of an adhesive polymer. Shear strength or creep resistance is determined by measuring the time it takes to pull an adhesive coated tape off a stainless steel plate when a specified weight is hung from the tape which pulls the tape in a direction parallel to the plate (Fig. 5.25).

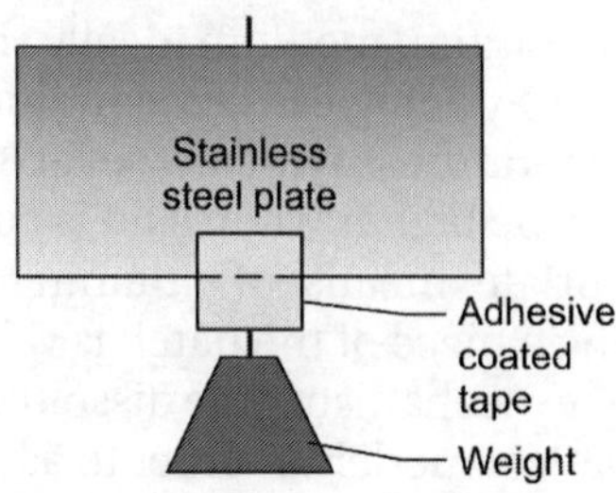


FIGURE 5.25: Shear strength test

*C. In vitro drug release study*

There are various methods available for determination of drug release rate of TDDS.

- **The paddle over Disk (USP apparatus 5)**: This method is identical to the USP paddle dissolution apparatus, except that the transdermal system is attached to a disk or cell resting at the bottom of the vessel which contains medium at 32 ±5°C.
- **The cylinder modified USP basket (USP apparatus 6)**: This method is similar to the USP basket type dissolution apparatus, except that the system is attached to the surface of a hollow cylinder immersed in medium at 32 ±5°C.
- **The reciprocating disk (USP apparatus 7)**: In this method, patches attached to holders are oscillated in small volumes of medium, allowing the apparatus to be useful for systems delivering low concentration of drug.
- **Diffusion cells, e.g. Franz diffusion cell and its modification Keshary-Chien cell**: In this method, transdermal system is placed in between receptor and donor compartment of the diffusion cell (Fig. 5.26). The transdermal system faces the receptor compartment in which receptor fluid, i.e. buffer is placed. The agitation speed and temperature are kept constant. The whole assembly is kept on magnetic stirrer and solution in the receiver compartment is constantly and continuously stirred throughout the experiment using magnetic beads. At predetermined time intervals, the receptor fluid is removed for analysis and is replaced with an equal volume of fresh receptor fluid. The concentration of drug is determined spectrophotometrically.

The pH of the dissolution medium ideally should be adjusted to pH 5–6, reflecting physiological skin conditions. For the same reason, the test temperature is typically set at 32°C (even though the temperature may be higher when skin is covered). The latter may be an appropriate means of attaining sink conditions, provided that cutting a piece of the patch is validated to have no impact on the release mechanism. The dissolution data obtained is fitted to mathematical models in order to ascertain the release mechanism.

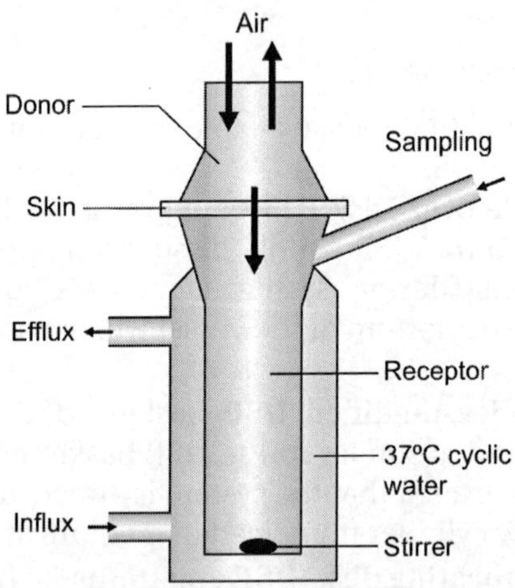


FIGURE 5.26: Franz diffusion cell

*D. In vitro permeation studies*

The amount of drug available for absorption to the systemic pool is greatly dependent on drug released from the polymeric transdermal films. The drug reached at skin surface is then passed to the dermal microcirculation by penetration through cells of epidermis, between the cells of epidermis through skin appendages.

Usually permeation studies are performed by placing the fabricated transdermal patch with rat skin or synthetic membrane in between receptor and donor compartment in a vertical diffusion cell, such as Franz diffusion cell or Keshary-Chien diffusion cell. The transdermal system is applied to the hydrophilic side of the membrane and then mounted in the diffusion cell with lipophilic side in contact with receptor fluid. The receiver compartment is maintained at specific temperature (usually 32 ± 5°C for skin) and is continuously stirred at a constant rate. The samples are withdrawn at different time intervals and equal amount of buffer is replaced each time. The samples are diluted appropriately and absorbance is determined spectrophotometrically. Then the amount of drug permeated per centimeter square at each time interval is calculated. Design of system, patch size, surface area of skin, thickness of skin and temperature, etc. are some variables that may affect the release of drug. So permeation study involves preparation of skin, mounting of skin on permeation cell, setting of experimental conditions like temperature, stirring, sink conditions, withdrawing samples at different time intervals, sample analysis and calculation of flux, i.e. drug permeated per $cm^2$ per second.

*Preparation of skin for permeation studies*: Hairless animal skin and human cadaver skin are used for permeation studies. Human cadaver skin may be a logical choice as the skin model because the final product will be used in humans. But it is not easily available. So, hairless animal skin is generally favored as it is easily obtained from animals of specific age group or sex.

*Intact full thickness skin*: Hair on dorsal skin of animal is removed with animal hair clipper, subcutaneous tissue is surgically removed and dermis side is wiped with isopropyl alcohol to remove residual adhering fat. The skin is washed with distilled water. The skin so prepared is wrapped in aluminum foil and stored in a freezer at –20°C till further use. The skin is defrosted at room temperature when required.

*Separation of epidermis from full thickness skin*: The prepared full thickness skin is treated with 2M sodium bromide solution in water for 6 hour. The epidermis is separated by using a cotton swab moistened with distilled water. Then epidermis sheet is cleaned by washing with distilled water and dried under vacuum. Dried sheets are stored in desiccators until further use.

## The future of transdermal therapy

Ten years ago, the nicotine patch had revolutionized smoking cessation; patients were being treated with nitroglycerin for angina, clonidine for hypertension, scopolamine for motion sickness and estradiol for estrogen deficiency, all through patches. The number of drugs formulated in patches has hardly increased, and there has been little change in the composition of the patch systems. Modifications have been mostly limited to refinements of the materials used.

*A. Molecular absorption enhancement*

Considerable research has been done on absorption enhancers, compounds that promote the passage of drugs through the stratum corneum. Terpene derivatives as well as certain phenols seem to improve transdermal absorption. For example, linalool, alpha terpineol, and carvacrol were studied in conjunction with haloperidol (a commonly prescribed neuroleptic drug). All three enhanced haloperidol absorption, but only linalool increased it to a therapeutic level. Limonene, menthone and eugenol were found to enhance transdermal absorption of tamoxifen. Phloretin, a polyphenol, enhanced the absorption of lignocaine.

*B. Absorption enhancement by energy input*

The above are potential adjuvants to the existing passive transdermal systems. There is also the possibility of active transfer of drugs through the skin by the action of electrical or other forms of energy. Iontophoresis, sonophoresis and electroporation have been gaining so much interest in this field.

**Iontophoresis**—It is a method of transferring substances across the skin by applying an electrical potential difference. It promotes the transfer of charged ionic drugs and possibly high molecular weight substances such as peptides.

Electric current is applied through two electrodes, placed on the patient's skin. The first, or donor, electrode (cathode) delivers the negatively charged therapeutic agent (e.g. an organic acid), whereas the second, or receptor, electrode (anode) serves to close the circuit (Fig. 5.27). This set up is named cathodal iontophoresis. For positively charged drugs (e.g. amines or peptides), the cell arrangement is reversed (anodal iontophoresis). The silver (anode) and silver chloride (cathode) electrode system—Utilized in both types of iontophoresis is favored largely because it does not affect the drug solution to the extent that other electrode systems can. Current commercial applications of iontophoresis include intradermal administration of lidocaine as a local anesthetic and dexamethasone for local inflammation.

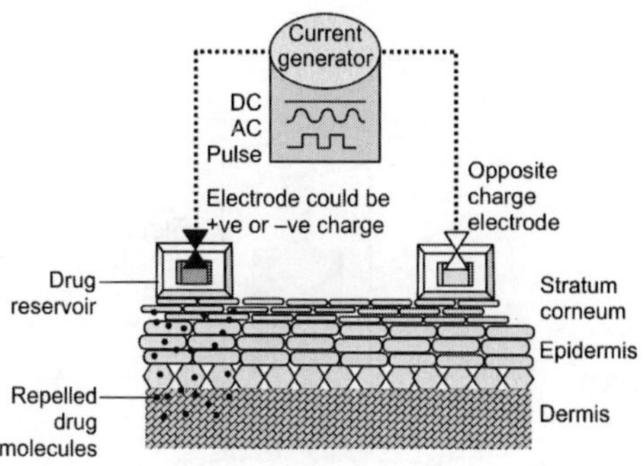


FIGURE 5.27: Iontophoresis

**Sonophoresis (phonophoresis, ultrasound) (Fig. 5.30)**—This is a technique for increasing the skin permeation of drugs using ultrasound (20 KHZ–16 MHZ) as a physical force. The drug is mixed with a coupling agent (may be a gel, cream, or ointment) which transfers the ultrasonic energy from device to skin. Drug is placed on the skin beneath the ultrasonic probe. Ultrasound pulses are passed through the probe and drug molecules are hypothesized to move into the skin through a combination of physical wave pressure and permeabilization of intercellular bilayers (Fig. 5.28).

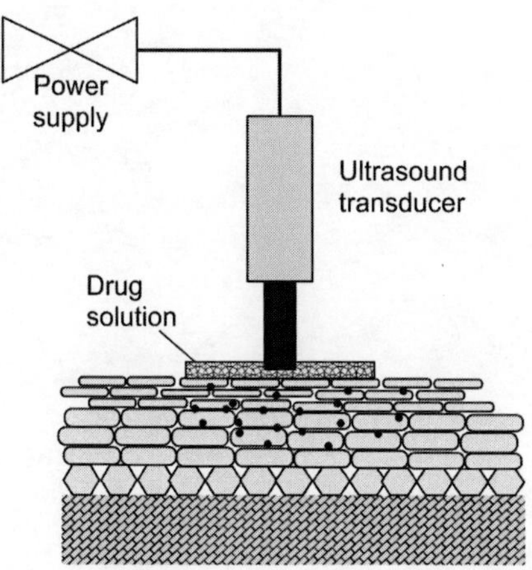


FIGURE 5.28: Sonophoresis

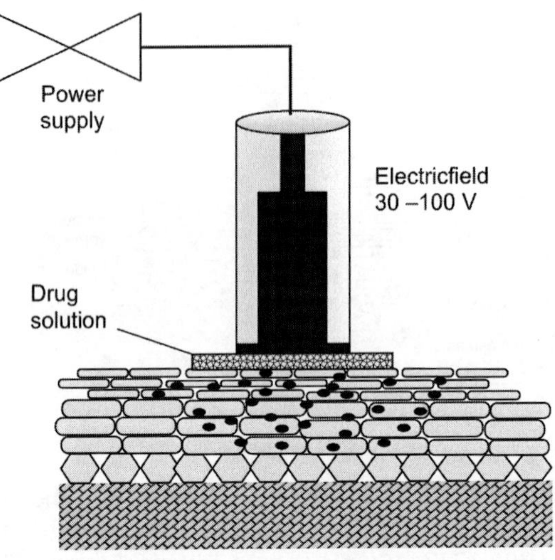


FIGURE 5.29: Electroporation

**Electroporation**—It is a technique that delivers high voltage pulses of micro-to-millisecond duration to the skin, causing transient changes in cell membranes or lipid bilayers (Fig. 5.29). It is hypothesized that pretreatment of the skin in this way would enable the passage of large, polar molecules such as heparin and peptides.

# Chapter 6

# Pharmaceutical Packaging

## INTRODUCTION

Packaging is the science, art and technology of enclosing products for distribution, storage, sale and use. It is also refers to the process of design, evaluation and production of packages. Packaging is a bridge connecting the production with marketing. It is an economical means of providing protection, presentation, identification, information and convenience for a pharmaceutical product from the moment of production until it is used or administered. Packaging is system or means by which the product will reach from production center to the consumer in a safe and sound condition with minimum loss. A package refers to the container closure system and labeling, associated components (e.g. dosing cups, droppers, spoons) and external packaging. In recent years, pharmaceutical manufacturing and packaging operations have struggled to respond quickly to market demand while overcoming operational inefficiencies. An increase in the number and complexity of product configurations, coupled with the demands of compliance with regulations in a time of growing market pressure, has made it a challenge to maintain a stable performance in the market place. New marketing strategies adopted by pharmaceutical companies have initiated the introduction of more packaging configurations to facilitate meeting customer requirements with greater precision. In an effort to compete under these circumstances, pharmaceutical manufacturers have seen the need to become lean and flexible, streamlining their operations and achieving a significant increase in quality, process and compliance management. Packaging is a critical tool in the pharmaceutical industry for product delivery and regulatory compliance; many pharmaceutical companies will do all their packaging within a contamination free environment or clean room. Some common pharmaceutical packaging techniques include foil and heat sealing; polyester and olefin package printing; polyethylene and polypropylene printing and flatbed die cutting.

## Importance of packaging

1. Protect against all adverse external influences that can alter the properties of the product.
2. Protect against biological contamination.
3. Protect against physical damage.
4. Carry the correct information and identification of the product.
5. Tamper evident/child resistance/anticounterfeiting.

## Objectives of packaging

Each package for any product basically serves upto 5 of the following purposes:
1. *Containment*: To hold the product directly.
2. *Information*: To identify the brand and any related companies, to explain how it should be used, to warn about the hazards for misuse and to reveal product contents.
3. *Protection*: To prevent spoilage, leakage, breakage, moisture changes, theft and tampering. These packages seal out contaminants in the environment (germs, dirt, dust, moisture, etc); protect against tampering, theft, breakage, and spoilage.
4. *Transportation*: To easily and safely move the product from the manufacturer, perhaps to a warehouse, then to the retailer and finally, to the consumer.
5. *Display*: To display attractively, to sell (a marketing tool). Size, cost, colors, brands, illustrations and shape are all considered for display. As this country changed from the sales person mode to self-service, the package was needed to inform and sell the product.

## Types of packaging (Table 6.1)

1. *Primary package*: It is the material that directly holds the product. That may be a can, bottle, jar, tube, carton, drum, etc. It is the package which is in direct contact with the contents.

2. *Secondary package*: It is outside the primary package. Any outer wrappings that help to store, transport, inform, display and protect the product are secondary package. The decorated carton is common examples.
3. *Tertiary package*: It is used for bulk handling, warehouse storage and transport shipping. The most common form is a palletized unit load that packs tightly into containers.

For any product, from one to all three types of packaging may be necessary depending on the intended purpose.

**Table 6.1**: Types of primary and secondary packaging material

| *Material* | *Type* | *Example of use* |
|---|---|---|
| Glass | Primary | Metric medical bottle, ampoule, vial |
| Plastic | Primary | Ampoule, vial, infusion fluid container, dropper bottle |
| Cardboard | Secondary | Box to contain primary pack |
| Paper | Secondary | Labels, patient information leaflet |

## PACKAGING AND STABILITY OF PRODUCT

The stability of drug shelf life depends on many factors and packaging is one of them. The selection of the package begins with the determination of the products' physical and chemical characteristics, its protective need and its marketing requirement. The stability of the pharmaceutical product may be totally dependent on proper functioning of package. Some of the selection criteria to be considered are as follows:

- It depends on the ultimate use of the product. The product may be used by skilled person in a hospital or may need to be suitable for use in the home by a patient.
- It depends on the physical form of the product. For example, solid, semisolid, liquids, or gaseous dosage form.
- It depends on the route of administration. For example, oral, parenteral, external, etc.
- It depends on the stability of the material. Moisture, oxygen, carbon dioxide, light, trace metals, temperature or pressure or fluctuation of these may have a deleterious effect on the product.

- It depends on the content. The product may react with the package such as the release of alkali from the glass or the corrosion of the metal and in turn the product is affected.
- It depends on cost of the product. Expensive product usually justifies expensive packaging.

## CONTAINERS FOR PHARMACEUTICAL USE

A container for pharmaceutical use is an article which contains or is intended to contain a product and is, or may be, in direct contact with it. The closure is a part of the container. The container is so designed that the contents may be removed in a manner appropriate to the intended use of the preparation. It provides a varying degree of protection depending on the nature of the product and the hazards of the environment, and minimizes the loss of constituents. The container does not interact physically or chemically with the contents in a way that alters their quality beyond the limits tolerated by official requirements.

### Types of containers

*a. Container used as primary packaging for liquid orals*

**Single dose containers**: Single dose containers hold the products that are intended for single use. An example of such a container is the glass ampule.
**Multidose containers**: Multidose containers hold a quantity of the material that will be used as two or more doses. An example of this system is the multiple doses vial or the plastic bottle.
**Well-closed containers**: Well-closed containers protect the product from contamination with unwanted foreign materials and from loss of contents during use.
**Airtight containers**: Airtight containers are impermeable to solids, liquids and gases during normal storage and uses. If the container is to be opened on more than one occasion, it must remain airtight after reclosure.
**Light-resistant container**: A light-resistant container protect the contents from the effect of radiation at a wave length between 290 nm and 150 nm.
**Sealed container**: A sealed container is a container closed by fusion of the material of the container.

**Tamper-proof container**: A tamper-proof container is a closed container fitted with a device that reveals irreversibly whether the container has been opened.

**Child-proof container**: A child-proof container is a container that is fitted with a closure that prevents opening by children.

*b. For solid dosage forms*

**Tamper-evident containers**: Tamper-evident containers are closed containers fitted with a device that irreversibly indicates if the container has been opened.

**Strip packages**: Strip packages have at least one sealed pocket of material with each pocket containing a single dose of the product. The package is made of two layers of film or laminate material. The nature and level of protection which is required by the contained product will affect the composition of these layers.

**Blister packages**: Blister packages are composed of a base layer, with cavities called blisters which contain the pharmaceutical product, and a lid. This lid is sealed to the base layer by heat, pressure or both. They are more rigid than strip packages and are not used for powders or semisolids. In tropical areas, blister packages with an additional aluminum membrane is used which provide greater protection against high humidity.

**Child-resistant containers**: Child-resistant containers, commonly referred to as CRCs, are designed to prevent the child accessing the potentially hazardous product.

*c. Containers for semisolid and pressurized products*

Semisolid dosage forms like ointments, creams, etc. are packed in metallic collapsible tubes. Plastic containers are also used for the packaging of creams. Pressurized packages expel the product through a valve. The pressure exerted for the expulsion of the product is an important consideration while selecting the packaging for any products.

## PHARMACEUTICAL PACKAGING MATERIALS

Packaging begins with the material selection. Material selection drives the choice and type of packaging equipment and, most importantly, the final package performance.

## Properties of packaging materials

To afford the necessary protection, the materials from which the container is to be made must show certain basic properties which can be divided into four groups.

### i. *Mechanical properties*

The materials used should possess sufficient mechanical strength to withstand while handling, filling, closing and processing. Typical care is needed during transport, storage and also at the time of usage by the consumer especially in case of glass containers. A glass container will have greater strength if all corners are rounded.

### ii. *Physical properties*

- The material should be impervious to any possible contaminants, for example, solids, liquids, gases, vapors or micro-organisms.
- The container must be able to withstand heat if the processing includes sterilization.
- The surface must be capable of clear labeling, often difficult, e.g. with plastics.
- The packaging must have a suitable size, thus, rubber may presents problems if it perishes.
- The material must protect from light if necessary, that is, it must be ultraviolet absorbent.
- The container must not absorb substances from the products, e.g. absorption of water from creams into cardboard box.

### iii. *Chemical properties*

- The container and the closure should not react together, either alone or in the presence of the product. This can occur with certain combination of dissimilar materials.
- The product should not react with the container or closure, as might happen if alkaline substances are placed in aluminum containers.
- Substances must not be extracted from the product, such as the loss of bactericides from injection solution to rubber.

- The container or closure must not yield substances to the product, e.g. alkali from glass, plasticizers from plastics, etc.

iv. ***Biological properties***

The material of the container must be able to withstand attack by insects if this hazard is likely to be encountered. The packing should not support mould growth. The risk is greatest with cellulosic substance and if the use of such materials is unavoidable, the attack may be minimized by impregnation.

## Packaging components

### *Paper and board*

The use of paperboard materials (cellulose fiber) remains a significant part of pharmaceutical packaging in spite of the facts that paper is rarely used on its own for a primary package. Cartons are used for a high percentage of pharmaceutical products for a number of reasons, increasing display area, providing better display of stock items and the collating of leaflets which would otherwise be difficult to attach to many containers. Cartons also provide physical protection especially to items such as metal collapsible tubes. Carton, therefore, tends to be a traditional of pharmaceutical packaging. Regenerated cellulose film (trade names cellophane and rayophane) are still used as an over wrapping material either for individual cartons or to collate a number of cartons. It is being substantially replaced by orientated polypropylene film. Although paper, even when waxed, has relatively poor protective properties against moisture, both paper and board (ointment, pill and tablets boxes) were once used widely for primary packages, particularly for dispensing operations.

### *Glass*

Glass is commonly used in pharmaceutical packaging because it possesses superior protective qualities.

Advantages

i. Economical.
ii. Readily available container of variety of sizes and shapes.

iii. Impermeability.
iv. Strength and rigidity.
v. FDA clearance.
vi. Does not deteriorate with age.
vii. Easy to clean.
viii. Effective closure and resolves are applicable.
ix. Colored glass, especially amber, can give protection against light when it is required.

### Disadvantages

i. Fragility
ii. Heavy weight.

### Composition of glass

Glass is composed principally of silica with varying amount of metal oxides, soda-ash, limestone and cullet. The sand is almost pure silica, the soda-ash is sodium carbonate and the limestone is calcium carbonate. Cullet is broken glass that is mixed with the batch and acts as a fusion agent for the entire mixture. The composition of glass varies and is usually adjusted for specific purposes. The most common cations found in pharmaceutical glassware are silicon, aluminum, boron, sodium, potassium, calcium, magnesium, zinc and barium. The only anion of consequence is oxygen. Many useful properties of glass are affected by the kind of elements it contains. Reduction in the proportion of sodium ions makes glass chemically resistant, however, without sodium or other alkalis, glass is difficult to melt and is expensive. Boron oxide is incorporated mainly to aid in the melting process through reduction of the temperature required.

Lead in small traces gives clarity and brilliance, but produces a relatively soft grade of glass. Alumina (aluminum oxide), however, is often used to increase the hardness and durability and to increase resistance to chemical action.

### Manufacture of glass

Four basic processes are used in the production of glass: blowing, drawing, pressing and casting.

i. **Blow molding process**: Blowing uses compressed air to form the molten glass in the cavity of a metal mold. Most bottles and jars are now made automatically by one of the two methods shown below.

a. *Blow and blow method (Fig. 6.1)*: In blow and blow process, molten 'gobs' (lump of soft substance) of glass are delivered into a mould known as a 'blank' or parison mould. A puff of compressed air blows the glass down into the base of the mould to form the neck or 'finish' part of the bottle or jar. A second blast of compressed air is then applied through the already formed neck of the container to form the 'parison' of pre form for the bottle against the walls of the parison mold cavity.

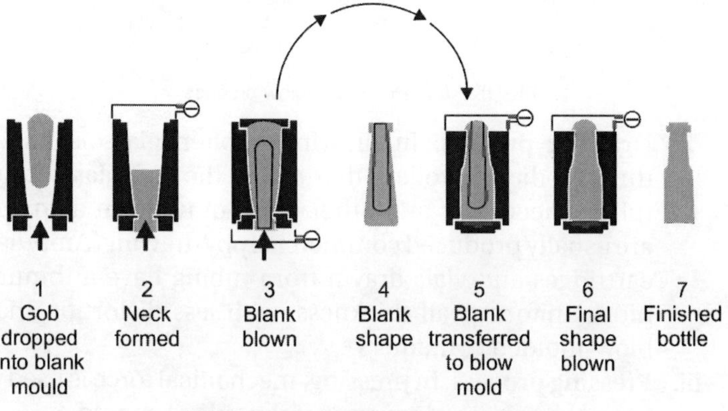


FIGURE 6.1: Blow and blow process

The thick-walled parison is then transferred to the final mold during which time the surface of the glass 'reheats' and softens again enough to allow the final container shape to be fully formed against the walls of the final mould cavity by the application of either compressed air or vacuum. The container is then removed and transferred to an annealing oven where it is reheated to remove the stresses produced during forming and then cooled under carefully controlled conditions.

b. *Press and blow method (Fig. 6.2)*: In press and blow method, molten 'gobs' of glass are delivered into the parison mould and a plunger is used to press the glass into the parison shape. The final mould stage of the process is the same as that described for the blow and blow process. Due to the first stage-pressing process the glass distribution overall is better controlled.

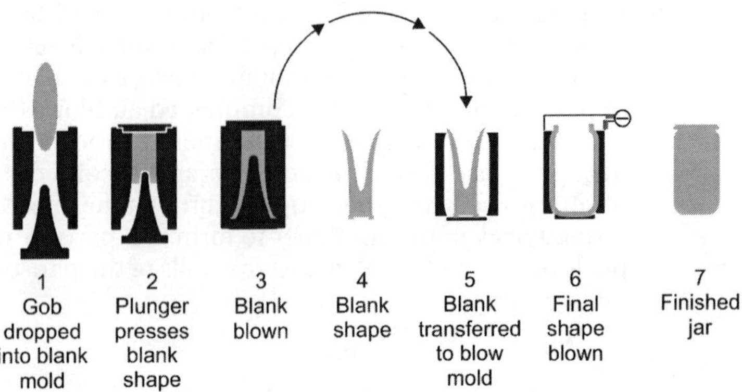


FIGURE 6.2: Press and blow process

ii. **Drawing process**: In drawing, molten glass is pulled through dies or rollers that shape the soft glass. Rods, tubes, sheet glass and other items of uniform diameter are usually produced commercially by drawing. Ampules, cartridges and vials drawn from tubing have a thinner, more uniform wall thickness, with less distortion than blow-molded containers.

iii. **Pressing process**: In pressing, mechanical force is used to press the molten glass against the side of a mold.

iv. **Casting process**: Casting uses gravity or centrifugal force to initiate the formation of molten glass in the cavity.

### Colored glass—Light protection

Glass containers for drugs are generally available in clear flint or amber color (Fig. 6.3). For decorative purposes, special colors such as blue, emerald green and opal may be obtained from the glass manufacturer. Only amber glass and red glass are effective in protecting the contents of a bottle from the effects of sunlight by screening out harmful ultraviolet rays. The USP specifications for light-resistant containers require the glass to provide protection against 2900–4500 Å of light. Amber glass meets these specifications, but the iron oxide added to produce this color could leach into the product. Therefore, if the product contains ingredients subject to iron catalyzed chemical reactions, amber glass should not be used. Manganese oxide can also be used for amber glasses.

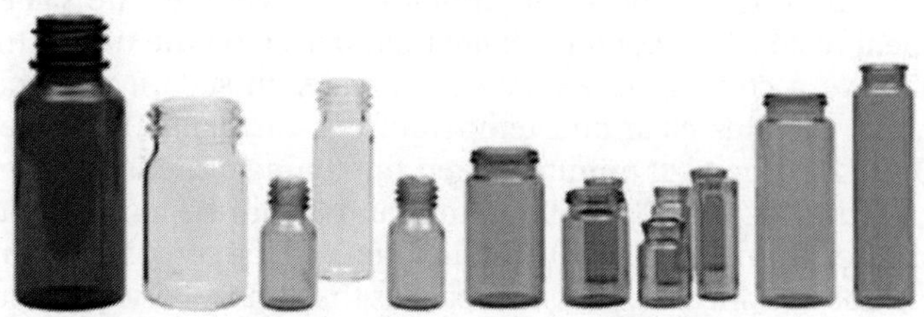

FIGURE 6.3: Types of glass containers

## Tests for glass containers

The USP and NF describe the various types of glass and provide the powdered glass and water attack tests for evaluating the chemical resistance of glass. The test results are measures of the amount of alkalinity leached from the glass by purified water under controlled elevated temperature conditions. The powdered glass test is performed on crushed glass of a specific size, and the water attack test is conducted on whole containers. The water attack test is used only with type II glass that has been exposed to sulfur dioxide fumes under controlled conditions.

a. **Test for surface hydrolytic resistance**: Surface hydrolytic resistance test is conducted on unused glass containers. The number of containers to be examined and the volume of the test solution necessary for final determination are indicated in Table 6.2.

**Table 6.2**: Nominal capacity, numbers of containers and volume of test solution to be used

| *Nominal capacity of container* | *Number of containers to be used* | *Volume of test solution to be used for titration (ml)* |
|---|---|---|
| 3 or less | At least 10 | 25.0 |
| 3 – 30 | At least 5 | 50.0 |
| More than 30 | At least 3 | 100.0 |

Initially, each container is rinsed three times carefully with carbon dioxide free water. Then the container is allowed to drain and it is filled with the carbon dioxide free water to the required volume. If vials and bottle are used, they are covered with neutral glass dishes or aluminum foil which is previously rinsed with carbon dioxide free water. If ampules are used, they are sealed by heat fusion. The containers are then placed on the tray of the autoclave a containing a quantity of water in such a way that the tray remains clear and temperature is maintained between 100°C–120°C over 20 minutes. Then the temperature is adjusted between 120°C–122°C for 60 minutes and finally the temperature is lowered from 120°C for 40 minutes. Remove the containers from the autoclave once the pressure reaches the atmospheric pressure and is cooled under running tap water. Combine the liquids obtained from the containers being examined. The following titration should be carried out within 1 hour after removing the container from the autoclave. Introduce the prescribed volume of liquid into a conical flask. Add 0.05 ml of methyl red solution for each 20 ml liquid. Titrate with 0.01 M hydrochloric acid taking as the end point the color obtained by repeating the operation using the same volumes of carbon dioxide free water. The result is not greater than the volume stated in Table 6.3.

**Table 6.3:** Test limits for surface glass test

| *Capacity of container* | *Volume of 0.01 M hydrochloric acid vs per 100 ml of test solution* | |
|---|---|---|
| | *Type I or II glass (ml)* | *Type III glass (ml)* |
| Not more than 1 | 3.0 | 20.0 |
| More than 1 but not more than 2 | 1.8 | 17.6 |
| More than 2 but not more than 5 | 1.3 | 13.2 |
| More than 5 but not more than 10 | 1.0 | 10.2 |
| More than 10 but not more than 20 | 0.80 | 8.1 |
| More than 20 but not more than 50 | 0.60 | 6.1 |
| More than 50 but not more than 100 | 0.50 | 4.8 |
| More than 100 but not more than 200 | 0.40 | 3.8 |
| More than 200 but not more than 500 | 0.30 | 2.9 |
| More than 500 | 0.20 | 2.2 |

b. **Test for hydrolytic resistance of powdered glass:** The containers to be tested are initially rinsed with water and dried in hot air oven. At least three containers are taken and broken with a hammer to get coarse fragments of about 100 gm size of which the largest fragment should not be greater than 25 mm. Transfer a part of the sample to a mortar and insert the pestle and strike heavily once with the hammer. Transfer the contents of the mortar to the coarsest sieve. Repeat the operation sufficient number of times until the entire fragment has been transferred to the sieve. The glass is sifted and the portion retained by the 710 µm and 423 µm sieve is taken and are further fractured. The operation is repeated until 20 gm of glass is retained by the 710 µm sieve. Reject this portion and the portion that passes through 250 µm sieve. Shake the nest of sieve manually or mechanically for 5 minutes. Glass grains that passes through 425 µm sieve is taken. Metal particles, are removed by suspending the glass grains in acetone and the supernatant liquid is decanted. The operation is repeated five times. Glass grains are speeded on an evaporating dish and allow the acetone to evaporate by drying in an oven at 110°C for 20 minutes and allow to cool. 20 gm of the glass grains to be treated is introduced into a 250 ml conical flask add 100 ml of carbon dioxide free water and weigh in the second flask 100 ml carbon dioxide free water serve as blank and weigh. Close the two flasks with neutral glass dish or aluminum foil rinsed with carbon dioxide free water. The flask is then placed in on autoclave and maintains the temperature at 121°C for 30 minutes and carry out the operations similar to those described in Test A for surface hydrolytic resistance. After cooling, remove the closure, wipe the flask and adjust the original weight by adding carbon dioxide free water. Transfer 50 ml (corresponding to 10 gm of glass grains) of the clear supernatant liquid into a conical flask. 50 ml of water is taken in other flask which is used as blank 0.1 ml methyl red solution, is added as indicator and titrated with 0.001 M hydrochloric acid until the color of the liquid is same as that obtained with blank. Subtract the value of the blank and express the result in milliliters of hydrochloric acid consumed per 10 gm of glass. Type I glass containers require not more than 2.0 ml, Type II or III requires not more than 17.0 ml and Type IV glass containers requires not more than 30.0 ml of 0.001 M hydrochloric acid (Table 6.4).

**Table 6.4:** Test limits for powdered glass test

| *Type* | *General description*[a] | *Type of test* | *Limits* | |
|---|---|---|---|---|
| | | | Size[b] (ml) | 0.020 N acid (ml) |
| I | Highly resistant, borosilicate glass | Powdered glass | All | 1.0 |
| III | Soda-lime glass | Powdered glass | All | 8.5 |

a—The description applies to containers of this type of glass usually available.
b—Size indicates the overflow capacity of the container.

## Types of glass

According to their hydrolytic resistance, glass containers are classified as (Table 6.5):

**Table 6.5:** Types of glass

| *Type* | *General description* | *Type of test* |
|---|---|---|
| I | Highly resistant, borosilicate glass | Powdered glass |
| II | Treated soda-lime glass | Water attack |
| III | Soda-lime glass | Powdered glass |
| IV | General-purpose soda-lime glass | Powdered glass |

### *a. Type I—Borosilicate glass*

Borosilicate glass is a highly resistant glass. In this type of glass, a substantial part of the alkali and earth cations is replaced by boron and/or aluminum and zinc. It is more chemically inert than the soda-lime glass, which contains either none or an insignificant amount of these cations. Although glass is considered to be a virtually inert material and is used to contain strong acids and alkalis as well as all types of solvents, it has a definite and measurable chemical reaction with some substances, notably water. The sodium is loosely combined with the silicon and is leached from the surface of the glass by water. Distilled water stored for one year in flint type III glass (to be described) picks up 10–15 parts per million (ppm) of sodium hydroxide along with traces of other ingredients of the glass. The addition of approximately 6% boron to form type I borosilicate glass reduces the leaching action, so that only 0.5 ppm is dissolved in a year.

*b. Type II—Treated soda-lime glass*

When glassware is stored for several months especially in a damp atmosphere or with extreme temperature variations, the wetting of the surface by condensed moisture (condensation) results in salts being dissolved out of the glass. This is called "blooming" or "weathering," and in its early stages, it gives the appearance of fine crystals on the glass. At this stage, these salts can be washed off with water or acid. Type II containers are made of commercial soda-lime glass that has been dealkalized or treated to remove surface alkali. The dealkalizing process is known as "sulfur treatment" and virtually prevents "weathering" of empty bottles. The treatment offered by several glass manufacturers exposes the glass to an atmosphere containing water vapor and acidic gases, particularly sulfur dioxide at an elevated temperature. This results in a reaction between the gases and some of the surface alkali, rendering the surface fairly resistant, for a period of time, to attack by water. The alkali removed from the glass appears on the surface as a sulfate bloom, which is removed when the containers are washed before filling. Sulfur treatment neutralizes the alkaline oxides on the surface, thereby rendering the glass more chemically resistant.

*c. Type III—Soda-lime glass*

The containers are untreated and made of commercial soda-lime glass of average or better-than-average chemical resistance.

*d. Type IV—General-purpose soda-lime glass*

The containers made of soda-lime glass are supplied for non-parenteral products, those intended for oral or topical use.

### Problems associated with glass containers

**Sorption**: When formulation components are removed by a package two different processes are involved—Adsorption onto the surface and absorption into the package wall by diffusion. A component may also desorb from the outer surface of the package and pass into the atmosphere if it is volatile enough. Strong adsorption or absorption requires a strong chemical interaction between the component and the packaging material in addition, for a high level of absorption the packaging material must be permeable to the component. Glass has a chemically active surface but is an absolute barrier so that while adsorption can be strong, no absorption occurs.

### Glass containers for injectable preparations

Glass containers intended for injectable preparations may be ampules, vials or bottles.

**Ampules**: Ampules are thin-walled glass containers, which after filling, are sealed by either tip sealing or pull sealing. The contents are withdrawn after rupture of the glass, or a single occasion only. These are great packaging for a variety of drugs. The filled in product is in contact with glass only and the packaging is 100% tamper proof. The break system OPC (one –point cut) or the color break ring offers consistent breaking force. There are wide variety of ampoule types from 0.5–50 ml. Upto 3 color rings can be placed the stem or body for identification purpose. Printed ampoules with heavy metal free colors are available. Some of them are:

- Type B straight –stem
- Type C funnel –tip
- Type D closed

**Bottles, vials and syringes**: These are more or less thick-walled containers with closures of glass or of material other than glass such as plastic materials or elastomers. The contents may be removed in several proportions on one or more occasions.

### *Plastic*

Plastics are the fastest-growing material used in pharmaceutical packaging. Plastics are replacing metal and glass containers for pharmaceutical end uses (Figs 6.4A to D). Plastics in packaging have proved useful for a number of reasons, including the ease with which they can be formed, their high quality and the freedom of design to which they lend themselves. Plastic containers are extremely resistant to breakage and thus offer safety to consumers along with reduction of breakage losses at all levels of distribution and use. Plastic containers for pharmaceutical products are primarily made from the following polymers—Polyethylene, polypropylene, polyvinyl chloride, polystyrene, and to a lesser extent, polymethyl methacrylate, polyethylene terephthalate, polytetrafluoroethylene, the amino formaldehydes and polyamides. Plastic containers consist of one or more polymers together with certain additives. Those manufactured for pharmaceutical purposes must be free of substances that can be extracted in significant quantities by the product contained. Thus, the hazards of toxicity or physical and chemical instability are avoided. The amount and nature of the additives are determined by the nature of the polymer, the process used to convert the plastic into the containers, and the service expected from the container. For plastic containers in general, additives may consist of antioxidants, antistatic agents, colors, impact modifiers, lubricants, plasticizers and stabilizers.

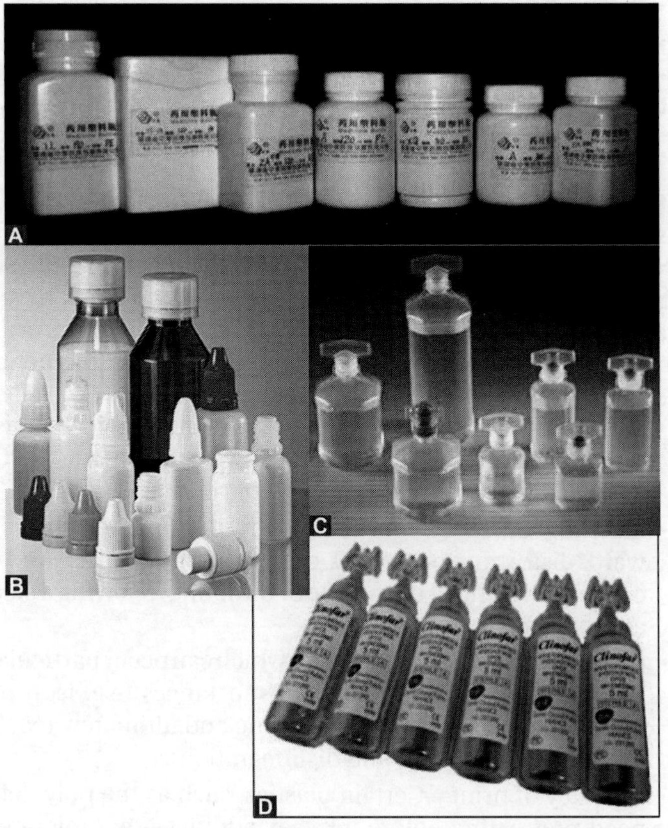


FIGURES 6.4A to D: Types of plastic containers

Mold release agents are not usually used unless they are required for a specific purpose.

### Advantages

Plastic containers have a number of inherent practical advantages over other containers or dispenses. They are as following:

- Low in cost
- Light in weight
- Durable
- Pleasant to touch
- Flexible facilitating product dispensing
- Odorless and inert to most chemicals
- Unbreakable
- Leak proof
- Able to retain their shape throughout their use
- They have a unique suck-back feature, which prevents product doze.

### Disadvantages

Plastics appear to have certain disadvantages like interaction, adsorption, absorption, lightness and hence poor physical stability. All are permeable to some degree to moisture, oxygen, carbon dioxide, etc. and most of them exhibit electrostatic attraction, allow penetration of light rays unless pigmented, black, etc. Other negative features include:

- Stress cracking—A phenomenon related to low density polythene and certain stress cracking agents such as wetting agents, detergents and some volatile oils.
- Paneling or cavitations—Whereby a container shows in ward distortion or partial collapse owing to absorption causing swelling of the plastic or dimpling following a steam autoclaving operation.
- Crazing—A surface reticulation which can occur particularly with polystyrene and chemical substances (e.g. isopropyl myristate which first causes crazing and ultimately reaches at total embitterment and disintegration).
- Poor key of print—Certain plastics, such as the polyolefins need pretreating before ink. Key additives that migrate to the surface of the plastic may also cause printing problem.

- Poor impact resistance—Both polystyrene and PVC have poor resistance. This can be improved by the inclusion of impact modifiers such as rubber in case of polystyrene and methyl methacrylate butadiene styrene for PVC.

Majority of these effects can be either minimized or can be overcome by one or another means. For example, it was required to pack a nasal spray formulation in a plastic squeeze bottle which was available worldwide. This immediately called for a low density polyethylene (LDPE) pack. The product, however, contained a volatile preservative system, which both dissolved in LPPE and was lost from it by volatilization, thereby immediately suggesting that a conventional squeeze pack was unsuitable. The LDPE bottle was enclosed in a PVC blister impermeable to the volatile preservative and fitted with a peelable foil lid (also impermeable). As a result of this combination the loss of preservative was restricted to less than 5% of the total, i.e. preservative soluble in the LDPE and preservative in the air space of the PVC blister reached a point where equilibrium was achieved between product, LDPE and the surrounding air space.

### Materials used for plastic containers

At present, a great number of plastic resins are available for the packaging of drug products. The more popular ones are:

#### *a. Polyethylene*

High-density polyethylene is the material most widely used for container by the pharmaceutical industry and will probably continues to be for the next several years. Polyethylene is a good barrier against moisture, but a relatively poor one against oxygen and other gases. Most solvents do not attack polyethylene, and it is unaffected by strong acids and alkalis. Polyethylene has certain disadvantages that it lacks clarity and a relatively high rate of permeation of essential odors, flavors and oxygen. Despite these problems, polyethylene in all its variations offers the best all-around protection to the greatest number of products at the lowest cost.

The density of polyethylene, which ranges from 0.91–0.96, directly determines the four basic physical characteristics of the blow-molded container: 1) stiffness, 2) moisture-vapor transmission, 3) stress cracking and 4) clarity or translucency.

As the density increases, the material becomes stiffer. It has a higher distortion and melting temperature. It becomes less permeable to gases and vapors, and becomes less resistant to stress cracking. The molecular structure of high-density material is essentially the same as that of low-density material, the main difference being fewer side branches. Since these polymers are generally susceptible to oxidative degradation during processing and subsequent exposure, the addition of some antioxidant is necessary. Usually levels of hundreds of parts per million are used. Antioxidants generally used are butylated hydroxytoluene or dilauryl thiodipropionate. Antistatic additives are often used in bottle grade polyethylenes. Their purpose is to minimize airborne dust accumulation at the surface bottle during handling, filling, and storage. These antistatic additives are usually polyethylene glycols or long chain fatty amides and are often used at 0.1– 0.2% concentrations in high-density polyethylene.

*b. Polypropylene*

Polypropylene has recently become popular because it has many good features of polyethylene, with one major disadvantage either eliminated or minimized. Polypropylene does not stress-crack under any conditions. Except for hot aromatic or halogenated solvents, which soften it, this polymer has good resistance to almost all types of chemicals, including strong acids, alkalis, and most organic materials. Its high melting point makes it suitable for boilable packages and for sterilizable products. Lack of clarity is still a drawback, but improvement is possible with the construction of thinner walls. Polypropylene is an excellent gas and vapor barrier. Its resistance to permeation is equivalent to or slightly better than that of high-density or linear polyethylene, and it is superior to low-density or branched polyethylene. One of the biggest disadvantages of polypropylene is its brittleness at low temperatures. In its purest form, it is quite fragile at 0°F and must be blended with polyethylene or other material to give it the impact resistance required for packaging.

*c. Polyvinyl chloride (PVC)*

Clear rigid polyvinyl chloride bottles overcome some of the deficiencies of polyethylene. PVC can be produced with crystal clarity, provide a fairly good oxygen barrier, and have greater stiffness. In its natural state, polyvinyl chloride is crystal clear and stiff, but has poor impact resistance. PVC can be softened with plasticizers. Various stabilizers, antioxidants, lubricants, or colorants may be incorporated. Polyvinyl chloride is seldom used in its purest form. PVC is an inexpensive, tough, clear material that is relatively easy to manufacture. PVC must not be overheated because it starts to degrade at 280°F, and the degradation products are extremely corrosive. Polyvinyl chloride yellows when exposed to heat or ultraviolet light, unless a stabilizer is included by the resin supplier. From the standpoint of clarity, the best stabilizers are the tin compounds, but the majority cannot be used for food or drug products. Dioctyltin mercaptoacetate and maleate compounds have been approved by the FDA, but these have a slight odor, which is noticeable in freshly blown bottles. Polyvinyl chloride is an excellent barrier for oil, both volatile and fixed alcohols, and petroleum solvents. It retains odor and flavors quite well and is a good barrier for oxygen. Rigid polyvinyl chloride is a fairly good barrier for moisture and gases in general, but plasticizers reduce these properties. Polyvinyl chloride is not affected by acids or alkalis except for some oxidizing acids. Its impact resistance is poor, specially at low temperatures.

*d. Polystyrene*

General-purpose polystyrene is a rigid, crystal clear plastic. Polystyrene has been used by dispensing pharmacists for years for containers for solid dosage forms because it is relatively low in cost. At present, polystyrene is not useful for liquid products. The plastic has a high water vapor transmission (in comparison to high-density polyethylene) as well as high oxygen permeability. Depending on the methods of manufacture and other factors, polystyrene containers are easily scratched and often crack when dropped. Polystyrene will build up static charge. Polystyrene has a low melting point (190°F) and therefore cannot be used for hot items or other high-temperature applications. Polystyrene is resistant to acids, except strong oxidizing acids, and to alkalis. Polystyrene is attacked by many chemicals, which cause it to craze and crack, and so it is generally used for packaging dry products only. To improve impact strength and brittleness, general-purpose polystyrene may be combined with various concentrations of rubber and acrylic compounds. Certain desired properties like clarity and hardness diminish with impact polystyrene. The shock resistance or toughness of impact polystyrene may be varied by increasing the content of rubber in the material, and often these materials are further classified as intermediate-impact, high-impact and super-impact polystyrene.

*e. Nylon (polyamide)*

Nylon is made from a dibasic acid combined with a di-amine. Variety of nylons can be made with different dibasic acids and amines. The type of acid and amine that is used is characteristic and denotes the type of acid and amine used, e.g. Nylon 6/10 has six carbon atoms in the di-amine and ten in the acid. Nylon and similar polyamide materials can be fabricated into thin-wall containers. Nylon can be autoclaved and is extremely strong and quite difficult to destroy by mechanical means. Important to the widespread acceptance of nylon is its resistance to a wide range of organic and inorganic chemicals. As a barrier material, nylon is highly impermeable to oxygen. It is not a good barrier to water vapor, but when this characteristic is required; nylon film can be laminated to polyethylene or to various other materials. Its relative high-water transmission rate and the possibility of drug-plastic interaction have reduced the potential of nylon for long-term storage of drugs. Some of the nylon approved by FDA is Nylon 6, Nylon 6/6, Nylon 6/10, Nylon 11, and certain copolymers.

*f. Polycarbonate*

Polycarbonate can be made into a clear transparent container. Polycarbonate is expensive and offers some advantage that it can be sterilized repeatedly. The containers are rigid, as is glass, and thus has been considered a possible replacement for glass vials and syringes. It is FDA-approved, although its drug-plastic problems have not been investigated adequately. It is only moderately chemically resistant and only a fair moisture barrier. The plastic is known for its dimensional stability, high impact strength, resistance to strain, low water absorption, transparency, and resistance to heat and flame.

Polycarbonate is resistant to dilute acids, oxidizing or reducing agents, salts, oils (fixed and volatile), greases and aliphatic hydrocarbons. It is attacked by alkalis, amines, ketones, esters, aromatic hydrocarbons and some alcohols. Polycarbonate resins are expensive and consequently are used in specialty containers. Since, the impact strength of polycarbonate is almost five times greater than other common packaging plastics, components can be designed with thinner walls to help reduce cost.

*g. Acrylic multipolymers (nitrile polymers)*

These polymers represent the acrylonitrile or methacrylonitrile monomer. Their unique properties of high gas barrier, good chemical resistance, excellent strength properties and safe disposability by incineration make them effective containers for products that are difficult to package in other plastic containers. Their oil and grease resistance and minimal taste transfer effects are particularly advantageous in food packaging. These types of polymers produce clear container and are less costly. The use of nitrile polymers for food and pharmaceutical packaging is regulated to standards set by the FDA. The present safety standard is less than 11 ppm residual acrylonitrile monomer, with allowable migration at less than 0.3 ppm for all food products.

*h. Polyethylene terephthalate (PET)*

Polyethylene terephthalate, generally called PET, is a condensation polymer typically formed by the reaction of terephthalic acid or dimethyl terephthalate with ethylene glycol in the presence of a catalyst. Although used as a packaging film since the late 1950s, its growth has recently escalated with its use in the fabrication of plastic bottles for the carbonated beverage industry. Its excellent impact strength and gas and aroma barrier make it attractive for use in cosmetics and mouth washes as well as in other products in which strength, toughness, and barrier are important considerations. Polyethylene terephthalate is used in food packaging and offers favorable environmental impact system.

## Product-plastic interactions

Product-plastic interactions have been divided into five separate categories: (1) permeation, (2) leaching, (3) sorption, (4) chemical reactivity and (5) modification.

*1. Permeation*

The transmission of gases, vapors, or liquids through plastic packaging materials can have an adverse effect on the shelf life of a drug. Permeation of water vapor and oxygen through the plastic wall into the drug can present a problem if the dosage form is sensitive to hydrolysis and oxidation. Temperature and humidity are important factors influencing the permeability of oxygen and water through plastic. An increase in temperature reflects an increase in the permeability of the gas. Great differences in permeability are possible, depending on the gas and the plastic used. Molecules do not permeate through crystalline zones; thus, an increase in crystallinity of the material should decrease permeability. Two polyethylene materials may, therefore, give different permeability values at various temperatures. Materials such as nylon, which are hydrophilic in nature, are poor barriers to water vapor, while such hydrophobic materials as polyethylene provide much better barriers. Studies have also revealed that formulations containing volatile ingredients might change when stored in plastic containers because one or more of the ingredients are passing through the walls of the containers. Often, the aroma of cosmetic products becomes objectionable, owing to transmission of one of the ingredients and the taste of medicinal products changes for the same reason. The physical system making up the product also may have an influence on the plastic container. For example, certain water-in-oil emulsions cannot be stored in a hydrophobic plastic bottle, since there is a tendency for the oil phase to migrate and diffuse into the plastic.

*2. Leaching*

Most plastic containers have one or more ingredients added in small quantities to stabilize or impart a specific property to the plastic and the prospect of leaching, or migration from the container to the drug product is present. Problems may arise with plastics when coloring agents in relatively small quantities are added to the formula. Particular dyes may migrate into a parenteral solution and cause a toxic effect. Release of a constituent from the plastic container to the drug product may lead to drug contamination and necessitate removal of the product from the market.

*3. Sorption*

This process involves the removal of drug content from the product by the packaging material. Sorption may lead to serious consequences and active ingredients are in solution. Since, drug substances of high potency are administered in small doses, losses due to sorption may significantly affect the therapeutic efficacy of the preparation. Sorption is seen mainly with preservatives. These agents exert their activity at low concentration, and their loss through sorption may be great enough to leave a product unprotected against microbial growth. Factors that influence characteristics of sorption from product are chemical structure, pH, solvent system, concentration of active ingredients, temperature, length of contact, and area of contact.

*4. Chemical reactivity*

Certain ingredients that are used in plastic formulations may react chemically with one or more components of a drug product. At times, ingredients in the formulation may react with the plastic. Even microquantities of chemically incompatible substances can alter the appearance of the plastic or the drug product.

*5. Modification*

The changes in physical and chemical properties of the packaging material by the pharmaceutical product are called modification. Such phenomena as permeation, sorption, and leaching play a role in altering the properties of the plastic and it may also lead to its degradation. Deformation in polyethylene containers is often caused by permeation of gases and vapors from the environment or by loss of content through the container walls. Some solvent systems have been found to be responsible for considerable changes in the mechanical properties of plastics. Oils, for example, have a softening effect on polyethylene; fluorinated hydrocarbons attack polyethylene and polyvinyl chloride. In some cases, the content may extract the plasticizer, antioxidant, or stabilizer, thus changing the flexibility of the package. Polyvinyl chloride is an excellent barrier for petroleum solvents, but the plasticizer in polyvinyl chloride is extracted by solvents. This action usually leaves the plastic hard and stiff. Sometimes, this effect is not immediately perceptible because the solvent either softens the plastic or replaces the plasticizer; later, when the solvent evaporates, the full stiffening effect becomes apparent.

## Constituents of plastic containers

The residues, additives and processing aids that may be used and therefore possibly extracted from plastic include:

- Monomer residues
- Catalysts
- Accelerators
- Solvents
- Extenders
- Fillers
- Slip additives
- Antislip additives
- Antistatic agents
- Antiblocking agents
- Release agents.

Most plastics include only a few of these constituents. Depending upon the additives used, other properties of the plastic can be changed, e.g. fillers such as chalk or talc are likely to increase moisture permeation.

## Quality control test for plastics

A. ***Tests on plastic container***—For parenteral and nonparenteral preparations:

   i. *Leakage test*: Fill ten containers with water. Fit with intended closures and keep them inverted at room temperature for 24 hours. There are no signs of leakage from any container.

   ii. *Collapsibility test*: This test is applicable to the container which is to be squeezed in order to remove the contents. A container by collapsing inwards during use yields at least 90% of its nominal contents at the required rate of flow at ambient temperature.

   iii. *Clarity of aqueous extract*: Select sufficient amount of unlabelled, unmarked and nonlaminated portions randomly from suitable containers, to yield a total area of sample required, taking into account the surface area of both sides. Cut these portions into strips, none of which has a total area of more than 20 $cm^2$. Wash the strips to make it free from extraneous matter by shaking them with at least two separate portions of distilled water for about 30 seconds in each case, then draining off the water thoroughly.

iv. *Transparency test*: Fill five empty containers to their nominal capacity with diluted suspension. The cloudiness of the diluted suspension in each container is detectable when viewed through the containers as compared with a container of the same type filled with water.

v. *Water vapor permeability test*: Fill five containers with nominal volume of water and heat seal the bottles with an aluminum foil-polyethylene laminate or other suitable seal. Weigh accurately each container and allow standing (without any overwrap) for 14 days at a relative humidity of 60% ± 5% and a temperature between 20°C and 25°C. Reweigh the containers. The loss in weight in each container is not more than 0.2%.

B. ***Biological tests***—The USP has provided its procedures for evaluating the toxicity of plastic materials. Essentially, the tests consist of three phases:

a. *Implantation test*: Implanting small pieces of plastic material intramuscularly in rabbits.
b. *Systemic injection test*: Injecting eluates using sodium chloride injection, with and without alcohol intravenously in mice and injecting eluates using polyethylene glycol 400 and sesame oil intraperitoneally in mice.
c. *Intracutaneous test*: Injecting all four eluates subcutaneously in rabbits. The reaction from test samples must not be significantly greater than nonreactive control samples.

### Plastic containers for injectable preparations

Only material, which is practically odorless, is used in the manufacture of containers. Additives such as antioxidants, lubricants, plasticizers, stabilizers, etc. It may be used but no pigment may be used for purposes of coloring.

The container is sufficiently transparent to allow adequate visual inspection of its contents. A filled container is to be sterilizable by heat or any other method without showing signs of shrinkage, distortion, discoloration, loss of transparency, cracking, tackiness, or any other kind of deterioration. The container is of a size, shape and design (including provisions for attachments where necessary) suitable for its intended use.

### Plastic containers for ophthalmic preparation

Plastic containers for ophthalmic preparations are made from plastic composed of a mixture of homologous compounds having a range of molecular weights. Such plastics frequently contain other substances such as residues from the polymerization process, plasticizers, stabilizers, antioxidants, lubricants and pigments. For deciding the suitability of a plastic for use as a container for ophthalmic preparations, factors such as the composition of the plastic, processing and cleaning procedures, contacting media, adhesives, adsorption and permeability of preservatives, conditions of storage, etc. must be considered.

### *Metal*

The collapsible metal tube is an attractive container that permits controlled amounts to be dispensed easily, with good reclosure and adequate environmental protection to the product. The risk of contamination of the portion remaining in the tube is minimal, because the tube does not "suck back." It is light in weight and unbreakable, and it lends itself to high-speed automatic filling operations.

### Advantages

i. Material strength (capable of withstanding internal pressure in aerosol containers).
ii. Impermeable to gases.
iii. Light barrier (opaque, this is both advantageous and disadvantageous).
iv. Lightweight (due to the strength of the material in thin cross-sections).
v. High heat transmission (metals conduct heat well, approximately 100 times better than glass and 400 times better than plastics).
vi. Mature manufacturing methods.
vii. Malleability, the materials can be tailored in hardness and flexibility to the container.

viii. Dead fold capability (only material with the strength and durability to act as the over-cap on vials with elastomeric closure).
ix. Low weight of finished package (a consequence of the high strength of the material).
x. Exterior decoration (both aluminum and tinplate can be highly decorated).
xi. Tamper evidence (breaking a metal seal cannot be reversed).

## Disadvantages

i. Potential interaction with product (the metal must be coated or insulated from the product).
ii. Limited shelf life (liquids).
iii. Container weight compared to glass (aluminum containers with density of approximately 2.7 can compete well with plastics; tinplate containers with density over 8 cannot compete against plastics).
iv. Cost to produce in small unit volumes (this is both advantageous and disadvantageous, depending on container specification).
v. Difficulty to produce small volume containers.

## Materials used for metal containers

The ductile metals used for collapsible tubes are tin (15%), aluminum (60%) and lead (25%). Tin is the more expensive than lead. Tin is the most ductile of these metals. Laminates of tin-coated lead provide better appearance and will be resistant to oxidation. They are also cheaper compared to tin alone. The tin that is used for this purpose is alloyed with about 0.5% copper for stiffening. When lead is used, about 3% antimony is added to increase hardness. Aluminum work hardens when it is formed into a tube, and must be annealed to give it the necessary pliability. Aluminum also hardens in use, sometimes causing tubes to develop leaks.

**Tin**: Tin containers are preferred for foods, pharmaceuticals, or any product for which purity is an important consideration. Tin is chemically inert of all collapsible tube metals. It offers a good appearance and compatibility with a wide range of products.

**Aluminum**: Aluminum tubes offer significant savings in product shipping costs because of their light weight. They provide good appearance.

**Lead**: Lead has the lowest cost of all tube metals and is widely used for nonfood products such as adhesives, inks, paints, and lubricants. Lead should never be used alone for anything taken internally because of the risk of lead poisoning. The inner surface of the lead tubes is coated and is used for products like fluoride toothpaste.

**Linings**: If the product is not compatible with bare metal, the interior can be flushed with wax-type formulations or with resin solutions, although the resins or lacquers are usually sprayed on. A tube with an epoxy lining costs about 25% more than the same tube uncoated. Wax linings are most often used with water-base products in tin tubes, and phenolics, epoxides, and vinyls are used with aluminum tubes, giving better protection than wax, but at a higher cost. When acidic products are packed, phenolics are used and for alkaline products, epoxides are used.

### Aerosol cans

Aerosol cans are unique applications for pharmaceutical containers. They deliver drugs for asthma and other inhalation products, sterile gases used as anesthetics and gas uncontaminated with other atmospheric gases to support the eye during ophthalmic surgery.

The application of antiseptics to wounds and the delivery of topical ointments are some additional uses of aerosols made possible by metal cans. Metal packages, particularly tinplate packages, are competing with plastic and composite materials, making their choice for packaging a cost/performance/consumer preference trade-off. Metal tubes are competing with plastic multilayer tubes in the same way. This is an example of a standard package being challenged for a number of different reasons, and in some cases, a decision being made to change from one material to another.

### *Rubber based components*

Rubber components may be made from either natural or synthetic sources. Natural rubber has got good resealing (multidose injection), fragmentation and coring (description for the means by which particles are created when a needle is passed through a rubber) when compared to synthetic rubber but is poor in respect to ageing and chances of moisture and gas permeation and the absorption of preservative systems is more. Sterilization by multiple autoclaving is also not possible. Synthetic rubbers tend to reverse all of these properties and some formulations actually contain natural rubber in order to improve resealability, fragmentation and coring. Most rubber formulation are relatively complex and may contain one or more of the vulcanizing agents, accelerators, fillers, activators, pigments, antioxidants, lubricants, softeners, or waxes. The main types of rubber used for pharmaceutical products include natural rubber, neoprene, nitrile, butyl, chlorobutyl, bromobutyl and silicone. Of these silicone is the most expensive and although the most inert, is readily permeable to moisture, gases and absorbent to certain preservatives. Rubber components are likely to contain more additives than plastics. Hence, product-package interactions should be properly tested before they are used for injectable or intravenous type products. Rubber gaskets are also sound in aerosols and metered-dose pump systems.

The closure is normally the most vulnerable and critical component of a container in so far as stability and compatibility with the product are concerned. An effective closure must prevent the contents from escaping and allow no substance to enter the container. The adequacy of the seal depends on a number of things, such as the resiliency of the liner, the flatness of the sealing surface on the container, and most importantly, the tightness or torque with which it is applied. In evaluating an effective closure system, the major considerations are the type of container, the physical and chemical properties of the product, and the stability-compatibility requirements for a given period under certain conditions.

## Closures

### *Function of a closure*

- It provides a totally hermetic seal
- It provides an effective seal which is acceptable to the products
- It provides an effective microbiological seal.

### *Characteristics of closure*

- It should be resistant and compatible with the product and the product/air space.
- If closure is of reclosable type, it should be readily operable and should be resealed effectively.

- It should be capable of high speed application where necessary for automatic production without loss of seal efficiency.
- It should be decorative and of a shape that blends in with the main containers.

*Types of closures*

Closures are available in five basic designs:

- Screw-on, threaded, or lug
- Crimp-on (crowns)
- Press-on (snap)
- Roll-on
- Friction.

Many variations of these basic types exist, including vacuum, tamper proof, safety, child resistant, and liner less types, and dispenser applicators.

i. *Threaded screw cap (Fig. 6.5)*: The screw cap when applied overcome the sealing surface irregularities and provides physical and chemical protection to content being sealed. The screw cap is commonly made of metal or plastics. The metal is usually tin plate or aluminum, and in plastics, both thermoplastic and thermosetting materials are used. Metal caps are usually coated on the inside with an enamel or lacquer for resistance against corrosion. Almost all metal crowns and closures are made from electrolytic tinplate, tin-coated steel on which the tin is applied by electrolytic deposition.

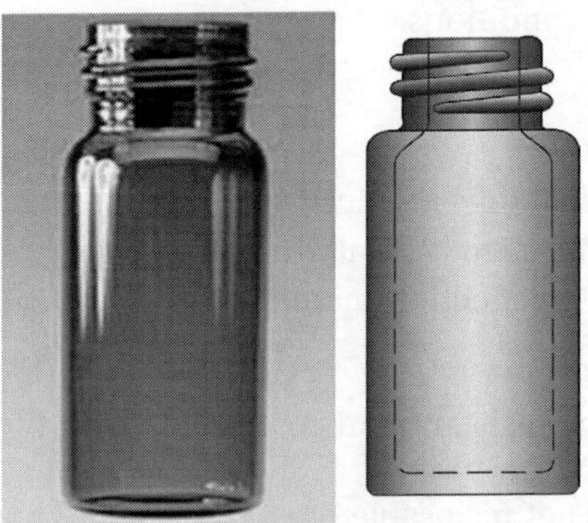

FIGURE 6.5: Threaded screw cap

ii. *Lug cap*: The lug cap is similar to the threaded screw cap and operates on the same principle. It is simply an interrupted thread on the glass finish, instead of a continuous thread. It is used to engage a lug on the cap sidewall and draw the cap down to the sealing surface of the container. Unlike the threaded closure, it requires only a quarter turn. The lug cap is used for both normal atmospheric-pressure and vacuum-pressure closing. The cap is widely used in the food industry because it offers a hermetic seal and handles well in sterilization equipment and on production lines.

iii. *Crown caps*: This style of cap is commonly used as a crimped closure for beverage bottles and has remained essentially unchanged for more than 50 years.

iv. *Roll-on closures (Fig. 6.6)*: The aluminum roll-on cap can be sealed securely, opened easily, and resealed effectively. It finds wide application in the packaging of food, beverages, chemicals, and pharmaceuticals. The roll-on closure requires a material that is easy to form, such as aluminum or other light-gauge metal. Resealable, nonresealable, and pilfer proof types of the roll-on closure are available for use on glass or plastic bottles and jars. The manufacturer purchases these closures as a straight-sided thread less shell and forms the threads on the packaging line as an integral part of the filling operation. The roll-on technique allows for dimensional variation in the glass containers, each roll-on closure precisely fits a specific container.

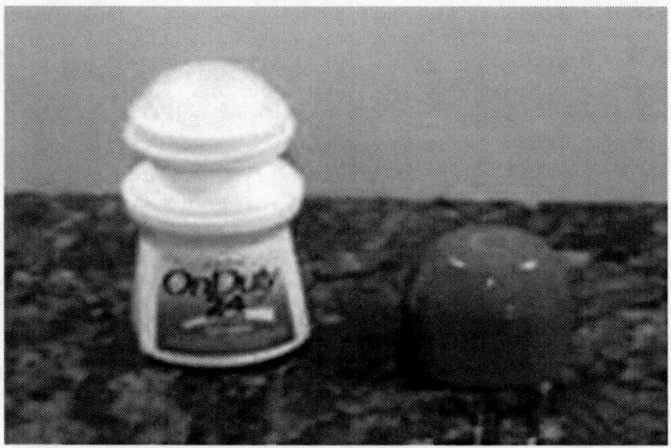

FIGURE 6.6: Roll-on closures

v. *Pilfer proof closures*: The pilfer proof closure is similar to the standard roll-on closure except that it has a greater skirt length. This additional length extends below the threaded portion to form a bank, which is fastened to the basic cap by a series of narrow metal "bridges." When the pilfer proof closure is removed, the bridges break, and the bank remains in place on the neck of the container. The closure can be resealed easily and the detached band indicates that the package has been opened. The torque is necessary to remove the cap.

### *Closure lines*

A liner may be defined as any material that is inserted in a cap to affect a seal between the closure and the container. Liners are usually made of a resilient backing and a facing material. The backing material must be soft enough to take up any irregularities in the sealing surface and elastic enough to recover some of its original shape when removed and replaced.

### Factors in selecting a liner

Many factors have to be considered before an effective liner can be selected. The most important consideration is that the liner be chemically inert with its product, so that the latter is protected against any possible change in purity or potency. Gas and vapor transmission rates are usually relative and depend chiefly on the shelf life required for the product. If the period between packing and consumer use is expected to be long, low transmission rates are necessary.

### Composition of closure

Closures are made of

a. Plastics
b. Rubber

a. **Plastic closures**: The two basic types of plastic generally used for closures are thermosetting and thermoplastic resins. They differ greatly in physical and chemical properties, and fundamentally different manufacturing methods are used for each type:
    i. *Thermosetting resins*: Phenolic and urea thermosetting plastic resins are widely used in threaded closures. The

thermosetting plastic first softens under heat and then curves and hardens to a final state. Shaping must occur in the first stage of softening, because after curving there is no further mobility, even upon reapplication of heat and pressure. During the molding process, thermosets undergo a permanent chemical change, and unlike thermoplastic material, they cannot be reprocessed. Since parts that are improperly molded must, therefore, be discarded, thermosetting materials are usually fabricated by compression molding. The manufacturing process is relatively slow, but allows better control and quick response to change in temperature and material is slow.

**Phenolics**: Phenolic molding compounds are available in different grades and in dark colors, usually black or brown. Phenolic compounds are used when a hard sturdy piece is needed and when dark colors are well-tolerated. Rigidity, heat, chemical resistance strengths are the outstanding properties of the phenolic compounds. Color limitation is the main drawback, although coatings are available at a premium price as a closure, the phenolic can withstand the torquing forces of the capping machines and maintains tight seal over a long period of time. The phenolic compounds are resistant to some dilute acids and alkalis. Organic acids and reducing acids usually do not have any effect. Strong alkalis decompose phenolic.

**Urea**: Urea is a hard translucent material. Urea is more expensive than the phenolic compounds, but the heat resistance and other properties of urea make it suitable for premium items. Elegant colors are obtained with urea because the translucency give brightness and color depth. Urea plastic is available in unlimited range of colors and is a hard, brittle material that is odorless and tasteless. Being a thermosetting plastic, urea can withstand high temperature without softening, but it chars at about 390°F. Urea absorbs water under wet conditions, but such absorption has no serious effect on the plastic. Urea is not affected by any organic solvents, but it is affected by alkalis and strong acids. Urea cannot be steam sterilized but can withstand elevated temperature. Parts may shrink as much as 0.003 inch after molding.

ii. *Thermoplastic resins*: Thermoplastic resins have become widely used in the manufacture of closures. Polystyrene, polyethylene and polypropylene are the materials used in 90% or more of all thermoplastic closures. Each material has specific performance advantage. The particular resins used depend on the physical and chemical properties desired for the particular products being packaged.

b. **Rubber closures**: Rubber is used in the pharmaceutical industry to make closures, cap liners and bulbs for dropper assemblies. The rubber stopper is used primarily for multiple dose vials and disposable syringes. The rubber polymers most commonly used are natural, neoprene and butyl rubber. Butyl rubber, nitrile rubber is some synthetic rubbers used for the manufacturing of closures.

In the manufacture of rubber closures the types of ingredients commonly found are:

- Rubber
- Vulcanizing agents
- Accelerator/activator
- Extended filer
- Reinforced filler
- Softener/plasticizer
- Antioxidant
- Pigment
- Waxes.

Since, the composition of rubber stopper is complex and the manufacturing process is complicated, it is common to encounter problems with certain rubber formulas. For example, when the rubber stopper comes in contact with parenteral solution, it may absorb active ingredient, antibacterial preservative or other materials and one or more ingredients of the rubber may be extracted into the liquid. These extractives could—

- Interface with chemical analysis of the active ingredient.
- Affect the toxicity or pyrogenicity of the injectable product.
- Interact with the drug preservative to cause inactivation.
- Affect the chemical and physical sterility of the preparation so that particulate matter appears in the solution.

*Pharmacopoeial requirements for rubber closures*

Rubber closures for containers used for aqueous parenteral preparations, powders and freeze dried products are made of materials obtained by vulcanization (cross-linking) of macromolecular organic substance (elastomers) with appropriate additives.

Tests to control quality of rubber caps: This include tests for –

i. *Quality*: The closures should not be tachy after:
   - Washing with detergent and rinsing several times.
   - Autoclaving at 121°C for half an hour in distilled water.

ii. *Penetrability*: The closure is sealed into a vial and the force required to make a hypodermic needle penetrate is measured using the piercing machine. The vial is moved on to the needle at a specified speed. The force must not exceed a stated value.

iii. *Fragmentation*: Test is carried out by using piecing machine with the vial. The vials are half-filled with particle free water. Each closure is penetrated with a hypodermic needle (0.08 mm external diameter) within a limited area and the last time the needle is washed to transfer fragments from bore to vial. Then the contents are filtered through paper (pore size 0.5 mm) of a color that contrasts with the rubber and the fragments are counted by eye. The test is carried out on 20 closures using a fresh needle for each if the previous one has become blunt. These must not be more than average of 3 fragments per closure.

iv. *Self-sealability*: Two tests are applied:
   - In the first, closed vials, half-filled with water are inverted and air, equal to the volume inside, is injected. Then the needle of water from the hole or more than a droplet on the surface.
   - In the second, methylene blue solution is used instead of water and 25 needle punctures are made evenly within a circle of 5 mm diameter to which a prescribed vacuum is applied (or reduced pressure of 27 kPa for 10 minutes, kept for 30 minutes in atmospheric pressure) for half an hour. There must be no signs of leakage in the water or on the closure.

v. *Acid or alkali treatment*: Specified number of closures is autoclaved with a given volume of freshly boiled and cooled distilled water of pH 6.8–7.2. The acid or alkali needed for the neutralization of this extract should be within the limit, i.e. not more than 0.3 ml of 0.01 M sodium hydroxide or 0.8 ml of 0.01 M hydrochloric acid.

vi. *Permeability to water vapor*: The increase in weight of vials containing dry fused calcium chloride is found after storage under the high humidity conditions and compared with the result for containers sealed with closures known to be satisfactory. Weighing are made fortnightly for 3 months.

vii. *Light absorption*: Rubber cap with 200 ml water is autoclaved. Filtered the autoclaved solution through 0.45 mm pore sized filter paper. Measure absorbance at 320–360 nm. Absorbance should not exceed 0.2 for type I and 4 for type II.

viii. *Limit test*: When treated with ammonium and heavy metals the limit must be not more than 2 ppm.

ix. *Titration*: Rubber in presence of 200 ml water for injection is autoclaved at 121°C for half an hour to 20 ml of 0.002 M potassium permanganate. Boil and cool (3 minutes). Add 1 g of potassium iodide and titrate with 0.01 M $Na_2S_2O_3$ using 0.25 ml of starch solution as indicator.

### *Rubber closures for injectable preparations*

A closure for an injectable preparation is a packaging components which are indirect contact with the drug. A rubber closure is made of materials obtained by vulcanization of elastomers. The elastomers are produced from natural or synthetic substances by polymerization, polyaddition or polycondensation. The nature of the principle components and of the various additives such as vulcanizers, accelerators, stabilizing agents, pigments, etc. depends on the properties required for the finished closure.

Rubber closures are used in a number of formulations and consequently different closures possess different properties. The closures chosen for use with a particular preparation should be such that the components of the preparation in contact with the closure are not absorbed onto the surface of the closure to an extent sufficient to affect the product adversely. The closure should not yield to the product substances in quantities sufficient to affect its stability or to present a risk of toxicity. The closures should be compatible with the preparation for which they are used throughout the shelf life of the product. It is impracticable to devise a set of standards which, if complied with, will ensure the compatibility of any closure with the preparation for which it is to be used. Therefore, a compatibility test has, to be carried out before a rubber composition is approved. The user of the closures must obtain an assurance from the supplier that the composition of the closure does not vary from supply to supply and that it is identical to that of the closure used during compatibility testing. When the user is informed of changes in the composition, compatibility testing must be repeated, totally or partly depending on the nature of the changes.

*Tamper resistant packaging*

The requirement for tamper resistant packaging is now one of the major consideration in the development of packaging for pharmaceutical products. As defined by the FDA "a tamper resistant package is one having an indicator or barrier to entry which, if breached or trussing, can reasonably be expected to provide visible evidence to consumers that tampering has occurred. Tamper resistant packaging may involve immediate container/closure systems or secondary container/carton systems or any combination thereof intended to provide a visual indication of package integrity when handled in a reasonable manner during manufacture, distribution, and retail display".

The following package configuration have been identified by the FDA as examples of packaging systems that are capable of meeting the requirements of tamper-resistant packaging as defined by FDA regulation are:

i. Film wrappers
ii. Blister package
iii. Strip package
iv. Bubble pack
v. Shrink seal and bands
vi. Foil paper or plastic pouches
vii. Bottle seals
viii. Tape seals
ix. Breakable caps

x. Sealed tubes
xi. Aerosol containers.

### i. Film wrapper

Film wrapping has been used extensively over the years for products requiring package integrity or environmental protection. Film wrapping can be accomplished in several ways and varies in configuration with packaging equipment.

Film wrapping machines can be generally categorized into the following types:

a. **End-folded wrapper (Fig. 6.7)**: The end-folded wrapper is formed by pushing the product into a sheet of over wrapping film, which forms the film around the product and folds the edges in a gift-wrap fashion. The folded areas are sealed by pressing against a heated bar. Because of the overlapping folding sequence of the seals, the film used must be heat-sealable on both surfaces. Materials commonly used for this application are cellophane and polypropylene. Cellophane, which is regenerated cellulose, is not inherently heat-sealable but requires a heat-seal coating to impart heat-sealing characteristics to the film. This is usually accomplished by coating the cellophane with either polyvinylidene chloride (PVDC) or nitrocellulose. The PVDC provides a durable moisture barrier, PVDC coated cellophane is often used for the over wrapping of products that are sensitive to moisture. To be tamper-resistant, the over wrap must be

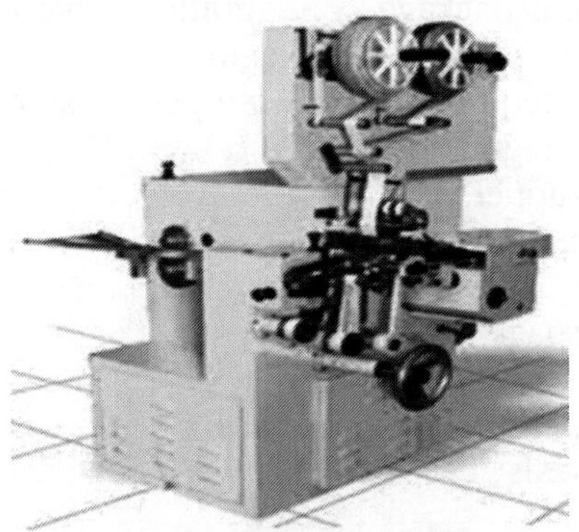

FIGURE 6.7: End-folded wrapper

well-sealed and must be printed or uniquely decorated. If the print of the carton being over wrapped, it is coated with a heat-sensitive varnish, it causes the over wrap to bond permanently to the paperboard carton during the sealing of the over wrap.

b. **Fin seal wrapper**: Unlike the end-folded wrapper configuration, fin seal packaging does not require the product to act as a bearing surface against which the over wrap is sealed. The seal are formed by crimping the film together and sealing together the two inside surfaces of the film, producing a "fin" seal. Since, the seals are formed by compressing the material between two heater bars rather than sealing against the package. When more consistent and greater sealing pressure is applied, better seal integrity can be accomplished. For this reason, fin sealing has primarily been used when protective packaging is critical. Since, the surface of the heat seal does not come in contact with the heated sealing bars on the packaging equipment, much more tenacious heat sealants such as polyethylene can be used. With good seal integrity, the over wrap can be removed or opened only by tearing the wrapper.

ii. Shrink wrapper (Fig. 6.8)

Film over wrapping can also be accomplished with the use of a shrink wrapper.The shrink wrap concept involves the packaging of a product in a thermoplastic film that has been stretched and oriented during its manufacture and that has the property of reverting back to its unstretched dimension once the molecular structure is "unfrozen" by the application of heat. The shrink wrap concept has a diversity of uses in packaging, one of which is its use as an over wrap. In this case, the shrink film is usually used in roll form, with the center folder in the direction of winding. As the film unwinds on the over wrapping machine, a pocket is formed in the center fold of the sheet, into which the product is inserted. An L-shaped sealer seals the remainder of the over wraps and trims off the excess film. The loosely wrapped product is then moved through a heated tunnel, which shrink the over wrap into a tightly wrapped unit. The material commonly used for this application are heat-shrinkable grades of polypropylene, polyethylene and polyvinyl chloride. Since the various heat-shrinkable grades of film have different physical characteristic such as tear and tensile strength, puncture resistance, and shrinking forces, selection of the particular material used must be based upon specific product consideration so that the shrink wrap provides suitable integrity without crushing or damaging the product. The major advantages of this type of wrapper are the flexibility and low cost of the packaging equipment required.

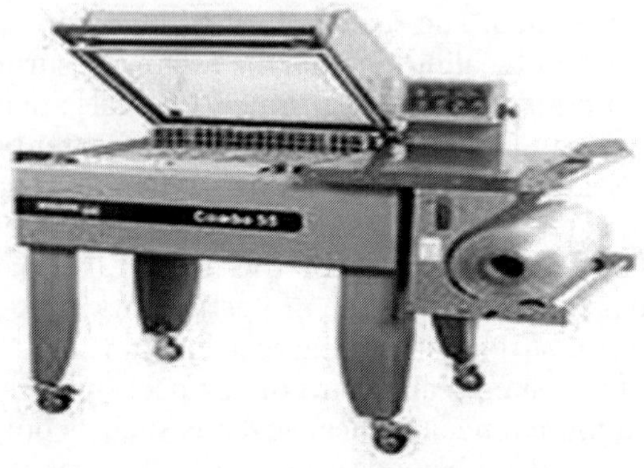

FIGURE 6.8: Shrink wrapper

### iii. Blister package

When one thinks of unit dose in pharmaceutical packaging, the package that invariably comes to mind is the blister package. This packaging mode has been used extensively for pharmaceutical packaging for several good reasons. It is a packaging configuration capable of providing excellent environmental protection, coupled with an aesthetically pleasing and efficacious appearance. It also provides user functionality in terms of convenience, child resistance and now, in tamper resistance.

The blister package is formed by heat-softening a sheet of thermoplastic resin and vacuum-drawing the softened sheet of plastic into a contoured mold. After cooling, the sheet is released from the mold and proceeds to the filling station of the packaging machine. The semirigid blister previously formed is filled with product and lidded with a heat-sealable backing material (Figs 6.9 and 6.10). The backing material, or lidding, can be of either a push-through or peelable type. For a push-through type of blister, the backing material is usually heat-seal-coated aluminum foil. The coating on the foil must be compatible with the blister material to ensure satisfactory sealing, both for product protection and for tamper resistance. Peelable backing materials have been used to meet the requirements of child-resistant packaging. This type of backing must have a degree of puncture resistance to prevent a child from pushing the product through the lidding and must also have sufficient tensile strength to allow the lidding to be pulled away from the blister even when the lidding is strongly adhered to it. To accomplish this, a material such as polyester or paper is used as a component of the backing lamination. Foil is generally used as a component of the backing lamination if barrier protection is a critical requirement; however, metalized polyester is replacing foil for some barrier applications. A peelable sealant compatible with the heat-seal coating on the blister is also required since the degree of difficulty of opening is a critical parameter for child-resistant packaging. The use of peelable backing materials for blister packaging must be carefully evaluated to ensure that peel strengths are sufficient to meet tamper-resistance objectives.

Materials commonly used for the thermoformable blister are polyvinyl chloride (PVC), PVC/polyethylene combinations, polystyrene and polypropylene. For commercial reasons and because of certain machine performance characteristics, the blisters on most unit dose packages are made of polyvinyl chloride. For added moisture protection, polyvinylidene chloride (saran) or polychlorotrifluoroethylene (aclar) films may be laminated to PVC. The moisture barrier of PVC/aclar is superior to that of saran-coated PVC, especially under prolonged and extremely humid storage conditions.

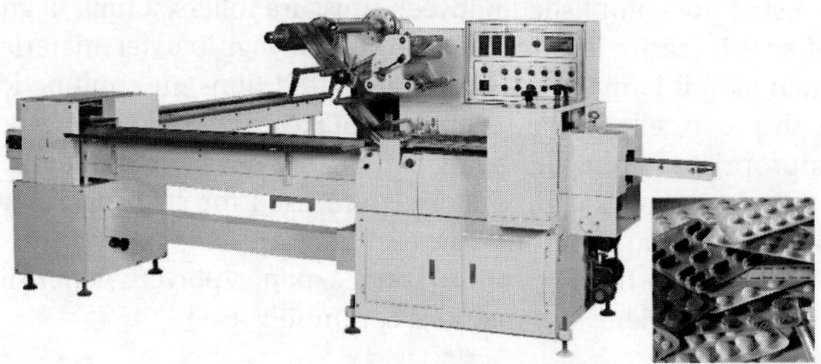

FIGURE 6.9: Blister packaging machine

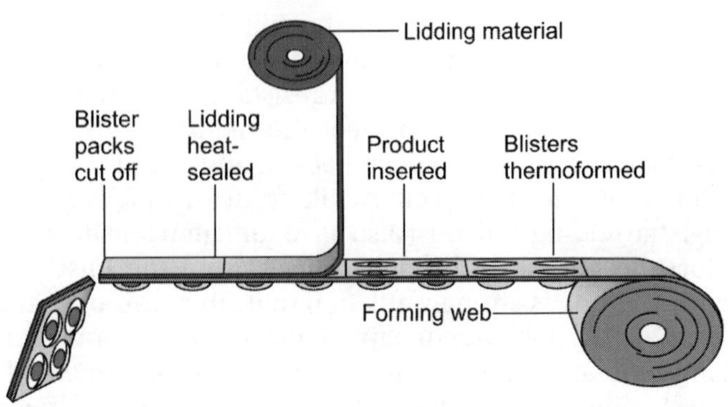


FIGURE 6.10: Diagrammatical representation of blister packaging system

### iv. Strip package

A strip package is a form of unit dose packaging that is commonly used for the packaging of tablets and capsules. A strip package is formed by feeding two webs of a heat-sealable flexible film through either a heated crimping roller or a heated reciprocating plate. The product is dropped into the pocket formed prior to forming the final set of seals (Figs 6.11 and 6.12). A continuous strip of packets is formed. The strip of packets is cut to the desired number of packets in length. The strips formed are usually collated and packaged into a folding carton. The product sealed between the two sheets of film usually has a seal around each tablet, with perforations usually separating adjacent packets. The seals can be in a simple rectangular or "picture-frame" format or can be contoured to the shape of the product. Since, the sealing is usually accomplished between pressure rollers, a high degree of seal integrity is possible. The use of high-barrier materials such as foil laminations or saran-coated films, in conjunction with the excellent seal formation, makes this packaging mode appropriate for the packaging of moisture-sensitive products.

Different packaging materials are used for strip packaging based on their properties. Few examples are cited below:

- For high-barrier applications, a paper/polyethylene/foil/polyethylene lamination is commonly used.

- When the visibility of the product is important, heat-sealable cellophane or heat-sealable polyester can be used.
- In some cases, the material used on each side of the strip package varies and the choice of material used depends on both the product and the equipment.

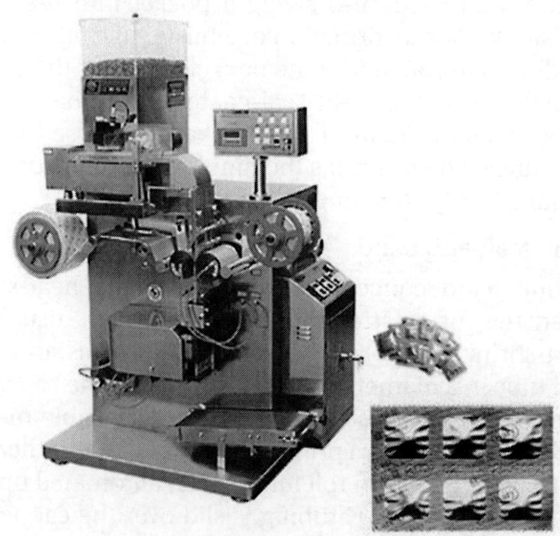

FIGURE 6.11: Strip packaging machine

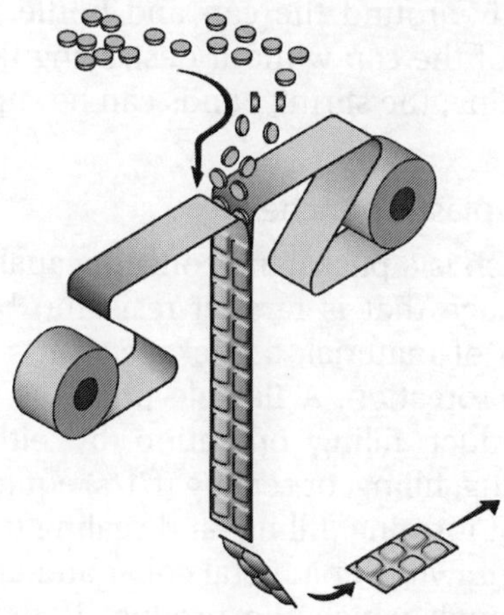

FIGURE 6.12: Diagrammatical representation of strip packaging system

### v. Bubble pack

The bubble pack can be made in several ways but is usually formed by sandwiching the product between a thermoformable, extensible, or heat-shrinkable plastic film and a rigid backing material. This is generally accomplished by heat-softening the plastic film and vacuum-drawing a pocket into the film in a manner similar to the formation of a blister in a blister package. The product is dropped into the pocket, which is then sealed to a rigid material such as heat-seal-coated paperboard. If a heat-shrinkable material is used, the package is passed through a heated tunnel, which shrinks the film into a bubble or skin over the product, firmly attaching it to the backing card.

### vi. Shrink seals and bands

The shrink band concept makes use of the heat-shrinking characteristics of a stretch-oriented polymer, usually PVC. The heat-shrinkable polymer is manufactured as an extruded, oriented tube in a diameter slightly larger than the cap and neck ring of the bottle to be sealed. The heat-shrinkable material is supplied to the bottler as a printed, collapsed tube, either pre-cut to a specified length or in roll form for an automated operation. The proper length of PVC tubing is slid over the capped bottle far enough to engage both the cap and neck ring of the bottle. The bottle is then moved through a heat tunnel, which shrinks the tubing tightly around the cap and bottle, preventing the disengagement of the cap without destroying the shrink band. For ease of opening, the shrink bands can be supplied with tear perforations.

### vii. Foil paper or plastic pouches

The flexible pouch is a packaging concept capable of providing not only a package that is tamper-resistant, but also, by the proper selection of material, a package with a high degree of environmental protection. A flexible pouch is usually formed during the product filling operation by either vertical or horizontal forming, filling, or sealing (f/f/s) equipment.

In the vertical forming, filling, and sealing (f/f/s) operation, a web of film is drawn over a metal collar and around a vertical filling tube, through which the product is dropped into the formed package. The metal filling tube also acts as a mandrel, which controls the circumference of the pouch and against which the longitudinal seal is made. The formation of this seal, which can be either a fin seal or an overlap seal, converts the packaging film into a continuous tube of film. Reciprocating sealers, orthogonal to the longitudinal seal, crimp off the bottom of the tube, creating the bottom seal of the package. The product drops through the forming tube into the formed package. The reciprocation sealer moves up the film tube a distance equal to the length of the package and forms the top and final seal of the package (Fig. 6.13).

The top seal of the package becomes the bottom seal of the next package and the process repeats itself. Since, vertical f/f/s machines are gravity-fed, they are primarily used for liquid, powder and granular products. The horizontal forming, filling and sealing (f/f/s) system is generally used for products of smaller volume, which are more amenable to the flatter format of the packages. In this system, the web of film is folded upon itself rather than around a tube. As the folded film is fed horizontally through the equipment, a reciprocating platen creates pockets in the film by making vertical separation seals. The product is then placed into each pocket and the final top seal is made. Packages formed on horizontal f/f/s equipment typically have a three-sided perimeter seal, but other variations are possible, depending on the type of equipment used. For moisture- and oxygen-sensitive products, foil is commonly used as part of

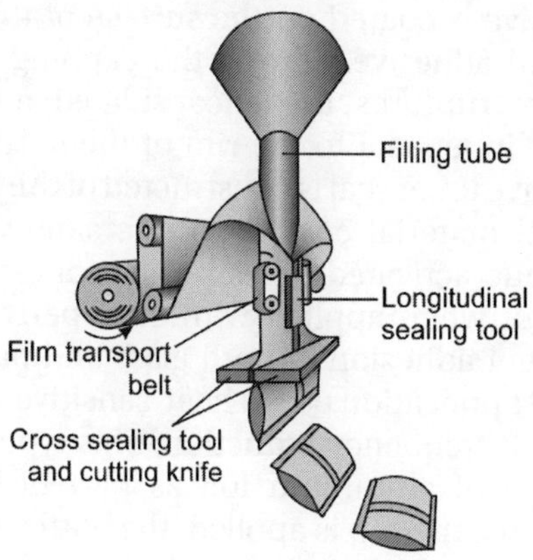


FIGURE 6.13: Vertical form, fill and seal pouch machine

the film lamination. Nowadays foil is replaced by metallized polyester which is used in the lamination for high barrier application and includes paper/polyethylene/foil/polyethylene and polyester/polyethylene/foil/polyethylene. They offer some advantages that they are of lower cost, excellent appearance, and flexural endurance.

### viii. Bottle seals

A bottle may be made tamper-resistant by bonding an inner seal to the rim of the bottle in such a way that access to the product can only be attained by irreparably destroying the seal. Various inner seal compositions may be used, but the structures most frequently encountered are glassine and foil laminations. Typically, glassine liners are two-ply laminations using two sheets of glassine paper bonded together with wax or adhesive. The inner seals are inserted into the bottle cap and held in place over the permanent cap liner either by applying friction or by a slight application of wax which temporarily adheres the seal to the permanent cap liner. If glue-mounted inner seals are to be used, glue is applied to the rim of the bottle prior to the capping operation. The application of the cap forces the inner seal into contact with the glued bottle rim and maintains pressure during glue curing and until the cap is removed. When the bottle cap is removed, the inner seal is left securely anchored to the bottle rim (Fig. 6.14).

Pressure-sensitive inner seals can also be used. The pressure-sensitive adhesive is coated on the surface of the inner seal as an encapsulated adhesive. During the capping operation, the torque pressure ruptures the encapsulated adhesive, which then bonds the inner seal to the rim of the bottle. One type of pressure-sensitive inner seal is constructed of thin-gauge styrene foam inner seal material coated on one side with a specially formulated torque-activated adhesive. The adhesive has minimal surface tack, but when applied with a properly torque cap, it provides excellent adhesion to both glass and plastic bottles. A third method of application uses a heat-sensitive adhesive that is activated by high-frequency induction. This type of application requires the use of aluminum foil as part of the inner seal composition. Once the cap is applied, the bottle is passed under an induction coil, which induces high-frequency resonation in the foil. The frictional heat that is generated activates the heat-seal coating and bonds the liner to the bottle. This type of seal can only be used with plastic caps since metal caps would interfere with the induction sealing of the inner seal. To meet the tamper-resistant criteria, the inner seals must be printed or decorated with a unique design. The seal must also be bonded sufficiently to ensure that its removal would result in destruction of the seal.

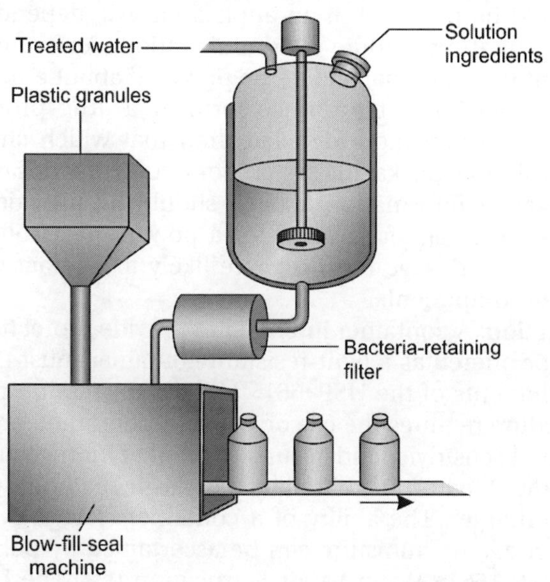


FIGURE 6.14: Overview of the blow, fill and seal process

### ix. Tape seals

Tape sealing involves the application of a glued or pressure-sensitive tape or label around or over the closure of the package, which must be destroyed to gain access to the packaged product. The paper used most often is a high-density lightweight paper with poor tear strength. Labels made of self-destructing paper are available; these cannot survive any attempt at removal once they have been applied. To reduce further the possibility of removing the label intact, perforation or partial slitting of the paper can be made prior to application so that the label tears readily along those weak points if any attempt is made to remove it.

## QUALIFICATION AND QUALITY CONTROL OF PACKAGING COMPONENTS

A packaging system found acceptable for one drug product is not automatically assumed to be appropriate for another. Each application should contain enough information to show that each proposed container closure system and its components are suitable for its intended use. The type and extent of information that should be provided in an application will depend on the dosage form and the route of administration. For example, the kind of information that should be provided about a packaging system for an injectable dosage form or a drug product for inhalation is often more detailed than that which should be provided about a packaging system for a solid oral dosage form. More detailed information usually should be provided for a liquid-based dosage form than for a powder or a solid, since a liquid-based dosage form is more likely to interact with the packaging components.

1. **Protection**: A container intended to provide protection from light or offered as a light-resistant container must meet the requirements of the USP<661> Light Transmission test. The procedure requires the use of a spectrophotometer, with the required sensitivity and accuracy, adapted for measuring the amount of light transmitted by the plastic materials used for the container. The ability of a container closure system to protect against moisture can be ascertained by performing the USP <661> Water Vapor Permeation test. The USP sets limits to the amount of moisture that can penetrate based upon size and composition of the plastic components (HDPE, LDPE, or PET). The integrity of the container can be evaluated in several ways. A couple of the most common tests are dye penetration and microbial ingress. Container closure systems stored in a dye solution and exposed to pressure and vacuum cycles are examined for dye leakage into the container. The microbial ingress is similar in fashion, but determines the microbial contamination of the contents when soaked in a media contaminated with bacteria. Other quantitative tests that can be run are vacuum/ pressure decay, helium mass spectrometry, and gas detection.
2. **Compatibility**: Components compatible with a dosage form will not interact sufficiently to change the quality of the

product or its components. A leachability study designed to evaluate the amount and/or nature of any chemical migrating from the plastic material to the pharmaceutical product should be implemented. The study should evaluate substances that migrate into the pharmaceutical product vehicle for the length of shelf life claim. The drug product should be evaluated at regular intervals, such as at one, three, or six months or at one or two years, until the length of the shelf life claim has been met.

Analytical techniques such as Liquid Chromatography/ Mass Spectrometry (LC/MS) to evaluate nonvolatile organics, Gas Chromatography/Mass Spectrometry (GC/MS) to evaluate semivolatile organics, and Inductively Coupled Plasma (ICP) spectroscopy to detect and quantitate inorganic elements should be a part of this study. Coupling MS to LC and GC methods provides a definitive and effective tool for identifying unknown impurities and degradation products. Other changes such as pH shifts, precipitates and discoloration, which may cause degradation of pharmaceutical product, must be evaluated. Changes in the physical characteristics of the container, such as brittleness must be evaluated using thermal analysis and hardness testing. An infrared (IR) scan of each plastic component should also be included. An IR scan can fingerprint the materials and also provide proof of identity, which will later become part of quality control.

3. **Safety**: All packaging components should be constructed of materials that will not leach harmful or undesirable amounts of substances to which a patient will be exposed during drug treatment. Determining the safety of a packaging component is not a simple process, and a standardized approach has not been established. However, an extraction study should be one of the first considerations. Isolation is accomplished through sample preparation, followed by incubation in solvents at well-defined and well-controlled times and temperatures. Sample preparation is an area in which an experienced chemist's knowledge of chemical procedures is indispensable.

   Prior to performing any of the chemical tests, it is important to have precise information on the synthesis of the polymer itself. This includes descriptions of the monomers used in the polymerization, the solvents used in the synthesis, and the special additives that have been added during material production. For containers used to package drugs ranked with a high degree of concern, such as inhalation aerosols and injectables, this type of information is imperative. Knowledge of degradation products that may be released into the drug product is also important. Some potential extractable chemicals from packaging materials are water soluble, while others are soluble only in nonpolar environments. For the packaging which is in contact with the drug products, extraction in both polar and nonpolar environments is relevant. The USP includes physicochemical tests for plastics based on water extracts; while water, alcohol and hexane extracts are required for polyethylene containers under controlled temperature and time parameters (70°C for 24 hours for water and alcohol and 50°C for 24 hours for hexane). These tests are particularly useful in defining materials as rich or poor in extractable chemicals. The tests categorize material extracts in general terms, such as non-volatile residue (total extractable), residue on ignition, buffering capacity, heavy-metals content and turbidity. Biological reactivity is the second part of safety testing and is designed to test extractable chemicals for toxicological properties. FDA's guidance document suggests that the USP biological reactivity tests can determine the safe level of exposure, via the label-specified route of administration.

4. **Performance**: The fourth attribute of suitability of the container closure system, performance and drug delivery, refers to its ability to function in the manner for which it was designed. There are two major considerations when evaluating performance. The first consideration is functionality that may be to improve patient compliance, minimize waste, or improve ease of use. The second consideration is drug delivery, which is the ability of the packaging system to deliver the right amount or rate. Packaging systems that address this consideration are prefilled syringes, transdermal patches, dropper or spray bottles and metered-dose inhalers.

## Package inspection

More critical part of packaging operation is package inspection. In the past, this was largely carried out by people under the head of quality control. With the increase in output of typical packaging lines the inspection task has become difficult for the human person to accomplish. Several important electronics techniques have been developed which allow the graphic inspection of a number of packaging variables and the rapid rejection of those which do not meet an established standard, and with the passing of those which do. One notable variable is the accuracy of weight or fill volume. Automatic check weight systems handle all of these. In the case a product sold by volume, a machine-vision system can determine whether the liquid level in a bottle is at the proper level. Labeling is another variable which is regulated. Again machine-vision systems are able to scan each label to be sure that it is correctly applied and that the text is correct for the product being packaged. Metal detection in a product and/or package can be accomplished with several techniques with an X-ray able to detect particulars as small as 0.01 mm at high line outputs. Leaking packages can be detected at high speed with helium leak detection.

## FDA Regulation

Food and Drug Administration evaluating a drug and the agency must be firmly convinced that the package for a specific drug will preserve the drug's efficacy as well its purity, identity, strength and quality for its entire shelf life. Under the provisions of the Food and Drug Administration Act, however, no specifications or standards for containers or container closures are provided. Under the Act, it is the responsibility of the manufacturer to prove the safety of a packaging material and to get approval before using it for any pharmaceutical product. The Food and Drug Administration does not approve containers as such, but only the materials used in the container are approved. A list of substances considered "Generally Recognized as Safe" (GRAS) has been published by the FDA. In the opinion of the qualified experts they are safe under specified conditions, assuming that they are of good commercial quality. A material that is not included under GRAS or prior sanction, and is intended to be used with food, must be tested by the manufacturer, and the data must be submitted to the FDA. The specific FDA regulation states that "containers, closures and other component parts of drug packages, to be suitable for their intended use, must not be reactive, additive or absorptive to an extent that the identity, strength, quality or purity of the drug will be affected." The packaging material must be approved for such use, along with the drug, before going to the market. The drug manufacturer must include data on the container and package components in contact with the pharmaceutical product in its New Drug Application (NDA). If the FDA can determine that the drug is safe and effective, and that the package is suitable, it approves the drug and package. Once approved, however, the package may not be altered in any manner without prior FDA approval. In the case of plastics, most resin manufacturers maintain master files on their resins with the FDA. Upon request from the resin manufacturer, the FDA uses this file as a reference to support a New Drug Application that which a drug manufacturer files.

### Child-resistant packaging

The definition of Child-Safe Packaging is "packaging that is difficult for a child to open within a reasonable period but that presents no difficulty for an adult to use properly and flexible packages with hidden tear starts or peel back and push blister packs did and still do present problems for elderly or handicapped people to use properly". The Child-Safe Packaging Group (CSPG) was formed 11 years ago and its objective is to promote the specification and success of child-resistant packaging systems for all products whose ingestion or other contact could prove seriously distressing to a child.

The Child-Safe Packaging Group has been a catalyst for the introduction to new standards: one British and the Pan-European which will help to create better flexible packs. A new standard for rigid packs has been published, this again will make them more acceptable to adults and help to banish, forever, the old quip about adults not being able to access their medicines when packed in child resistant packs because child-resistant packaging remains the only packaging for any product which has to be tested for openability by adults. It has already and will continue to make for a more consumer acceptable pack and the system of testing for adult openability could well be applied to packaging generally.

The report of the inquest into the circumstances surrounding the death of three year old Yaqoob Lookman, published in most national newspapers on 2000, has been described by members of the Child-Safe Packaging Group as predictable, avoidable and the result of pure negligence. Briefly, the child swallowed 44 ferrous sulfate tablets, which he extracted from two blister packages. The Child-Safe Packaging Group had declared this type of packaging to be dangerous since its own research was published in 1995. Blister packages are tested for child resistance in the United States, Canada and Germany. Pharmaceuticals and other hazardous products are packaged in either rigid or flexible containers. Rigid packaging systems, bottle and child-resistant closure, are subject to testing for child resistance and have been so since 1975.

The Child-Safe Packaging Group consists of the greater part of the supply industry for reclosable packaging systems for pharmaceutical or other hazardous products. The Child-Safe Packaging Group commissioned research in 1995 that conclusively proved that blister packages in common use in the United Kingdom and other European countries were not child-resistant. The results of this research were announced in the press then and have subsequently been referred to in papers published by the group and debated in the packaging and pharmaceutical industries.

# Chapter 7

# Surgical Dressings

## INTRODUCTION

Surgical dressing is a term applied to a wide range of materials used for dressing of wounds or injured or diseased tissues.

### Function of dressings

i. Provide an environment for moist wound healing
ii. Promote hemostasis
iii. Protect the wound from further damage
iv. Reduce heat loss
v. Promote autolysis
vi. Promote healing
vii. Provide support
viii. Reduce pain, increase patient comfort.

## CLASSIFICATION OF SURGICAL DRESSINGS

Functionally, the simplest method of classification uses the term primary and secondary dressing. A primary dressing directly contacts the wound. It may provide absorptive capacity and may prevent desiccation, infection and adhesion of the secondary dressing to the wound.

A secondary dressing is placed over a primary dressing, providing further protection, absorptive capacity and compression on occlusion. Although some dressings are solely primary or secondary in nature, others have the characteristic of both. The following classification is used here:

*Nonofficial dressings*

- Primary wound dressing

- Primary/secondary wound dressings
- Secondary wound dressings
- Protectives.

*Official dressings:*

- Sutures and ligatures.

*Selection of surgical dressings*

Dressing selection should be made on the basis of the degree of exudation, presence or likelihood of infection, presence of necrotic tissues and anatomical site. The correct selection of a wound dressing depends not only on the type of wound but also on the stage of repair.

## NONOFFICIAL DRESSINGS

### Primary wound dressings

These dressings are directly placed on a wound surfaces and are usually reinforced by materials of various types to absorb the wound secretions.

Types of primary wound dressings:

a. Plain gauze
b. Impregnated gauze
c. Film dressings.

a. **Plain gauze**: Plain gauze has been used as a primary dressing but will stick to the incised wounds. Although this property has been used to debride exudative, infected and necrotic wounds but this practice may be painful and is often counterproductive, causing the removal of granulation tissue and new epithelium.
b. **Impregnated gauze**: They are used to reduce its adherence to wound, e.g. cotton, rayon, or cellulose acetate gauze impregnated with a variety of substances such as petrolatum or paraffin, paraffin emulsion, zinc saline, etc. With these types of dressings, secondary dressings should be used to prevent desiccation, provide absorbency and prevent entrance of pathogens.
c. **Film dressings**: They are transparent films, occlusive or semi-occlusive films of polyurethane with acrylic or polyether adhesive that provides a semipermeable membrane to water

vapor and oxygen. These dressings will adhere to intact skin and have a low adherence for wound tissue. They should not be used on infected or heavily exuding wounds.

### Primary/Secondary wound dressings

They are classified into following types

a. Composite dressings
b. Hydrogels
c. Hydrocolloid dressings
d. Calcium alginate dressings.

a. **Composite dressings**: These types of dressings have primary and secondary component that prevent adherence to the wound, with the same degree of absorbency. It consists of lightly absorbent rayon or cotton pad sandwiched between porous polyethylene films.
b. **Hydrogels**: These are nonadherent dressings that through semipermeable film allow a high rate of evaporation without compromising wound hydration. This makes them useful in burn treatment. These are generally made from typically cross-linked polymers such as polyvinylpyrrolidone (PVP), polyethylene oxide gel, polyamide, etc.
c. **Hydrocolloid dressings**: Such type of dressings has combined benefits of occlusion and absorbency. These types of dressings consist of gum like materials such as karaya gum, sodium carboxymethyl cellulose, pectin bound by an adhesive such as polyisobutylene.
d. **Calcium alginate dressings**: These fibrous dressings are highly absorbent and used on moderate to highly absorbent wounds. They may be held in place with gauze or film dressings.

### Secondary wound dressings

They are classified into following types:

a. Absorbents
b. Bandages
c. Adhesive tapes.

a. **Absorbents**: An absorbent refers to a substance that absorbs or promotes absorption.
   They are classified into:
   i. Surgical cotton
   ii. Surgical gauze.

i. **Surgical cotton**: Cotton is the basic surgical absorbent. The balls (fruits) contain numerous seeds with cotton fibers. Each cotton fiber is a minute hair-like tube. It is flattened and twisted. The raw cotton fiber, after seeds have been removed by grin is mechanically cleaned of dirt and compressed into balls of various sizes. This form is non-absorbent cotton.

   ***Nonabsorbent cotton***: Raw cotton fiber mechanically cleaned of dirt and carded into layers but not otherwise treated and has a limited use for padding and covering of unbroken surface. It is used as cotton plugs in the bacteriological laboratory because of its absorbency.

   ***Absorbent cotton***: Absorbent cotton is prepared from the raw fiber by a series of processes that remove natural waxes and all impurities and foreign substances and render the fiber absorbent. It is a practically pure, white cellulose fiber.

   ***Absorbent balls***: They are made of uniform viscose-rayon fiber. They absorb fluids faster and retain their shape better than cotton balls.

   ***Nonabsorbent cotton***: They are prepared by a modified bleaching process that retains the water repellent natural oils and waxes.

ii. **Surgical gauzes**: Their function is to provide an absorbent material of sufficient tensile strength for surgical dressings. It is known as absorbent gauze.

*Procedure*

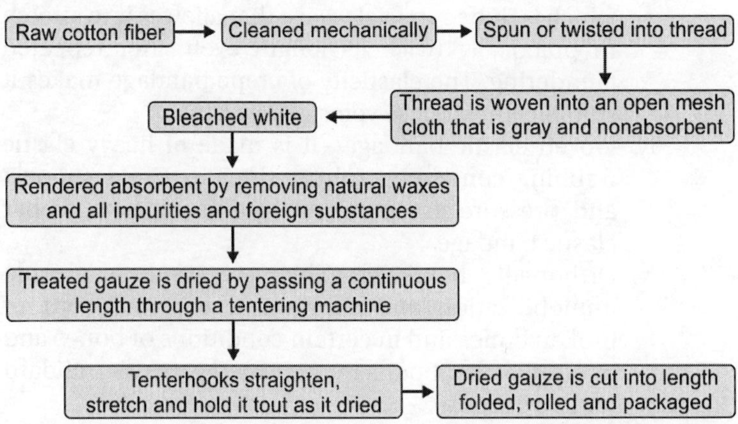

Gauze is classified according into its mesh or number of threads per inch. Various forms of pads, compresses and dressings are made from surgical gauze alone or in conjunction with absorbent cotton, tissue fiber and other materials:

- Filmated gauze
- Nonwoven surgical sponges
- Selvage edge gauze strips
- Gauze pads or sponges
- X-ray detectable gauze pads
- Eye pads.

b. **Bandages**: Their function is to hold the dressing in place by providing pressure or support. They may be elastic, inelastic or become rigid on shaping for immobilization.

Various types of bandages, common in use, are listed here:

i. Common gauze roller bandages—It is prepared from absorbent gauze in various width and length. Each bandage is one continuous piece tightly rolled and free from loose threads and raveling.

ii. Muslin bandage rolls—They are made of close mesh nonabsorbent gauze. They are supplied in the same width as the regular gauze bandage. Muslin bandages are strong and are used wherever normal gauze bandage does not provide sufficient strength or support. They are frequently used to hold splints or bulky compression dressings in place.

iii. Crepe bandage—Such types of bandage have elasticity which is due to special weave that allowes it to stretch to practically twice its length even after repeated laundering. The elasticity of crepe bandage makes it suitable for varicose veins and sprains.

iv. Woven elastic bandage—It is made of heavy elastic webbing containing rubber threads. Good support and pressure are provided by this type of rubber elastic bandage.

v. Orthopedic bandages—They are used to provide immobilization and support in the treatment of broken bones and in certain conditions of bones and joints. Plaster of paris impregnated gauze is standard for this purpose.

   vi. Stockinette bandages—They are made of stockinette material knitted or woven in tubular form. Surgical stockinette is unbleached. It is soft and stretched readily to conform comfortably to the arms, legs, or body.

c. **Adhesive tape**: These are pressure sensitive or self adhesive. Their adhesive action is due to presence of rubber based or acrylate adhesives. Surgical adhesive tapes are made in many different forms varying both in the type of backing and in the formulation of adhesive mass according to specific needs and requirements.

*Adhesive tapes are divided into two categories:*

   i. *Rubber based adhesives*: Rubber-based adhesives composed of an elastomer (pale rubber or synthetic elastomer made from polymers of isobutylene, alkyl acrylate and similar materials) resins or modified resins, antioxidants, plasticizer (naphthalene) fillers (kiselgur) and coloring agent to give desired tint or whiteness.

      They are used on cloth or plastic backing. They are used where heavy support and superior adhesion required.

   ii. *Acrylate adhesives*: Acrylate adhesives are unipolymeric system and eliminate the use of large number of components. They are used on nonwoven or fabric backing. They are widely used in a surgical dressing application where reduced trauma is required as in operative or post-operative procedures.

### Protective

They include only the various impermeable materials intended to be used adjunctively with other dressing components to prevent the loss of moisture or heat from a wound site or to protect clothing or bed liners from wound exudates. Protectives are also employed to cover wet dressings and hot or cold compresses.

## OFFICIAL DRESSINGS

**Sutures and ligatures**: Although the term suture and ligature are often used in same sense and they are of the same material, there is never a technical difference.

A ligature is a thread used to constrict and tying off blood vessels, vein and artery.

The thread is a suture when it is used to stitch together the edges of various tissues, e.g. skin, fascia, muscle, tendon, peritoneum, etc.

Hence, a needle is always used for a suture (sewing) but not for a ligature.

Sutures and ligatures are classified as absorbable and non-absorbable depending on materials from which they are made.

a. **Absorbable sutures/ligatures**: They are prepared from collagen derived from healthy mammal or from a synthetic polymer. They are sterile.

***Collagen suture or catgut***: The classic absorbable suture catgut derived from collagen rich animal tissues. It is proteinaceous in nature and it appears that certain proteolytic enzymes are responsible for the digestion of *catgut* and its disappearance from the wound area.

Collagen suture is designated as either plain suture or chromic suture. Both types consist of processed strand of collagen, but chromic suture is processed by physical and chemical means so as to provide greatest resistance to absorbance in living mammalian tissues. Plain suture is digested by enzymes at a faster rate than chromic gut. The surgeon chooses either plain or chromic suture depending on the type of tissue involved, the condition of the patient and the estimated healing time of the wound.

***Synthetic suture***: Some absorbable sutures are made from synthetic polyesters such as polyglycolic acid, copolymers of lactide and caprolactone and a blend of glycolide, trimethylene carbonate and dioxanone. Sutures prepared from synthetic polymer may be in either monofilament or multifilament form. It is capable of being absorbed by living mammalian tissue but may be treated to modify its resistance to absorption.

b. **Nonabsorbable suture/ligature**: They are prepared from natural or synthetic materials such as polyester, nylon, polypropylene, etc. They are nonsterile. Such materials are relatively resistant to attack by normal tissue fluids. Several of these materials remain apparently unchanged for many years in tissue and usually will be found encapsulated in a thin sheath of fibrous connective tissues. When nonabsorbable sutures are used for skin closure, they usually are removed after the incision or wound has healed to the point where suture support is no longer necessary. Nonabsorbable sutures are used frequently for cardiovascular, ophthalmic and neurological procedure.

Nonabsorbable sutures are classified as:

a. Class I: They composed of silk or braided silk, polyester or nylon, monofilament nylon or polypropylene.
b. Class II: They composed of cotton or linen fibers or coated natural or synthetic fibers.
c. Class III: They composed of monofilament or multifilament metal wire.

## CELLULOSIC HEMOSTASIS

Hemorrhage is the most difficult part of neurological procedures. Surgeon must constantly battle pooling and oozing blood when performing dissection and manipulation in or near the spinal cord, brain, or nerve. Neurosurgeons employ several techniques and devices to gain control of unrelenting bleeding such as use of ligature, endovascular therapies and bone wax. However, when conventional means of controlling bleeding fail, neurosurgeons often turn to absorbable cellulosic hemostasis devices.

Absorbable cellulosic hemostasis devices are classified as:

a. Oxidized cellulose
b. Gelatin foams
c. Microfibrillar collagen.

### a. *Oxidized cellulose*

Oxidized cellulose is an absorbable hemostatic agent prepared from cellulose by a special process that converts it into polyanhydroglucuronic acid (cellulosic acid). Oxidation of cellulose by nitrogen dioxide is controlled to yield an absorbable product of known acidity, soluble in alkali. In appearance and texture it resembles ordinary surgical gauze or cotton. It provides hemostatic action when applied to sites of bleeding. On contact with blood, oxidized cellulose becomes a dark reddish-brown or almost black, tenacious, adhesive mass. By this transformation oxidized cellulose conforms and adheres readily to the bleeding surface. After 24–48 hours, oxidized cellulose becomes gelatinous and can be removed usually without causing additional bleeding.

If left in situ, absorption of oxidized cellulose depends on several factors including the amount used, degree of saturation with blood and the tissue bed. Oxidized cellulose swells upon contact with blood and the resultant pressure adds to its hemostatic action. It does not enter into the normal clotting mechanism but, on contact with blood, forms an artificially produced clot in the bleeding area within a few minutes.

**b. *Gelatin foams***

These sponges were first introduced for use in neurosurgical cases. It is made from animal skin gelatin, whipped and baked into sponge foam. It is available as gelatin sponge or compressed sponge. It absorbs 45 × its weight in blood and expands as much as 200% of its initial volume. It is applied after wetting with saline or thrombin. The over-packing of such foams are avoided, otherwise it may cause undesirable pressure on surrounding structure, i.e. nerves.

Absorbable gelatin sponges such as Surifoam and Gelfoam are used in conjunction with thrombin which generates fibrin from fibrinogen and promote platelet aggregation. Gelatin sponge absorbs within 4–6 weeks and is capable of holding within their mesh many times their weight in whole blood.

**c. *Microfibrillar collagen***

This type of collagen causes aggregation of platelets. It is prepared from purified bovine corium collagen and shredded into fibrils. On contact with blood it causes platelet aggregation, denaturation and the release of coagulation factors that along with plasma factors enable the formation of fibrin. It causes minimal swelling. It absorbs within 8–10 weeks.

# Bibliography


1. Akers MJ, Larrimor DS, Guazzao MD. Parenteral Quality Control. Basel, New York: Marcel Deckker Inc.
2. Ansel H, Allen L, Popovich N. Pharmaceutical Dosage Forms and Drug Delivery Systems (8th ed). Philadelphia: Lippincott Williams & Wilkins.
3. Aulton ME. Pharmaceutics—The Science of Dosage Form Design (1st ed). Edinburgh: Churchill Livingstone.
4. Avis KE, Lieberman HA, Lachman L. Pharmaceutical dosages forms—Parenteral Medications (2nd ed). Basel, New York: Marcel Deckker Inc. Vol. I.
5. Banker GS, Rhodes CT. Modern Pharmaceutics (4th ed). New York: Marcel Deckker Inc.
6. Bansode SK, Banarjee DD, Gaikwad SL, Jadhav RM. Microencapsulation: A Review. International Journal of Pharmaceutical Sciences Review and Research 2010;1(2).
7. Benita S. Microencapsulation—Methods and Industrial Applications (2nd ed). London and New York: Tylor and Francis.
8. Brahmanker DM, Jaiswal SB. Biopharmaceutics and Pharmacokinetics (1st ed). New Delhi: Vallabh Prakashan.
9. Chien YW. Novel Drug Delivery System (2nd ed). Basel, New York: Marcel Deckker Inc.
10. Dean DA, Evans ER, Hall IH. Pharmaceutical Packaging Technology. London and New York: Tylor and Francis.
11. Hartburn K. Quality Control of Packaging in Pharmaceutical Industry. Basel, New York: Marcel Deckker Inc.
12. Heller J. Polymers for Controlled Parenteral Delivery of Peptides and Proteins. Advanced Drug Delivery Review 1993;10.
13. Indian Pharmacopoiea, Indian Pharmacopoieal Commission, Ghaziabad 2007;Vol. I.
14. Jain NK. Advances in Controlled and Novel Drug Delivery System. CBS Publishers and Distributors.
15. Jain NK. Controlled and Novel Drug Delivery. New Delhi: CBS Publishers and Distributors.
16. Kawashima Y. Nanoparticulate Systems for Improved Drug Delivery. Advanced Drug Delivery Reviews 2001;47.

17. Kumaresh S, Soppimath TM, Aminabhavi AR, Kulkarni WE. Biodegradable Polymeric Nanoparticles as Drug Delivery Devices. Journal of Controlled Release 2001;70.
18. Lieberman HA, Lachman L, Schwartz JB. Pharmaceutical dosages forms – Tablets (2nd ed). Basel, New York: Marcel Deckker Inc.
19. Lieberman HA, Lachman L, Schwartz JB. Pharmaceutical dosages forms – Tablets (2nd ed). Basel, New York: Marcel Deckker Inc.
20. Manato RI. Pharmaceutical Dosages Forms and Drug Delivery. London and New York: CRC Press, Tylor and Francis.
21. Martin A. Physical Pharmacy (4th ed). New Delhi: Lippincott Williams & Wilkins. B. I. Publication Pvt. Ltd.
22. Mohanraj VJ, Chen Y. Nanoparticles—A Review, Tropical Journal of Pharmaceutical Research 2006;5(1).
23. Parikh DM. Handbook of Pharmaceutical Granulation Technology (2nd ed). London and New York: Tylor and Francis.
24. Rawlins EA. Bentley Textbook of Pharmaceutics (8th ed). New Delhi: All India Traveler Book Seller (AITBS).
25. Robinson JR, Lee VHL. Controlled Drug Delivery—Fundamentals and Applications (2nd ed). Basel, New York: Marcel Deckker Inc.
26. Swarbrick J, Boylen JC. Encyclopedia of Pharmaceutical Technology. New York: Marcel Deckker Inc. Vol. 2.
27. Troy DB. Remington—The Science and Practice of Pharmacy (21st ed). Philadelphia: Lippincott Williams & Wilkins. Vol. I.
28. Troy DB. Remington—The Science and Practice of Pharmacy (21st ed). Philadelphia: Lippincott Williams & Wilkins. Vol. II.
29. Uchegbu IF. Parenteral Drug Delivery. Journal of Pharmaceutical Sciences 1999;263.
30. USP 32 (the official compendia of standards) United State Pharmacopieal Convention, Maryland 2009;Vol. I.
31. Vyas SP, Khar RK. Controlled Drug Delivery Concepts and Advances (1st ed). New Delhi: CBS Publishers and Distributors.
32. Vyas SP, Khar RK. Targeted and Controlled Drug Delivery (Novel Carrier Systems). New Delhi: CBS Publishers and Distributors.
33. Wilmer A, Jenkinns, KR. Packaging Drugs and Pharmaceutical. Lancaster Basel, New York: Technomic Publishing Co. Inc.
34. Wise DL. Handbook of Pharmaceutical Controlled Release Technology. Basel, New York: Marcel Deckker Inc.

# Index

## Q



## R



## S



## T



## V



## W